MK 100

ATLAS OF CLINICAL
ENDOCRINOLOGY

ATLAS OF CLINICAL
ENDOCRINOLOGY

Series Editor
Stanley G. Korenman, MD

Professor and Associate Dean
Department of Medicine
UCLA School of Medicine
UCLA Medical Center
Los Angeles, California

Volume V
HUMAN NUTRITION
AND OBESITY

Volume Editor
David Heber, MD, PhD

Professor
Department of Medicine
UCLA School of Medicine;
Director, UCLA Center for Human Nutrition
Los Angeles, CA

With 20 contributors

b

Blackwell
Science

Developed by Current Medicine, Inc., Philadelphia

Current Medicine

CM 400 Market Street
Suite 700
Philadelphia, PA 19106

Developmental Editor:	*Marian A. Bellus*
Editorial Assistant:	*Forrest Rian Perry*
Design and Layout:	*Christopher Allan*
Illustrators:	*Paul Schiffmacher, Debra Wertz, Anne Rains, Larry Ward, Arlene Ligori, Marie Dean, Beth LaRow, Lisa Weischedel, Teresa Mulley*
Managing Editor:	*Mary Kinsella*
Art Director:	*Jerilyn Kauffman*
Art Department Manager:	*Debra Wertz*
Production:	*Lori Holland, Amy Giuffi*
Indexing:	*Dorothy Hoffman*

Human nutrition and obesity / [edited by] David Heber
    p. cm.—(Atlas of clinical endocrinology; 5)
    Includes bibliographical references and index.
    ISBN 0-632-04401-2
    1. Nutrition disorders Atlases.   2. Obesity Atlases.   3. Nutrition
Atlases.   I. Heber, David.   II. Series
    [DNLM: 1. Nutrition Atlases.   2. Diet Atlases   3. Obesity
Atlases.   WK 17 A8806 1999 v. 5]
    RC620.5.H846   1999
    616.3'9—dc21
    DNLM/DLC
    for Library of Congress   99—34471
                                        CIP

Printed in Hong Kong by Paramount Printing Group Limited

10 9 8 7 6 5 4 3 2 1

DISTRIBUTED WORLDWIDE BY BLACKWELL SCIENCE, INC.

Series Preface

The human body depends on information even more than energy. The means of information transfer are chemical, whether at synapses or through the mediation of hormones at a distance (endocrine), between adjacent cells (paracrine), or within a single cell (autocrine). The body seems to be able to utilize any available molecule for signaling, including gases like nitric oxide and nutrients such as calcium and glucose. In endocrinology, the physician deals with signaling and its disorders, and in nutrition and metabolism, both signaling and energetics.

Endocrinology has been at the forefront of scientific medicine because the molecules involved are so potent that they produce measurable responses at low concentration, and the syndromes produced by an absence or an excess of hormones are relatively dramatic. Furthermore, researchers purified hormones and elucidated their properties very early, which led to their introduction as pharmaceuticals for both diagnostic and therapeutic purposes. As new hormones, signaling pathways and molecular responses are elucidated, endocrinology continues to expand and become more sophisticated. Because the available knowledge is so extensive, it is relatively simple to place new information in context. Providing information to clinicians in an atlas format is particularly suitable for the field of endocrinology because the syndromes are often dramatic, molecular and metabolic pathways are well described, and algorithms for diagnosis and therapy can be developed. In fact, the reader will be struck by the remarkable thoroughness achievable in depicting this field in an atlas, namely, the *Atlas of Clinical Endocrinology*.

The Atlas of Clinical Endocrinology series includes five volumes: Thyroid Diseases, Diabetes, Osteoporosis, Neuroendocrinology and Pituitary Diseases, and Human Nutrition and Obesity. In each field, outstanding experts have contributed not only "state of the art" information but also their expert perspectives on the problems they cover. Throughout the field of endocrinology, major advances have strengthened the scientific base, the diagnostic armamentarium, and the therapeutic options.

In the Thyroid Diseases volume, the recent advances in our understanding of the thyroid hormone economy shed light on the alterations that occur with chronic illness, drugs, and aging. The contributors thoroughly illustrate the dilemmas associated with the management of thyroid nodules and thyroid cancer as well as thyroid disease in pregnancy and the complications of Graves' disease.

Advances in diabetes research and treatment have been dramatic. The volume on Diabetes illustrates the great advances in our understanding of the regulation of insulin secretion and the multiple mechanisms of its action. These advances, as well as the epidemiologic and genetic research that is covered, provide a strong foundation for understanding and managing the consequences of long-term hyperglycemia on the eye, kidney, nerves, and lipids, and on the cardiovascular system. Algorithms are provided for clinical treatment of deficient insulin action with newer agents as well as insulin in both types of diabetes.

Therapy to prevent osteoporotic fractures has become a mainstay in the health care of older women and now older men as well. The Osteoporosis volume describes the bone economy and illustrates the various syndromes leading to loss of bone mineral and the consequences of osteoporotic fracture. The authors describe and justify approaches to preventive and post-fracture therapy, using both medications and non-pharmaceutical means.

In the Neuroendocrinology and Pituitary Diseases volume, major advances in understanding of the interrelationships between the central nervous system and control of pituitary and hypothalamic function are illustrated. Individuals with disorders of growth are characterized. The role of medical treatment in the management of acromegaly and prolactinomas and the approach toward the diagnosis of Cushing's syndrome are elucidated.

Disorders of nutrition, particularly obesity, are the most common disorders in advanced societies. In the Human Nutrition and Obesity volume, the regulation of appetite and eating is addressed; the nutritional requirements for growth and development are characterized; and the impact of diet on clinical conditions such as diabetes, hypertension, cardiovascular disease, cancer, aging and digestive diseases is discussed. The growing use of nutritional supplements is addressed and an integrated program for the management of obesity given.

We are grateful to Current Medicine and especially to Abe Krieger who saw the *Atlas of Clinical Endocrinology* as a dramatic and efficient medium for providing information about endocrinology and metabolism.

Stanley G. Korenman, MD

Preface

The most common nutritional disorder in the United States today is obesity, affecting between 30% and 50% of Americans. This disease has resulted from an imbalance of energy expenditure and energy intake superimposed on the background of metabolic pathways which are very well-adapted to starvation but poorly adapted to overnutrition. It is estimated that between 300 and 900 years or approximately 30 generations are required for significant adaptations to occur in the human genome. Our diets have changed rapidly in the last 100 years with increased fat, sugar, and decreased fiber and micronutrients. The ability of modern food production methods to produce good tasting but nutritionally poor snack foods has contributed significantly to the imbalance between food intake and our inherited metabolic pathways that are designed to process a plant-based diet rich in fiber and phytochemicals.

The endocrine system translates environmental signals of overnutrition at a cellular and tissue level that lead to a number of long-term consequences. Obesity is an independent risk factor for heart disease and contributes to the development and progression of obesity in the vast majority of the millions of non-insulin dependent diabetics in this country. Obesity also contributes to hypertension and many forms of osteoarthritis. Gynecologic disorders, including polycystic ovarian syndrome and many forms of dysmenorrhea, are associated with obesity. Large population-based studies have also shown an association of obesity with many common forms of cancer, including breast cancer, prostate cancer, colon cancer, ovarian cancer, uterine cancer, kidney cancer, and gallbladder cancer. Many of these disease associations are believed to be due to the lifelong effects of diet, making the emerging epidemic of obesity among school children particularly troubling. Adult height is a biomarker for prepubertal nutrition and is increased over time in populations where the incidence of obesity is on the rise, such as the Japanese population. In many developing countries both undernutrition and obesity co-exist in different socioeconomic groups.

Today the treatment of obesity is based on an improved understanding of nutrition, human behavior, the regulation of appetite, and metabolism. The discovery of leptin and other neuropeptides that regulate food intake and metabolism in the hypothalamus and the fat cell has provided exciting new avenues for developing pharmacotherapeutic approaches to obesity. Increased experience with gastric surgery for severe or morbid obesity has provided a lifesaving alternative for high-risk obese patients for whom medical nutritional therapy has failed.

During much of the last 50 years, the efforts of nutrition scientists have been focused on the treatment of undernutrition, including the development of technical innovations such as total parenteral nutrition and specialized approaches to patients with renal or liver failure. These applications of nutrition science have now become routine therapy administered by various specialists caring for patients in acute-care facilities. Multidisciplinary teams including pharmacists, nurses, and dietitians have controlled costs and complications in the hospital and critical care setting. Multivitamin and multimineral supplementation has become accepted mainstream practice in this country, with about one third of the population taking daily vitamin and mineral supplements on the basis of the publicized benefits for heart disease, cancer prevention, and age-related disorders. Botanical dietary supplements are growing in popularity, and an accumulating body of scientific evidence suggests that many of these supplements may have health benefits.

As the description of the entire human genome sequence is completed early in the next century, the science of nutrition will become increasingly relevant to the understanding and treatment of chronic diseases involving the expression of multiple genes, and with the development of new treatment strategies, nutrition should become an integral part of the practice of primary care medicine as well as endocrinology.

David Heber, MD, PhD

Contributors

SHALENDER BHASIN, MD

Professor
Department of Internal Medicine
UCLA School of Medicine;
Chief, Division of Endocrinology
Charles R. Drew University
Los Angeles, California

GEORGE L. BLACKBURN, MD, PhD

Associate Professor of Surgery
S. Daniel Abraham Chair
Department of Medicine
Division of Nutrition
Harvard Medical School;
Director of Nutrition Support Service
Division of Surgical Nutrition
Beth Israel Deaconess Medical Center
Boston, Massachusetts

JEFFREY B. BLUMBERG, PhD

Professor of Nutrition
Tufts University School of Nutrition, Science and Policy
Medford, Massachusetts;
Associate Director/Senior Scientist
Jean Mayer USDA Human Nutrition Research Center on Aging
    at Tufts University
Boston, Massachusetts

BENJAMIN BONAVIDA, PhD

Professor
Department of Microbiology and Immunology
UCLA School of Medicine
Los Angeles, California

SUSAN BOWERMAN, MS, RD

Executive Assistant to the Director
UCLA Center for Human Nutrition
Los Angeles, California

RACHELLE BROSS, PhD

Research Associate
Division of Endocrinology, Metabolism, and Molecular Medicine
Charles R. Drew University of Medicine and Science
Los Angeles, CA

ANN M. COULSTON, MS, RD

Nutrition Consultant
Stanford University
Stanford, California

JOHANNA DWYER, DSc, RD

Professor
Department of Medicine
Tufts University Schools of Medicine and Nutrition;
Director, Frances Stern Nutrition Center
New England Medical Center Hospitals
Boston, Massachusetts

JENNIFER R. ELIASI, MS, RD

Dietetic Intern
Frances Stern Nutrition Center;
Graduate Student
Tufts University School of Nutrition, Science and Policy
Boston, Massachusetts

VAY LIANG W. GO, MD

Professor of Medicine
Department of Medicine
UCLA School of Medicine;
Associate Director, UCLA Center for Human Nutrition
Los Angeles, California

CHARLES H. HALSTEAD, MD

Professor
Department of Internal Medicine
University of California, Davis, School of Medicine
Davis, California;
University of California, Davis, Medical Center
Sacramento, California

DAVID HEBER, MD, PhD

Professor
Department of Medicine
UCLA School of Medicine;
Director
UCLA Center for Human Nutrition
Los Angeles, California

LALITA KHAODHIAR, MD

Fellow in Clinical Nutrition
Department of Nutrition/Medicine
Harvard Medical School;
Fellow in Clinical Nutrition
Beth Israel Deaconess Medical Center
Boston, Massachusetts

Contributors, *continued*

DAVID KRITCHEVSKY, PhD

Professor Emeritus
Department of Biochemistry
University of Pennsylvania School of Veterinary Medicine;
Professor, Caspar Wistar Scholar
Wistar Institute
Philadelphia, Pennsylvania

MANOJ MALOO, MD

Fellow
Department of Surgery
Harvard Medical School;
Fellow
Department of Surgery
Beth Israel Deaconess Medical Center
Boston, Massachusetts

MORTON MAXWELL, MD

Clinical Professor
Department of Medicine
UCLA School of Medicine;
Co-director
UCLA University Obesity Center
Los Angeles, California

DIANE MCKAY, PhD

Graduate Research Assistant
Jean Mayer USDA Human Nutrition Research Center on Aging
     at Tufts University
Boston, Massachusetts

NAOMI D. NEUFELD, MD

Clinical Professor
Department of Pediatrics
UCLA School of Medicine;
Medical Director
Kidshape, Inc.
Los Angeles, California

ATAM B. SINGH, MD

Clinical/Research Fellow
Division of Endocrinology, Metabolism, and Molecular Medicine
Charles R. Drew University of Medicine and Science
Los Angeles, CA

SUSAN STANGL, MD

Assistant Professor
Department of Family Medicine
UCLA School of Medicine;
Assistant Dean for Student Affairs
UCLA School of Medicine
Los Angeles, California

Contents

Contents, *continued*

Contents, *continued*

Color Plates

Fundamentals of Human Nutrition

David Heber and Susan Bowerman

Human nutrition comprises a wide variety of disciplines and requires the integration of a number of different conceptual models for research and clinical purposes. Nutrition begins with food choices, which are determined by availability as well as individual and social factors. Whole foods are the expression of eating behaviors; however, they also can be analyzed in terms of their provision of macronutrients, micronutrients, and fiber. Nutrition can be further reduced to considerations of carbohydrate metabolism, quality of individual amino acids and proteins, and lipid composition and fatty acid metabolism.

In the United States today, vitamin, mineral, and nutrient deficiencies are rare as a result of food fortification. The challenge for the future is to combat the problems of obesity and overnutrition with fat and calories. To understand these problems, it is important to realize that all food components can be interconverted and stored as fat when less calories are ingested. In addition, the efficiency with which extra calories are converted to fat is determined genetically. Therefore, a gene-nutrient interaction is of importance in every nutritional disorder.

The basic processes of oxidant stress have influenced both plant and human evolution. Plants contain a number of natural antioxidants. Humans have developed endogenous enzyme systems, as well as antioxidants produced endogenously, that are relevant to the nutritional environment. For example, humans do not manufacture vitamin C as do most other animal species owing to its abundance in a plant-based human diet. Scurvy only occurred once man moved to the food supplies of the past few hundred years. These supplies are significantly less diverse when compared with the ancient biodiverse diet of fifty to one hundred thousand years ago.

Plants also contain a number of unique phytochemicals not available as supplements. These phytochemicals, which are beneficial, nonnutritive substances in plants, stimulate the cells of our bodies to develop enzymes to metabolize these substances. For example, someone taking 500 mg daily of vitamin C has a different panel of metabolizing enzymes in the liver than does someone taking only 20 mg daily of vitamin C. The interaction of the nutritional environment and human body occurs at the molecular genetic, cellular, organ, and whole-body levels.

Modern dietary recommendations need to consider the basic science of nutrition and the current problems of overnutrition, obesity, and chronic disease. Recommendations for dietary intake among populations often take the form of pyramids, with the base of the pyramid being the basis of the diet.

The base of the pyramid developed in the late 1980s by the United States Department of Agriculture (USDA) consists of cereals and grains without emphasis on the fiber content of those grains. The fruits and vegetables appear on the second level and are comprised of two separate groups. In a new pyramid developed in 1997 by the Center for Human Nutrition at the University of California at Los Angeles, a modified plant-based diet is recommended. The base consists of fruits and vegetables to provide unique phytonutrients for prevention of chronic diseases. The second level emphasizes high-fiber cereals and grains to provide the benefits of fiber from these foods as well as from fruits and vegetables. The protein level is made up of low-fat protein choices from both plants and animals. The top tier of the USDA pyramid has only dots representing fats and sweets with the mixed message "use sparingly." The top tier of the new California pyramid emphasizes taste enhancers including olives, avocados, garlic, onion, nuts, cheese, chili peppers, and small amounts of mono-unsaturated or omega-3-rich oils. The overall fat recommendation of the USDA pyramid is 30% or less of calories from fat. In contrast, the California pyramid reflects the decreased fat intake in the population and recommends 20% or less of calories from fat.

Food Choices

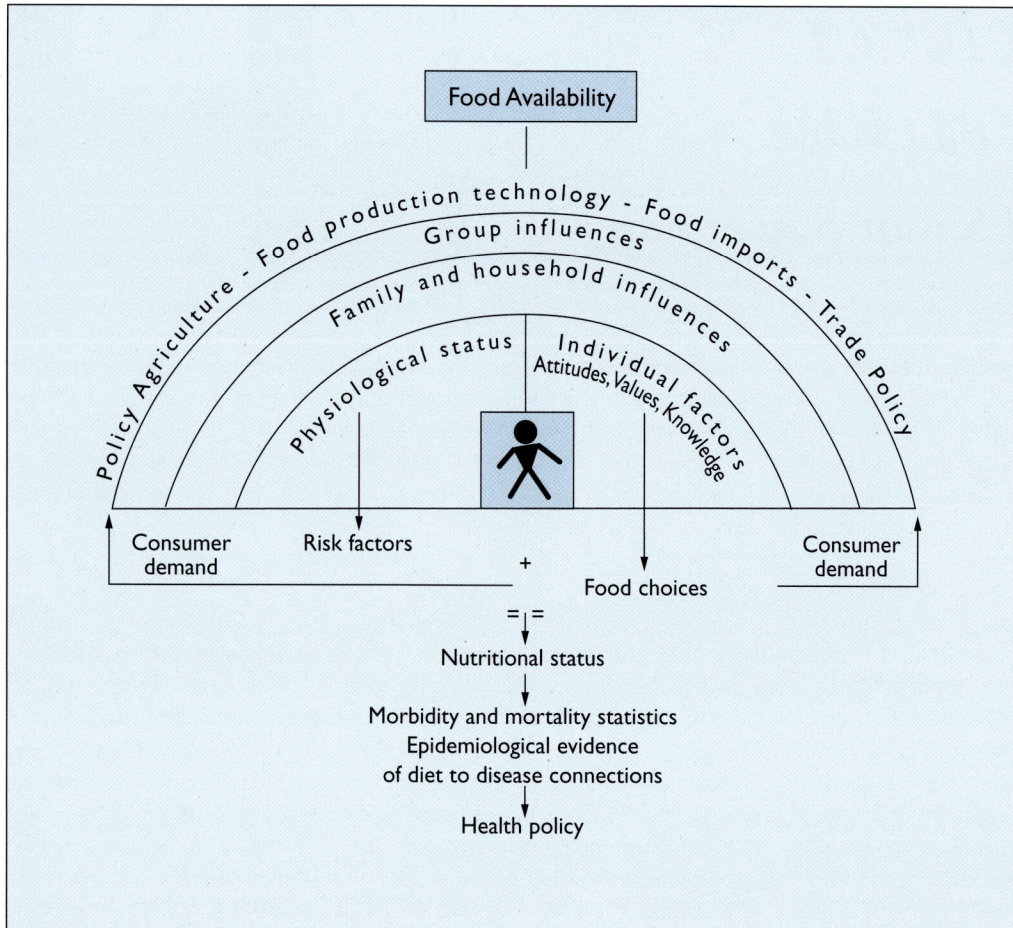

FIGURE 1-1. Food choices. The choice of foods is a complex product of multiple influences, including culture, family, and availability. Food choices clearly affect the nutritional value of the diet. Although foods are purchased by consumers primarily based on taste, cost, and convenience, many of the specific factors noted also influence food choices. These factors can be used to influence healthier food choices within the constraints of a free food economy. (*Adapted from* Sims [1].)

Macronutirents and Micronutrients

COMPONENTS OF DIET

Macronutrients
  Carbohydrates
  Fats and oils
  Proteins and amino acids
  Water
Micronutrients
  Minerals
  Phytochemicals
  Vitamins
Nonnutrients
  Insoluble fibers
  Some soluble fibers

FIGURE 1-2. Macronutrients and micronutrients make up the nutritional landscape. Micronutrients derive their name from the fact that they are needed in relatively small amounts compared with macronutrients. The nonnutrient components of diet such as fiber play an important role in human nutrition.

ELEMENTS ESSENTIAL TO LIFE

Major Elements	Macrominerals*	Microminerals†
Carbon	Calcium	Arsenic
Hydrogen	Chlorine	Boron
Nitrogen	Magnesium	Chromium
Oxygen	Phosphorus	Cobalt
	Sodium	Copper
	Sulfur	Fluorine
		Iodine
		Iron
		Manganese
		Molybdenum
		Nickel
		Selenium
		Silicon
		Tin
		Vanadium
		Zinc

*More than 0.005% body weight, over 100 mg needed daily.

†Less than 0.005% body weight, a few milligrams or less needed daily.

FIGURE 1-3. Chemical elements essential to life are classified as major, macrominerals, and microminerals. These elements are derived from the diet or dietary supplements. As the diet becomes refined and processed the risk of depletion of some of these elements is increased. In more biodiverse diets, the risk of dietary deficiency is decreased.

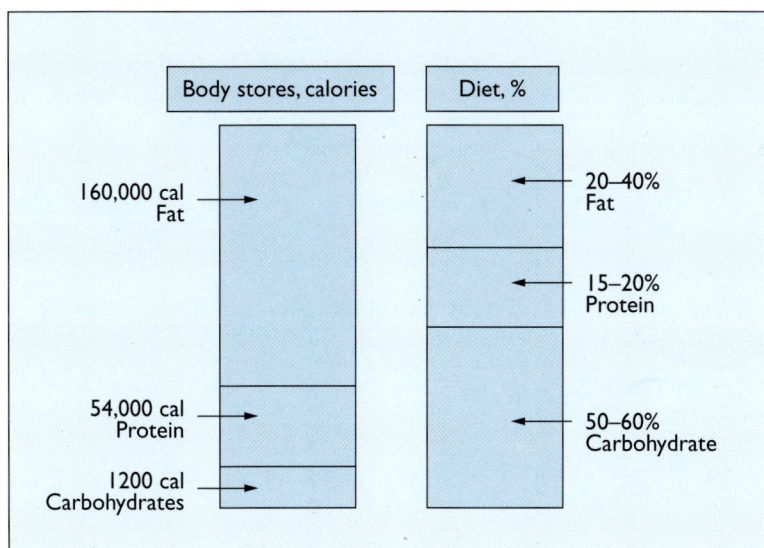

FIGURE 1-4. Storage of macronutrients. The human body stores macronutrients in a very different proportion from those found in the human diet. Whereas the daily diet may be 30% fat, 50% carbohydrate, and 20% protein, the body stores 160,000 calories as fat (about 13.5 kg in a typical man weighing 70 kg), and 54,000 calories (about 13.5 kg) as protein. Surprisingly, only 1200 calories of carbohydrate are stored as 300 g of glycogen in the liver and muscle. These storage fractions are correlated with the portability of the energy stored. Fats are the most portable, and carbohydrates are the least portable because they require water of hydration.

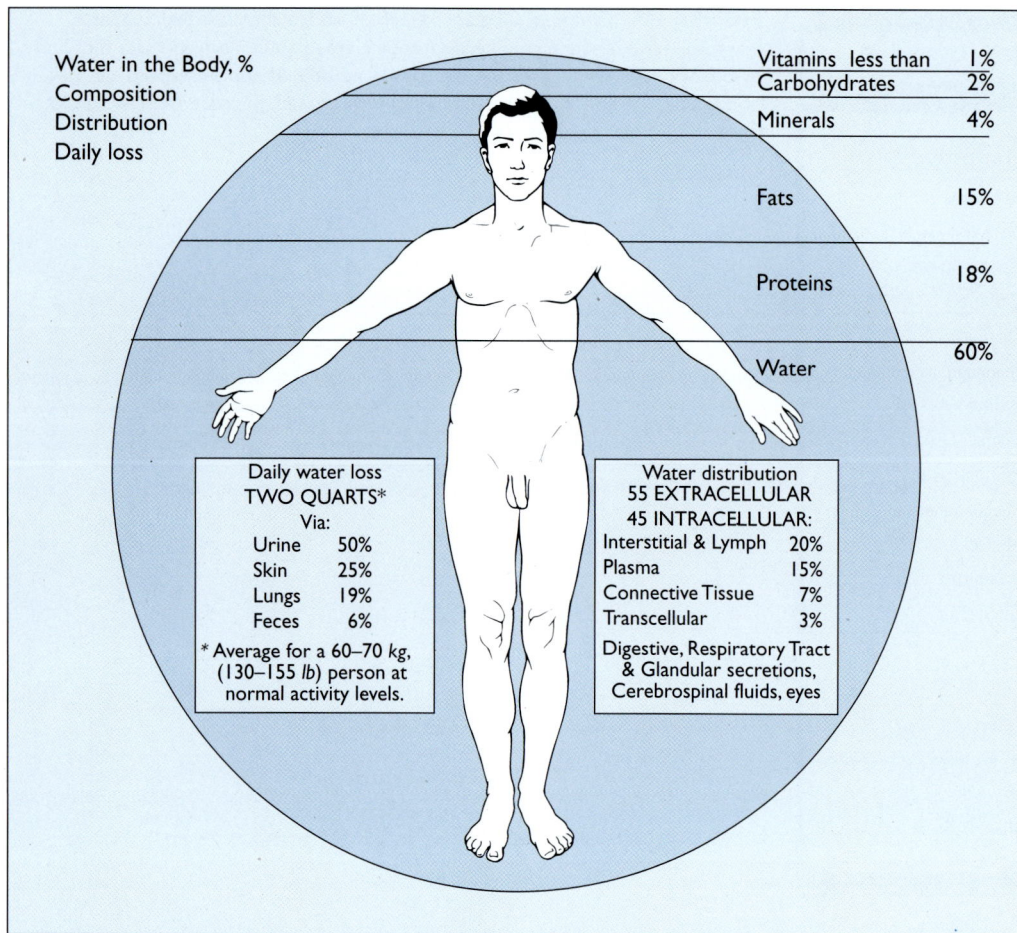

Water in the Body, %
Composition
Distribution
Daily loss

Vitamins less than	1%
Carbohydrates	2%
Minerals	4%
Fats	15%
Proteins	18%
Water	60%

Daily water loss
TWO QUARTS*
Via:
Urine   50%
Skin   25%
Lungs   19%
Feces   6%

* Average for a 60–70 *kg*,
(130–155 *lb*) person at
normal activity levels.

Water distribution
55 EXTRACELLULAR
45 INTRACELLULAR:
Interstitial & Lymph   20%
Plasma   15%
Connective Tissue   7%
Transcellular   3%

Digestive, Respiratory Tract
& Glandular secretions,
Cerebrospinal fluids, eyes

FIGURE 1-5. Water composition, distribution, and daily loss. Water is the most prevalent of the macronutrients in the body. An average man weighing 70 kg is comprised of 45 L of water divided among intracellular (30 L), interstitial (12 L) and blood plasma (3 L). A moderately active adult cycles about 2.5 L of water daily. Body water is derived mainly from beverages, food, and metabolic products (60%, 30%, and 10%, respectively). Excretion occurs in urine, skin, perspiration, and feces (60%, 28%, 8%, and 4%, respectively). (*Adapted from* Haas [2].)

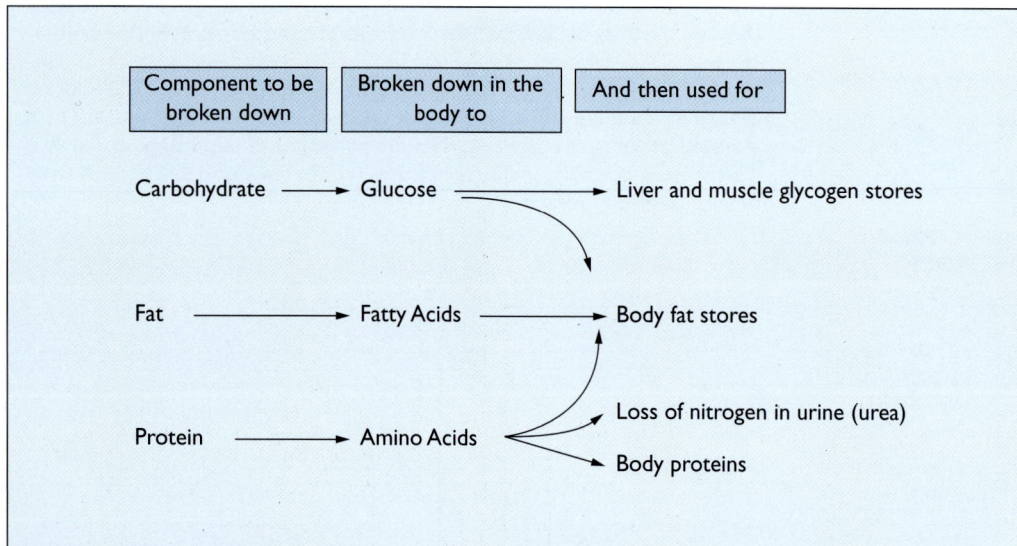

| Component to be broken down | Broken down in the body to | And then used for |

Carbohydrate → Glucose → Liver and muscle glycogen stores

Fat → Fatty Acids → Body fat stores

Protein → Amino Acids → Loss of nitrogen in urine (urea)
Body proteins

FIGURE 1-6. Metabolism in the fed state. The metabolism of carbohydrates, fats, and proteins, is interconnected. This interrelationship provides essential flexibility to humans when faced with dietary restriction or starvation. In fact, the body can interconvert to a greater or lesser degree macronutrients, proteins, fats, and carbohydrates during starvation or overfeeding. (*Adapted from* Whitney and Rolfes [3].)

AMINO ACIDS

Essential Amino Acids
  Histidine
  Isoleucine
  Leucine
  Lysine
  Methionine
  Phenylalanine
  Threonine
  Tryptophan
  Valine
Nonessential Amino Acids
  Alanine
  Arginine
  Asparagine
  Aspartic acid
  Cysteine
  Glutamic acid
  Glutamine
  Glycine
  Proline
  Serine
  Tyrosine

FIGURE 1-7. Proteins are composed of amino acids, which are classified as essential or nonessential. Essential amino acids must be obtained from the diet. Nonessential amino acids can be synthesized in the body from the essential amino acids. The quality of dietary proteins is based on the content of essential and nonessential amino acids. Proteins with the highest utilization efficiency are said to have the highest biologic value.

PROTEIN DIGESTIBILITY CORRECTED AMINO ACID SCORE VALUES

Protein Source	Value*
Casein (milk)	1.00
Egg whites	1.00
Soybeans (isolate)	0.99
Beef	0.92
Pea flour	0.69
Kidney beans (canned)	0.68
Garbanzo beans (canned)	0.66
Pinto beans (canned)	0.63
Rolled oats	0.57
Lentils (canned)	0.52
Peanut meal	0.52
Whole wheat	0.40

*1.0 is the maximum value a food protein can receive.

FIGURE 1-8. The protein-digestibility-corrected amino acid score (PDCAAS) method of evaluating the quality of a protein compares its amino acid content with human amino acid requirements and corrects for digestibility. Amino acid scoring is a method of evaluating protein quality by comparing the amino acid patterns of a test protein with that of a reference protein. Once the amino acid score is derived, it is compared against the amino acid requirements of preschool-aged children. The rationale behind using the requirements of this age group is that if a protein will effectively support a young child's growth and development, it will meet or exceed the requirements of older children and adults. (*Adapted from* Whitney and Rolfes [3].)

MAJOR LIPIDS

Type	Function
Fatty acids	Metabolic fuel; transport
Fatty acid derivatives:	
Triglycerides	Fatty acid storage; transport
Phospholipids	Membranes
Cholesteryl esters	Cholesterol storage
Steroids:	
Cholesterol	Membranes; transport
Bile acids	Fat digestion
Hormones	Metabolic regulation

FIGURE 1-9. Lipid classes include fatty acids, fatty acid derivatives, and steroids. The lipid class has many functions from acting as a metabolic fuel to membrane function and metabolic regulation. Fatty acids are an essential component of the diet albeit at a low level of 10% of the total calories in the diet to ensure that 6% comes from a combination of linoleic and linolenic acids.

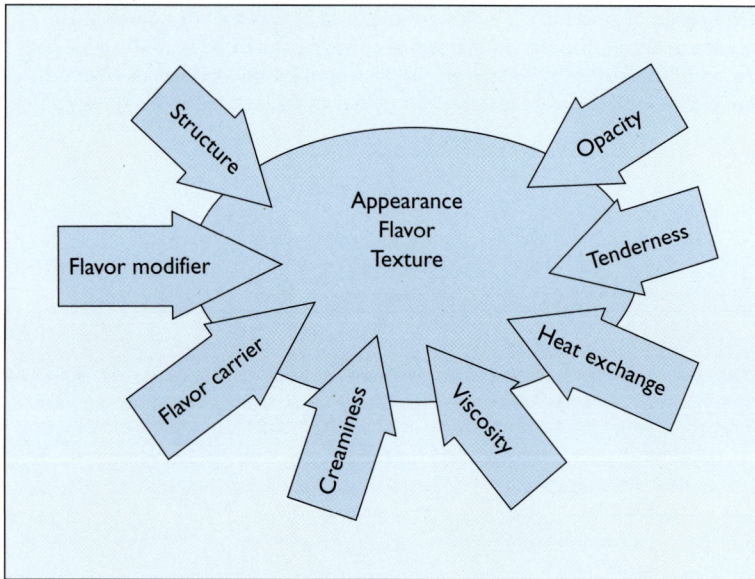

FIGURE 1-10. Qualities of food. Fats impart many qualities to foods: flavor, texture, aroma, and appearance. Many of the compounds that provide flavor are fat soluble, and fats transport these substances to sensory cells in the mouth, providing taste and aroma. Fats also provide a creamy sensation in foods such as ice cream and tenderness in marbled meats. In baked goods, fats provide structure and tenderness. Food manufacturers have introduced thousands of fat-free and low-fat foods into the marketplace. Consumer demand has created the challenge of reducing fat content while preserving the taste and textural qualities that fat provides. (*Adapted from* Sims [1].)

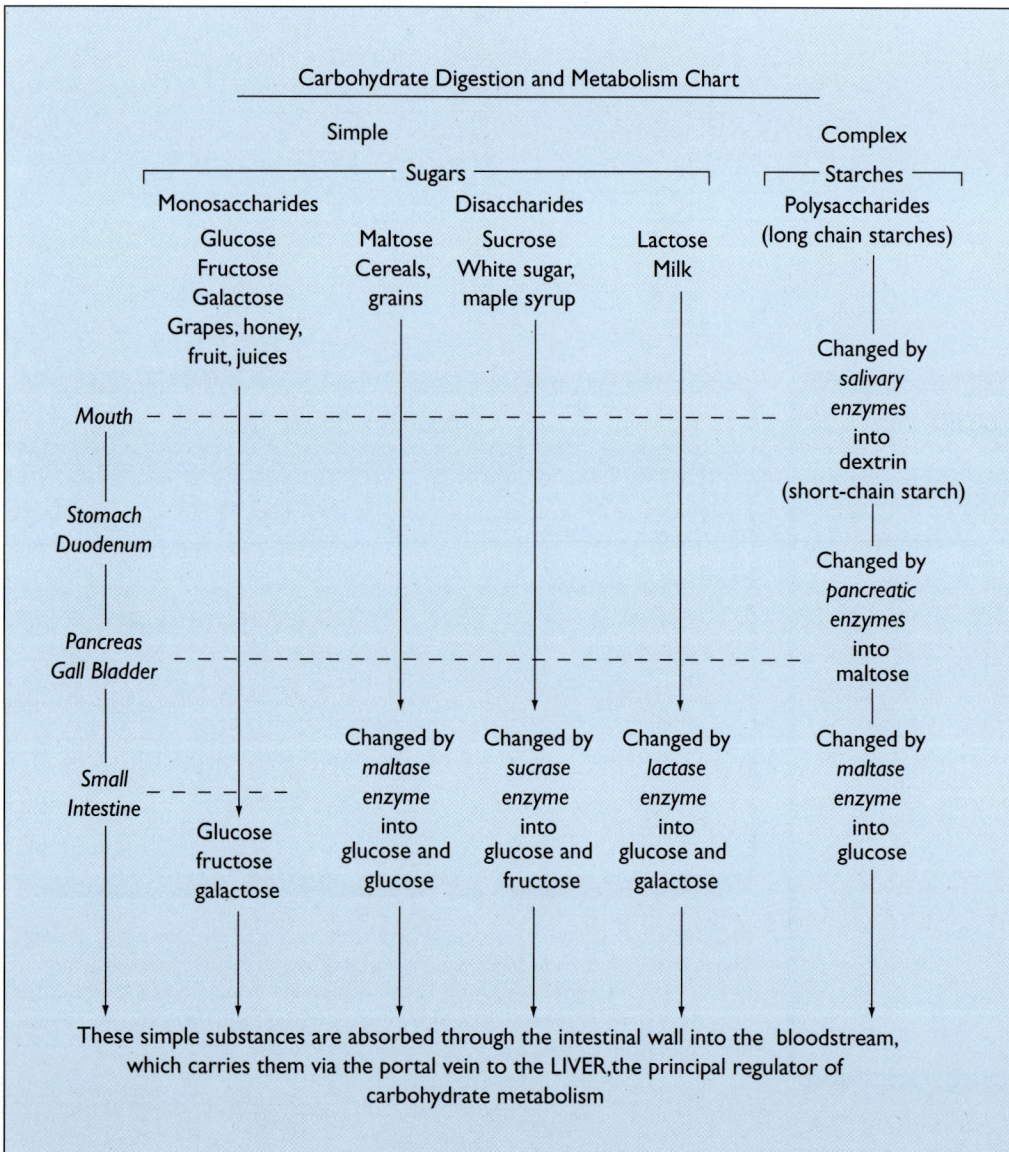

FIGURE 1-11. Carbohydrate digestion and metabolism. Carbohydrates are classified as simple or complex. Simple carbohydrates include the monosaccharides (glucose, fructose, and galactose) and disaccharides (maltose, lactose, and sucrose). Complex carbohydrates are composed of many monosaccharides linked together to form starch and fiber. An anomalous group classified as complex by labeling law are the polysaccharides. These dissolve in the stomach and essentially act like simple carbohydrates except for their effects on intestinal osmolality, which may influence bowel motility. (*Adapted from* Haas [2].)

SOURCE AND ACTION OF FIBERS

	Soluble Fibers	Insoluble Fibers
Food sources	Fruit such as apples and citrus	Wheat bran
	Oats	Whole grain breads and cereals
	Barley	Vegetables
	Legumes	
Action in the body	Delays gastrointestinal transit	Accelerates gastrointestinal transit
	Stimulates colonic fermentation	Increases fecal weight
	Delays glucose absorption	Slows starch hydrolysis
	Lowers blood cholesterol	Delays glucose absorption
Examples	Gums	Cellulose
	Pectins	Lignins
	Some hemicelluloses	Many hemicelluloses
	Mucilages	

FIGURE 1-12. Fiber is an important nonnutrient constituent of food such as cereals, grains, fruits, and vegetables. Fiber can be classified as soluble or insoluble. (*Adapted from* Whitney and Rolfes [3].)

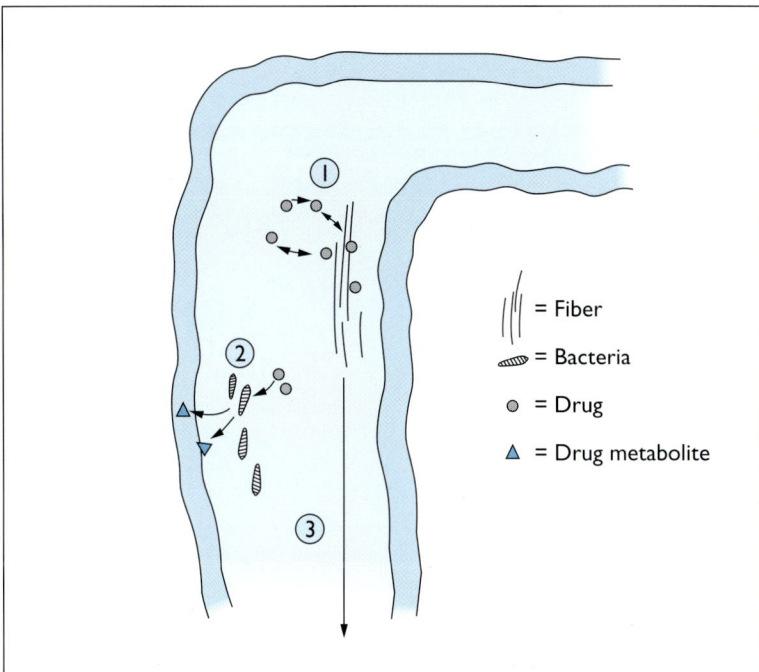

|||| = Fiber

= Bacteria

○ = Drug

△ = Drug metabolite

FIGURE 1-13. The effects of fiber on drug metabolism in the colon. Fiber has a number of actions in the colon. In addition to the binding of certain drugs (1) fiber can have effects on drug metabolism through the actions of colonic bacteria that, in turn, can be influenced by the fiber content of the diet (2). Studies have demonstrated that dietary differences correlate with differences in colonic bacteria species. Some of these species differences have functional implications for nutrient and hormone metabolism. Finally, fiber can affect transit time of nutrients in the colon that, in turn, can affect absorption of drugs through the colonic mucosa [3].

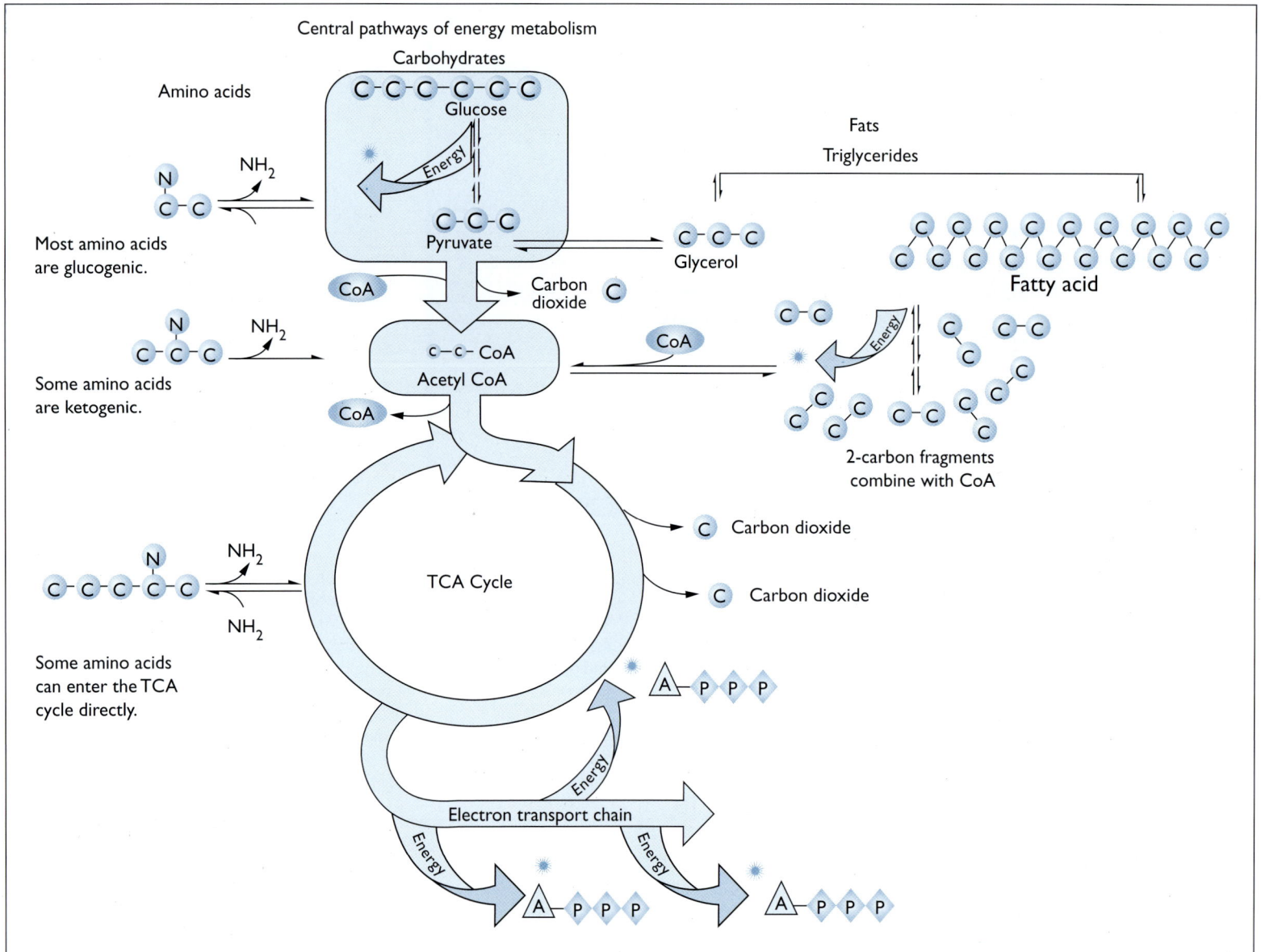

FIGURE 1-14. Central pathways of energy metabolism. The digestion of carbohydrate yields glucose. Some of the glucose is stored as glycogen and some is taken into the brain and other cells to be broken down to provide energy. The digestion of fats yields glycerol and free fatty acids. Some fats are reassembled into triglycerides and stored as fat; others are broken down to provide energy. Protein digestion yields amino acids, some of which are used to build body protein. When a surplus of amino acids exists, or when there is inadequate carbohydrate or fat to meet energy needs, amino acids also can provide energy. Of the energy-containing nutrients, fat provides the most energy by weight. A— adenosine; C—carbon; CoA— coenzyme A; N— nitrogen; NH_2— amino group; P— phosphate; TCA— tricarboxylic acid. (*Adapted from* Whitney and Rolfes [3].)

Oxidation Stress

REACTIVE OXYGEN SPECIES	
$O_2^{\bullet-}$, superoxide anion	One electron reduction product of O_2
$HO_2^{\bullet}$, perhydroxy radical	Protonated form of $O_2^{\bullet-}$
H_2O_2, hydrogen peroxide	Two-electron reduction product of O_2
$^{\bullet}OH$, hydroxyl radical	Three-electron reduction product of O_2
$RO^{\bullet}$, alkoxyl radical	Example: lipid radical ($LO^{\bullet}$)
$ROO^{\bullet}$, peroxyl radical	Example: lipid peroxyl radical ($LOO^{\bullet}$)
$^1\Delta gO_2$ (also $^1O_2$)	Singlet molecular oxygen

FIGURE 1-15. Oxidation is a basic chemical reaction essential to energy metabolism in the mitochondrion. However, oxidation also can result in damage to the structures of proteins, lipids, carbohydrates, and nucleic acids. Quite a few chemical species can lead to oxidant damage. The body has a number of anti-oxidant defense mechanisms to counteract oxidant stress. In addition, phyto-chemicals such as flavonoids also can act as scavengers of oxygen radicals.

hNQO₁

471   -452

GCAGTCA CAG TGACTCAGCA

ARE   ATG   TGA

-1850 —————————— E1 -- E2 -- E3 -- E4 -- E5 -- E6

100 bp (Exon-intron 3' flank)
E1–E7 exons

-936   -917   hNQO₂

TGACTGC AAA TGAGGTGGCA

ARE   ATG   TAA

-1336 —————————— E1 -- E2 -- E3 -- E4 -- E5 -- E6 -- E7

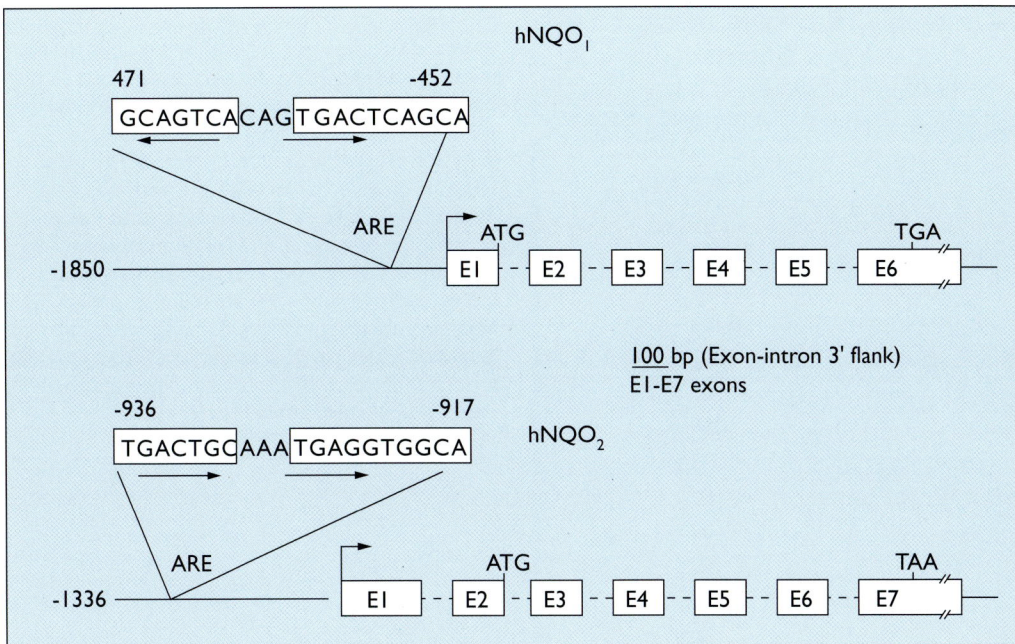

FIGURE 1-16. The anti-oxidant response gene. This gene involves at least six genes on at least two different chromosomes and is a coordinated response to oxidant stress. Shown here are the nicotinamide adenine dinucleotide phosphate (NADPH) quinone oxidoreductase I and II (hNQO₁ and hNQO₂) genes with the antioxidant response element. These complex gene responses evolved to deal with the ubiquitous oxidant stress to which cells are exposed. There are both endogenous antioxidants, such as the tripeptide glutathione, and exogenous antioxidants ingested from the diet, such as vitamin E, vitamin C, and the carotenoids. The endogenous and exogenous systems work together to reduce oxidant stress. ARE— antioxidant response element; ATG— adenine, thymine, guanine. (*Adapted from* Jaiswal [4].)

Vitamins and Minerals

WATER-SOLUBLE AND FAT-SOLUBLE VITAMINS

	Water-Soluble Vitamins	Fat-Soluble Vitamins
Absorption	Directly into blood	Into lymph, then into blood
Transport	Travel freely	May require protein carriers
Storage	Freely circulate in aqueous media	Trapped in cells associated with fat
Excretion	Kidneys remove excess	Less readily excreted; tend to remain in fat storage
Toxicity	Unlikely to reach toxic levels when consumed in excess	Could reach toxic levels when consumed in excess
Requirements	Small, frequent dosages	Needed in periodic doses

FIGURE 1-17. Vitamins are organic compounds that largely serve as coenzyme factors. Their name derives from *vita,* Latin for life, and *amine,* signifying a protein because early vitamin researchers assumed these factors must be proteins. In fact, the vitamins are defined operationally by their necessity for the maintenance of life. Some vitamins such as A and D really are steroid hormones unrelated to the many enzyme cofactors found among the vitamins.

The fat-soluble vitamins are A, D, E, and K. Because they are stored by the body, fat-soluble vitamins are less readily excreted than are water-soluble vitamins. Thus, fat-soluble vitamins are needed in periodic doses. The water-soluble vitamins include the B vitamins (B₁ [thiamin], B₂ [riboflavin], B₃ [niacin] B₆ [pyridoxine], folic acid, and B₁₂ [cyanocobalamin]) and vitamin C (ascorbic acid). These vitamins are absorbed directly into the bloodstream and circulate freely. Because the kidneys detect excesses in the blood and excrete them into the urine, water-soluble vitamins are needed in more frequent doses. In addition to these vitamins, fruits and vegetables provide a large number of phytochemicals. These phytochemicals include carotenoids, isoflavones, terpenoids, isothiocyanate, organic sulfides, and polyphenols, which have various physiologic effects. The functions of many of these compounds have not been fully elucidated. (*Adapted from* Whitney and Rolfes [3].)

ELEMENTAL COMPOSITION OF THE HUMAN BODY
AT AN AVERAGE WEIGHT OF 70 KG, OR 155 LB

	Key Function	Amount
Macrominerals		
Oxygen	Cell and tissue respiration, water	43,000 g
Carbon	Protoplasm	12,000 g
Hydrogen	Water, tissue	6300 g
Nitrogen	Protein tissue	2000 g
Calcium	Bones and teeth	1100 g
Phosphorus	Bones and teeth	750 g
Potassium	Intracellular electrolyte	225 g
Sulfur	Amino acids, hair and skin	150 g
Chloride	Electrolyte	100 g
Sodium	Extracellular electrolyte	90 g
Magnesium	Metabolic electrolyte	35 g
Silicon	Connective tissue	30 g
Microminerals		
Iron	Hemoglobin, oxygen carrier	4200 mg
Fluoride	Bones and teeth	2600 mg
Zinc	Metallo-enzymes	2400 mg
Strontium	Bone integrity	320 mg
Copper	Enzyme cofactor	90 mg
Cobalt	Vitamin B_{12} core	20 mg
Vanadium	Lipid metabolism	20 mg
Iodine	Thyroid hormones	15 mg
Tin	Unknown	15 mg
Selenium	Enzyme, antioxidant, detoxification	15 mg
Manganese	Metallo-enzymes	13 mg
Nickel	Unknown	11 mg
Molybdenum	Enzyme cofactor	8 mg
Chromium	Glucose tolerance factor	6 mg

FIGURE 1-18. Minerals are inorganic compounds. They are classified as either major minerals or trace minerals, depending on the amounts present in the body. The major minerals are calcium, phosphorus, potassium, sulfur, sodium, chloride, and magnesium. They are present in amounts over 5 g. The major minerals provide structure to the body and help maintain fluid balance. The trace minerals function primarily as coenzymes in energy metabolism. The trace minerals are iron, zinc, copper, manganese, iodine, and selenium. They are found in the human body in amounts under 5 g. Some foods contain binders, such as phytic acid and oxalic acid, that can form complexes with minerals and prevent their absorption. (*Adapted from* Haas [2].)

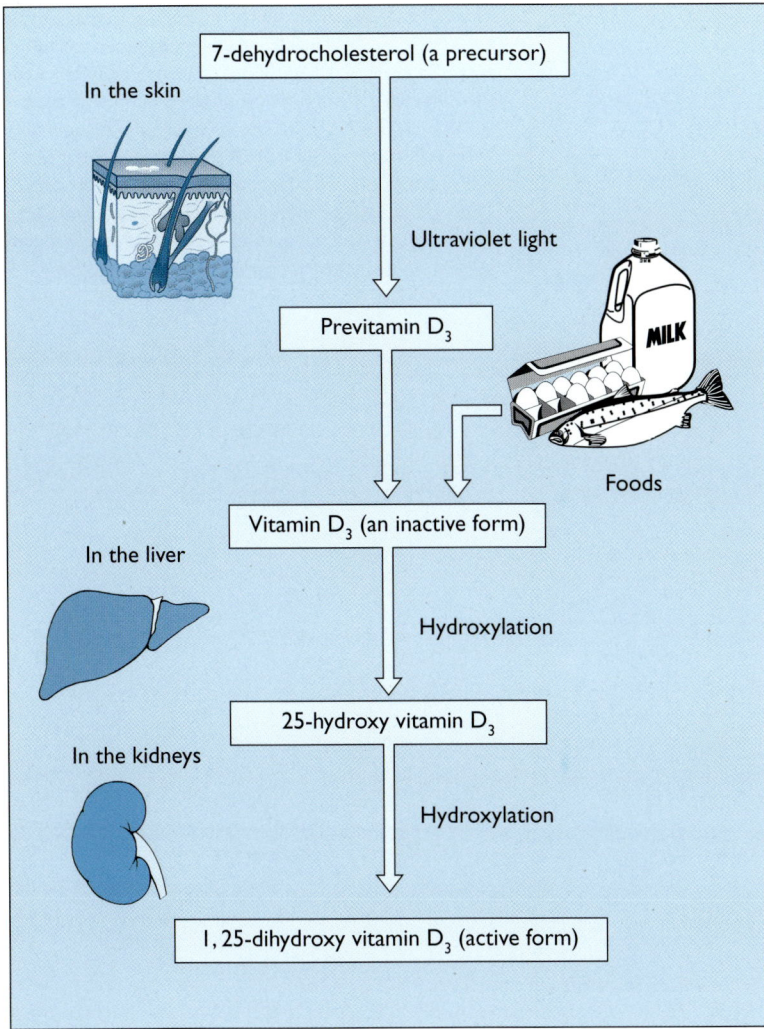

FIGURE 1-19. Vitamin D synthesis and activation. Vitamin D is different from all the other nutrients because it can be synthesized from 7-dehydrocholesterol in the skin in the presence of sunlight. Ergosterol also can be ingested from plants and converted to active forms of vitamin D. Vitamin D functions as a hormone, with the intestines, kidneys, and bones as target organs. These organs respond to vitamin D by making calcium available for bone growth. Ultraviolet rays from the sun convert 7-dehydrocholesterol into previtamin D_3. The liver hydroxylates the compound to 25-hydroxy-vitamin D_3, and within the kidney further hydroxylation yields either active (1,25-dihydroxy-vitamin D_3) or inactive (24,25-dihydroxy-vitamin D_3) forms of the vitamin. This important branch-point regulation is critical in the regulation of calcium metabolism. (*Adapted from* Whitney and Rolfes [3].)

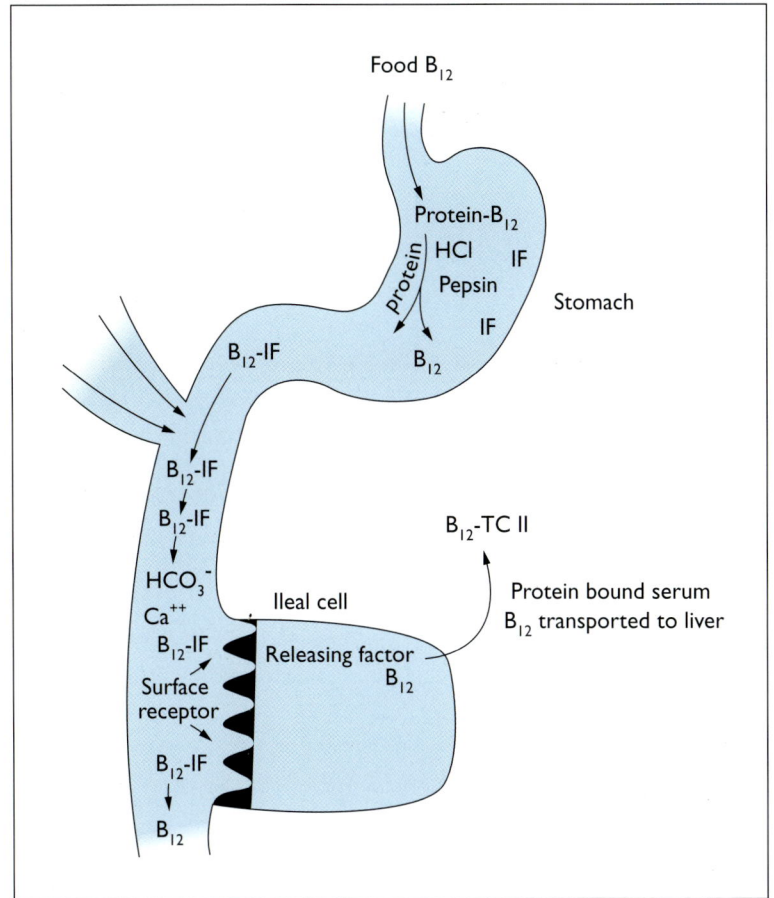

FIGURE 1-20. Vitamin B_{12} absorption. Vitamin B_{12} illustrates an example of complex regulation of vitamin absorption. After ingestion, the vitamin B_{12} present in protein foods is released from the proteins by hydrochloric acid (HCl) and pepsin in the stomach. Absorption of the vitamin requires another protein (intrinsic factor) that is secreted by parietal cells in the stomach to bind to B_{12} and travel to the ileum. There the complex is absorbed. Ca^{2+}— calcium ion; HCO_3^-— bicarbonate; IF— intrinsic factor; TC II— transcobalamin II. (*Adapted from* Roe [5].)

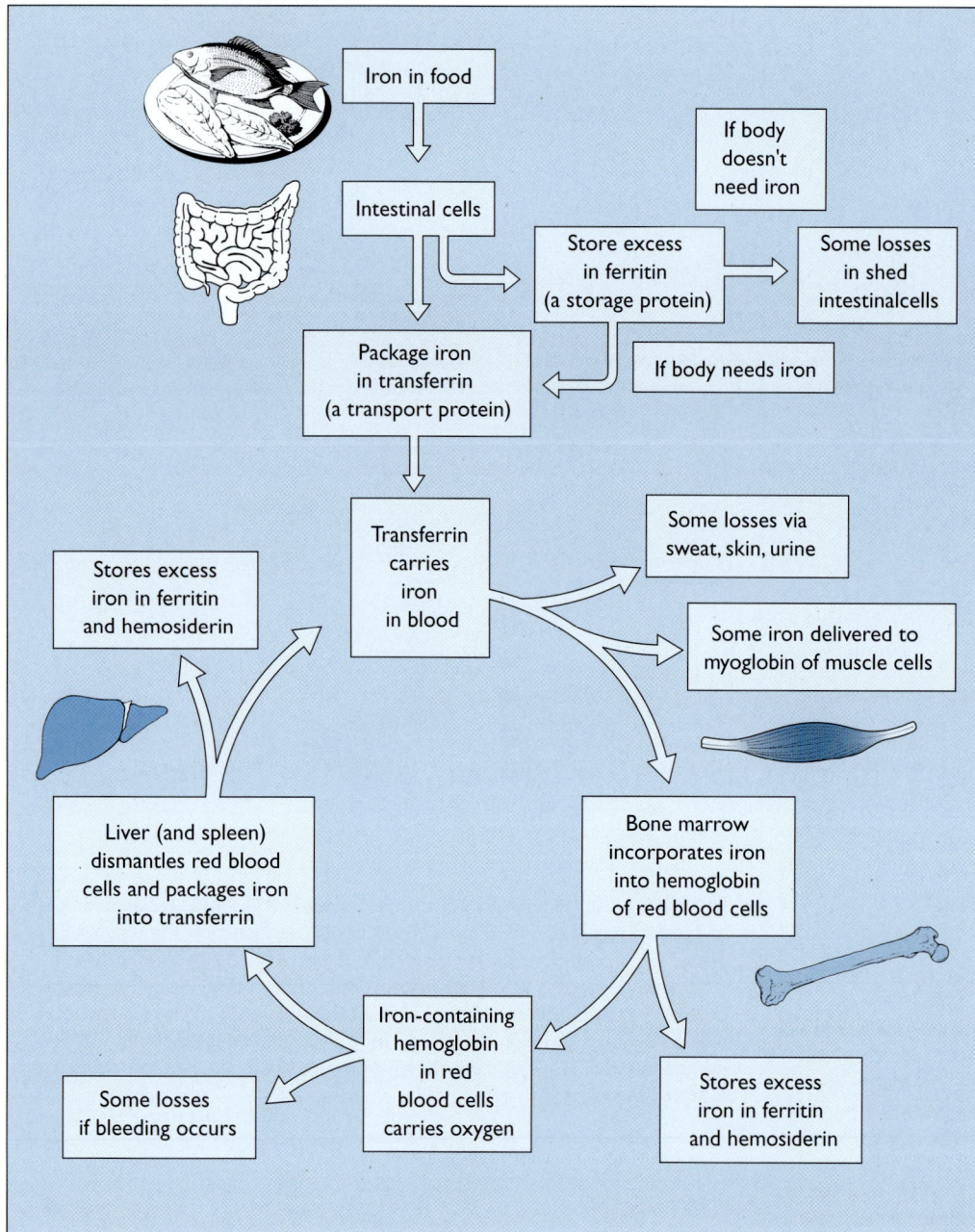

FIGURE 1-21. The routes of iron in the body. Iron metabolism illustrates a carefully regulated system at the intracellular level. When there is deficient iron, the cell triggers production of transferrin receptor at the cell membrane to transport iron into the cell. When there is excess iron available, the cell triggers the production of ferritin, an iron-storage protein. The iron response element (IRE) is responsible for both of these environmental signals at the molecular genetic level. (*Adapted from* Whitney and Rolfes [3].)

Phytochemicals

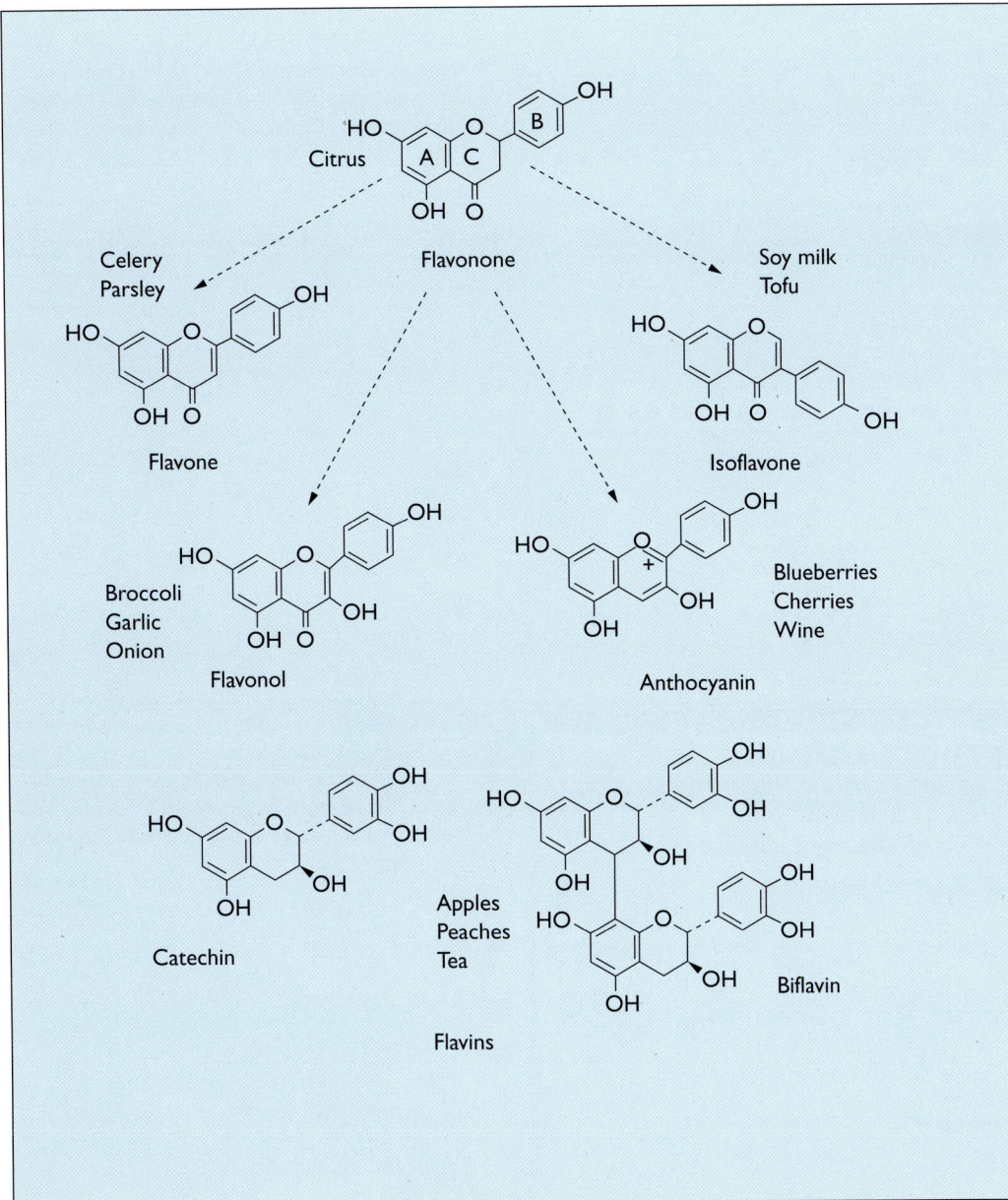

FIGURE 1-22. Hormone-like substances found in plants. There are many active hormone-like substances found in plants such as isoflavones in soy protein. The isoflavones genistein and daidzein are selective estrogen response modifiers. These isoflavones are proestrogenic in bone and brain, and they are anti-estrogenic in breast and uterus. Isoflavones also are antioxidants and tyrosine kinase inhibitors capable of inhibiting the growth of breast and prostate tumor cells *in vitro*.

Xenobiotics

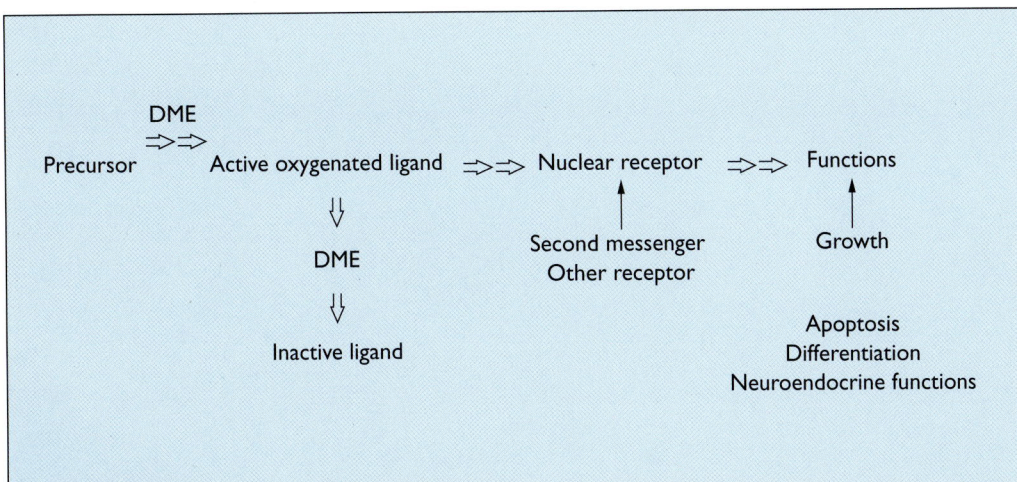

FIGURE 1-23. Xenobiotic metabolism and cellular signaling. Xenobiotics are external elements providing a signal to the cell. Often these xenobiotics have a precursor form that requires activation by oxidation. These reactions are carried out by so-called drug metabolizing enzymes (DMEs). Other DMEs carry out inactivation of the oxygenated ligand, providing a regulatory mechanism. *Apoptosis*, or cell death, differentiation, and neuroendocrine functions can be carried out in response to the expression of specific genes triggered by active oxygenated ligands derived from xenobiotics. (*Adapted from* Heber et al. [6].)

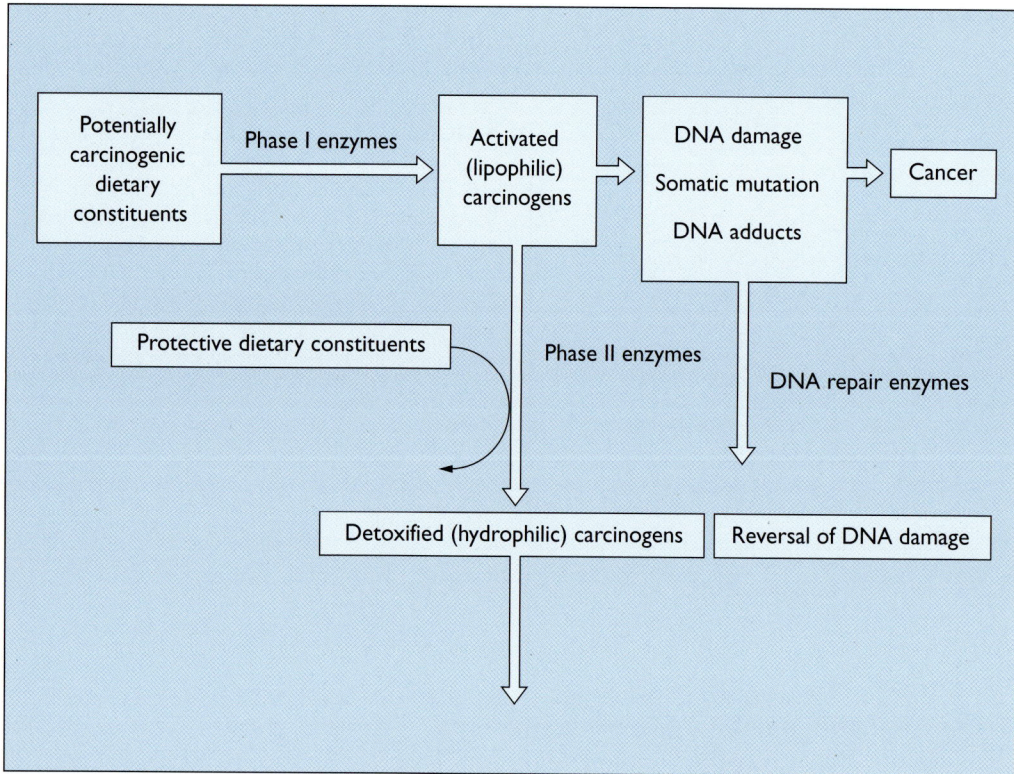

FIGURE 1-24. Xenobiotic metabolisms and cancer. Potentially carcinogenic and potentially protective dietary constituents interact in pathways of DNA oxidation and cause damage, leading to carcinogenesis. These pathways have been well studied in smoking-related carcinogens. Evidence is emerging about the applicability of this common pathway to drugs and food constituents. (*Adapted from* Heber *et al.* [6].)

DIETARY AND ENVIRONMENTAL CONSTITUENTS

Potential Carcinogens	Protective Dietary Constituents
Polycyclic aromatic hydrocarbons (benzopyrene) in tobacco smoke	Isoflavones (soy protein)
Heterocyclic amines (fired meats and fish)	Dithiolthiones, indoles (cruciferous vegetables)
Arylamines (cigarette smoke)	Isothiocyanates (cruciferous vegetables)
Nitrated polycyclic aromatic hydrocarbons (diesel exhaust)	Flavonoids (fruits and vegetables)
Aflatoxin (fungus)	Polyphenols (fruits, vegetables, and tea)
Alcohol	Terpenoids (citrus fruits)
Nitrosamines (tobacco smoke)	

FIGURE 1-25. Potentially carcinogenic and potentially protective dietary constituents co-exist in the food supply. Pesticides are considered a potential source of carcinogens. The protective substances found in foods may counteract the harmful effects of other toxins. (*Adapted from* Heber *et al.* [6].)

METABOLISM OF EFFECTOR LIGANDS

Retinol → Retinal → Retinoic acid

Hydroxylation of retinoic acid

Glucuronidation of retinoic acid

Hydroxylation, dehalogenation of thyroxine, thyroid hormone

20-Hydroxylation of ecdysone

1-Alpha-hydroxylation of 25-hydroxy-vitamin D_3

24-Hydroxylation of 1-alpha, 25-dihydroxy-vitamin D_3

7-Alpha-hydroxylation of cholesterol

Conversion of androstanedione to estrone

Aromatization of estrone to estradiol

Aromatization of testosterone to estradiol

Numerous interconversions of adrenal steroids

Glucuronide, GSH, and SO_4 conjugation of steroids

Epinephrine → Norepinephrine → Isoproterenol

Tryptamine → Serotonin (5HT) → Melatonin

Eicosanoid metabolism

FIGURE 1-26. Metabolism of effector ligands by drug metabolizing enzymes comprises some of the most important hormone interconversions known, as well as neuroendocrine and cell growth signaling. GSH—reduced glutathionine. (*Adapted from* Heber *et al.* [6].)

Gene-Environment Interactions

NUTRITIONAL EVOLUTION

Then (50,000 BC)	Now
Fruits, nuts, seeds, roots, tubers, flowers, leaves, stalks, and beans	Potatoes, refined pasta, flour, cereal, rice, corn, and beans
One to two times the fat	Added fat and sugar
Two to three times the protein	Chicken, red meat, fish, seafood, and pizza
0 dairy and refined flour	Ice cream and yogurt
0 processed foods	Cheese and whole milk
0 alcohol and tobacco	

FIGURE 1-27. Nutritional evolution. Man evolved on earth about fifty to one hundred thousand years ago. In contrast, the drug metabolizing enzymes were developed hundreds of millions of years ago in simple bacteria. For example, cytochrome P450 has over 150 isoforms in different species. Agriculture only evolved ten thousand years ago, and modern Western diets have been in existence only a few hundred years. There is a gene-environment imbalance for persons eating a typical high-fat diet.

PIMA INDIANS AND GENE-ENVIRONMENT INTERACTION

	Mexico	Arizona
Weight, *kg*	64.2 ± 13.9	90.2 ± 21.1
Height, *cm*	160 ± 8	164 ± 8
Body mass index, *kg/m²*	24.9 ± 4	33.4 ± 7.5
Cholesterol, mg/dL	146 ± 30	174 ± 31
Incidence of non–insulin-dependent diabetes mellitus:		
Males	6% (1/16)	54%
Females	11% (2/19)	37%

dependent diabetes mellitus (NIDDM). Pima Indians in Arizona have the highest reported prevalence of obesity and NIDDM, whereas the incidence is low in Pima Indians living in Northern Mexico. Pima Indians living in the mountains of Northern Mexico were separated some 700 to 1000 years ago from the Pima Indians living today in Arizona and continue to live a traditional lifestyle. They eat a diet with much less animal fat and more complex carbohydrates, and have higher activity levels than do the Pima Indians in Arizona. This population demonstrates increased body weight, height (which is a biomarker of prepubertal nutrition), increased body mass index, increased cholesterol, and increased incidence of NIDDM. The "thrifty gene" hypothesis states that genes for conserving energy, while adaptive in a traditional environment, are responsible for the high prevalence of obesity and diabetes in persons exposed to overnutrition and underactivity. (*Adapted from* Ravussin *et al.* [7].)

FIGURE 1-28. Gene-environment interactions. The Pima Indians of Northern Mexico and Southern Arizona demonstrate the impact of nutrition on genetic expression of chronic diseases such as obesity and non–insulin-

Food Pyramids

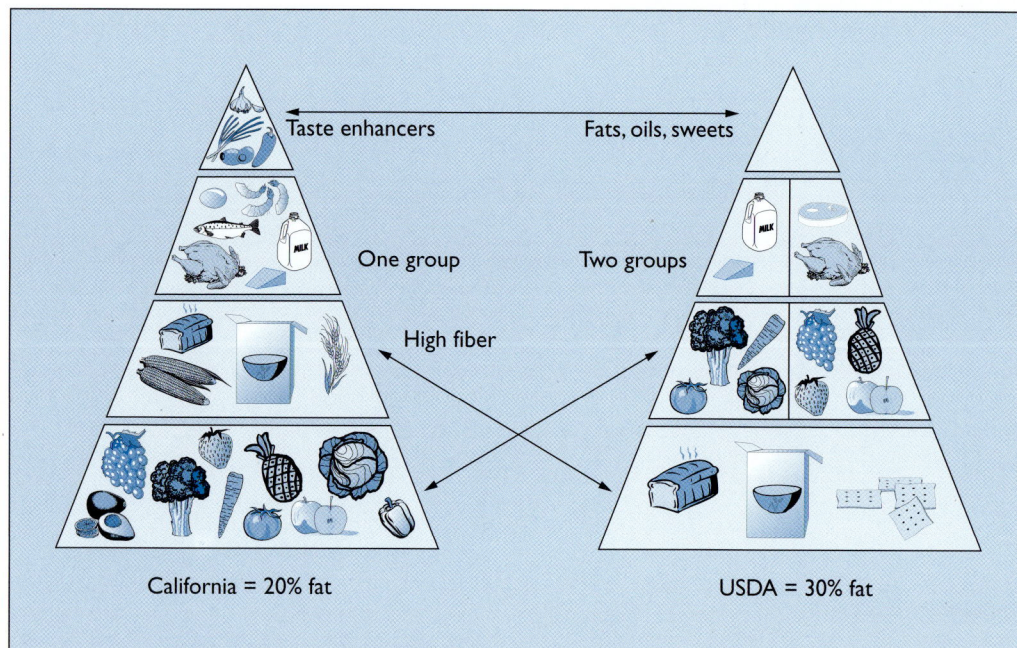

FIGURE 1-29. Pyramid comparisons. Recommendations for dietary intake among populations often take the form of pyramids, with the base of the pyramid determining the basis of the diet. In the pyramid developed by the United States Department of Agriculture (USDA) in the late 1980s the base consists of cereals and grains, without an emphasis on the fiber content of those grains. The fruits and vegetables appear on the second level and are two separate groups. In a new pyramid developed in 1997 by the Center for Human Nutrition at the University of California at Los Angeles, a modified plant-based diet is recommended. The base consists of five to 11 servings of fruits and vegetables to provide unique phytonutrients for prevention of chronic diseases. The second level consists of six to nine servings of high-fiber cereals and grains to provide the benefits of fiber from this level as well as from fruits and vegetables. The protein level is made up of low-fat protein choices, including protein from plants (beans, rice, and soybeans) and animals (egg whites, chicken breast, turkey, low-fat fish, other seafood, and nonfat milk products). The top tier of the USDA pyramid has only dots representing fats and sweets with the mixed message "use sparingly." The top tier of the new California pyramid emphasizes taste enhancers including olives, avocados, garlic, onion, nuts, cheese, chili peppers, and monounsaturated or omega-3-rich oils. The overall fat recommendation of the USDA pyramid is 30% or less of calories from fat. The new pyramid reflects the decreased fat intake in the population by recommending 20% or less of calories from fat. This exercise illustrates how the science of nutrition can be used to influence dietary recommendations (also see Chapter 13). (*Adapted from* Heber [8].)

References

1. Sims LS: *The Politics of Fat: Food and Nutrition Policy in America.* Armonk, NY. ME Sharpe; 1998:9.

2. Haas EM: *Staying Healthy with Nutrition.* Berkeley, CA: Celestial Arts; 1992:29.

3. Whitney EN, Rolfes SR: *Understanding Nutrition,* edn 7. Minneapolis-St. Paul: West Publishing Company, 1996:261.

4. Jaiswal AK: Antioxidant response element (ARE) and the regulation of gene expression. In *Oxygen, Gene Expression and Cellular Function.* Edited by Clerch, Massaro.

5. Roe DA: *Drug-Induced Nutritional Deficiencies.* Westport, CN: The Avi Publishing Company; 1983:14.

6. Heber D, Blackburn GL, Go VLW (eds): *Nutritional Oncology.* San Diego: Academic Press; 1999:615–617.

7. Ravussin E, Valencia ME, Esparza J, *et al.*: Effects of a traditional lifestyle on obesity in Pima Indians. *Diabetes Care* 1994, 17:1067–1074.

8. Heber D: The Resolution Diet. Garden City Park, NY: The Avery Publishing Group; 1999.

2

NUTRITION IN GROWTH AND DEVELOPMENT

Naomi D. Neufeld

What makes pediatrics unique is the dynamic nature of growth and development that traces the human being from birth through the developmental stages to become a man or woman at the end of puberty. To this end, hormones are important but nutrition is limiting.

Growth is a continuous phenomenon; however, the rate of growth is always changing. The rate of growth not only determines maximum height, but is also responsible for the differences in height observed among children of the same age.

Multiple factors are involved in the regulation of growth and development from infancy through childhood and finally adulthood. The main elements include the following: (1) genetic factors that determine the basis of the developmental process, (ie, the programming of the organism): this is most clearly seen in the estimate of mid-parental height; (2) hormonal factors that translate the genetic information into a physiologic control mechanism: the role of hormones appears to be the regulation of the rate of growth, particularly after the newborn period and the presence or absence of adequate hormonal secretion is reflected in the rate of growth in comparison to normal; (3) environmental (primarily nutritional) factors that serve to promote or severely distort programmed growth: both severe limitation and overabundance of calories relative to basal requirements is associated with differences in final height.

The relative importance of these various factors to the growth process is dependent upon the stage of development. Broadly considered, growth in childhood is divided into three phases, determined by the important regulating factor: Nutrient dependent, in the first to second year of life; growth and thyroid hormone dependent; and finally, at puberty, sex-steroid dependent. At any stage however, an excess or restriction of calorie and macronutrient intake can alter the rate at which growth proceeds.

The newborn period, in particular, is one that sees the greatest caloric need. This is due primarily to the requirement to generate heat in order to maintain temperature stability. This in turn results from the much greater surface area relative to body mass in the infant, which promotes greater heat loss per unit of mass than seen in the adult. As a result, normal neonates require up to 120 kcal/kg/24 h, whereas the calorie requirement falls dramatically after the first year of life. By mid-childhood, children require no more than 50–60 kcal/kg/24 h.

Studies of the relation of genetic factors to the development of muscle mass and fat mass show that the former is strongly heritable and that the latter has little association with genetic makeup. Development of adipose tissue is most strongly related to environmental factors, particularly those that limit or promote nutritional intake.

Nowhere is this more evident than in the United States today, where an epidemic of childhood obesity has emerged as the most important nutritional disorder in pediatrics. Nearly one out of four children is considered overweight, and many are at risk for developing diseases previously seen only in older individuals: hypertension, dyslipidemias, and type 2 diabetes mellitus. Obesity occurs disproportionately among ethnic minorities, including African-Americans, Native Americans and Hispanic-Americans, who are also at risk for developing the serious complications of obesity already mentioned. In many cases, obesity is associated with the development of hyperinsulinemia and insulin resistance. It is believed that hyperinsulinemia promotes growth by the same pathways identified for growth hormone–dependent insulin-like growth factors. Thus obesity, which is the result of excess caloric intake above basal requirements and lack of normal caloric expenditure, is also associated with rapid growth and early maturation. Children who are overweight are taller than would be expected for their genetic potential and mature earlier than other family members who are not obese. This predisposes the individual to a higher risk of certain cancers, particularly breast and uterine cancer for females and prostate and colon cancer in males.

Despite the dramatic increase in the rates of childhood obesity over the past 15 years, the trend continues unabated. The reasons for this are not clear, but the statistics suggest that clinicians may not have adequate information related to effective diagnosis and intervention [1]. The definition of childhood overweight for children ages 6 to 10 years old is a weight-for-height greater than the 85th percentile; obesity is defined as weight-for-height greater than the 95th percentile. In children above age 10, overweight is defined as BMI (body mass index) greater than the 85th percentile for age and obesity comparably as BMI greater than 95th percentile [2].

The data on the success of treatment regimens in children with morbid obesity are sparse. In early studies, some attempts using severe calorie restriction and protein-sparing diets showed short-term success, but data on the long-term efficacy of such methods are lacking. Given the disastrous outcome in adults with commercial programs using appetite suppressant therapy, there has been a (justifiable) reluctance on the part of practitioners to use these methods in children [3].

The best "treatment" for childhood obesity is actually prevention, with intervention beginning when a child is overweight, ie, BMI > 85th percentile. Successful treatment regimens for childhood obesity should start early and should involve the family in helping the child to make reasonable food choices, based on the Food Guide Pyramid at calorie intakes appropriate for age, to incorporate daily physical activity at a minimum of 35–45 min/d, and to limit television and computer time to one hour per day. In the most severe cases of childhood obesity, ie, when the child's weight is more than 200% of ideal body weight, other forms of treatment, including gastric stapling, have been proposed.

Additional emphasis on supportive parenting is necessary, in order to promote and to encourage self-esteem, necessary to prevent eating disorders, including anorexia and bulimia. These disorders affect nearly 5% of adolescents. In response to the growing epidemic of childhood obesity, some children respond by severe restriction in calorie intake. In its most severe form, anorexia nervosa (AN) is associated with an extreme fear of becoming fat and the subsequent need to reduce calorie intake. While a detailed description of this disorder is beyond the scope of this text, the short-term consequences of AN include endocrine disorders such as growth failure, delayed onset of puberty, and absent or irregular menses. More recently, the Centers for Disease Control showed that adolescents (particularly girls) are using cigarette smoking as a means of preventing weight gain. Restrained eating in adolescents is also associated with a decrease in bone density and the later development of osteoporosis.

PHASES OF GROWTH

Phase	Main Determinants
Infancy	Nutrient dependent
Childhood	Growth hormone dependent
Puberty	Gonadal hormone dependent

FIGURE 2-1. Phases of growth. The main determinant of growth in childhood varies depending on the stage being examined. During the first two years of life, nutrition is the dominant factor that determines growth. It is at this time that one often sees evidence of failure to thrive, due to lack of adequate caloric intake, as well as growth and maturation in advance of normal. During childhood, from age s 2 through 10, growth is dependent on growth hormone secretion; subnormal growth rates often characterize growth hormone deficiency. On the other hand, nutrient excess during this stage can also stimulate growth and promote early puberty and maturation. Finally, during the pubertal phase, from ages 11 through 15, gonadal steroids are the predominant factors in determine growth rate. During this period, excess nutrition, may alter the age at which puberty occurs.

Nutrition in Infancy

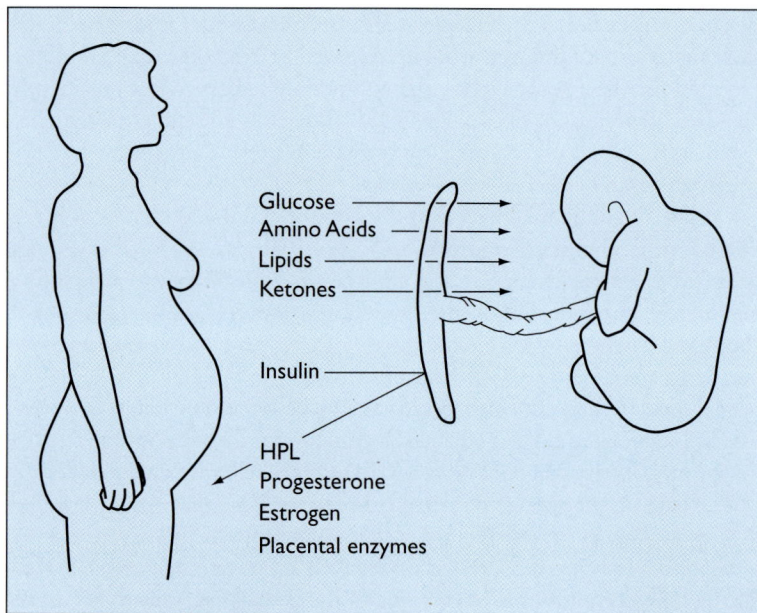

Glucose
Amino Acids
Lipids
Ketones

Insulin

HPL
Progesterone
Estrogen
Placental enzymes

FIGURE 2-2. Neonatal and fetal link: Infants of diabetic mothers are far more likely to be large at birth, as well as to demonstrate a greater rate of obesity later in life. The mechanism through which this occurs is through the delivery of substrates (including glucose, fatty acids and proteins) from the maternal circulation to the developing fetus. In the face of an increased glucose load, the fetal pancreas is stimulated to release more insulin, which subsequently promotes growth and fat deposition[4].

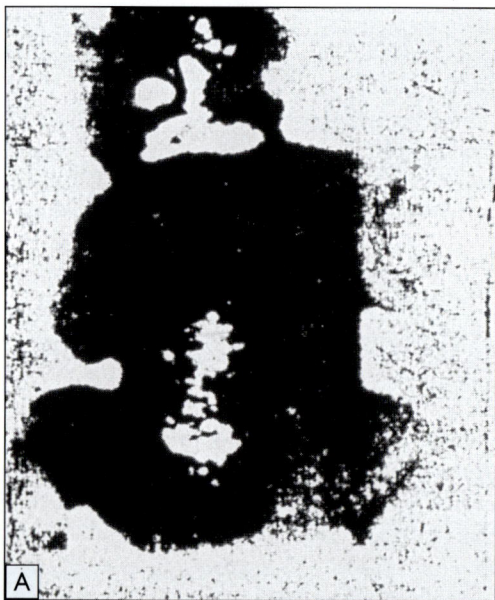

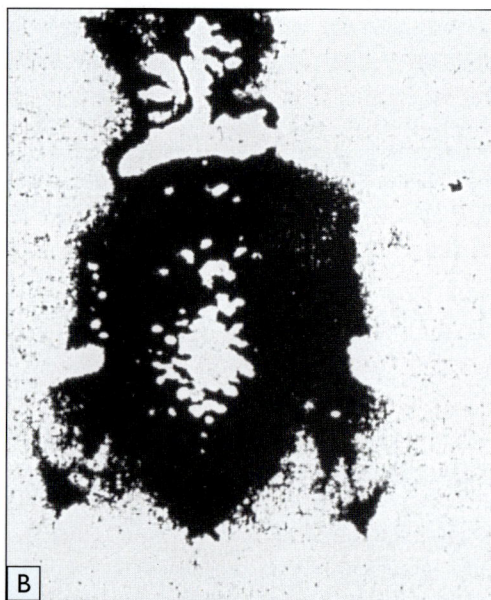

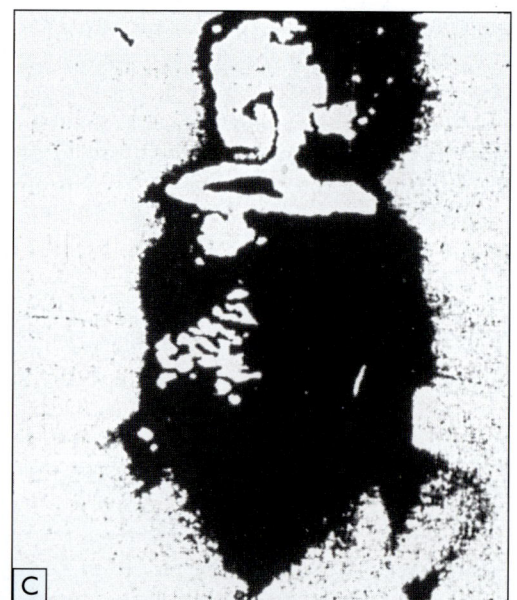

A   B   C

FIGURE 2-3. (see Color Plate) Brown adipose tissue (BAT) and exposure to cold. Brown adipose tissue, rich in heat-generating mitochondria is important in the process of nonshivering thermogenesis, and permits adaptation of the newborn infant to the extrauterine environment. This tissue is critical to permit heat generation and temperature stability. In the process of heat production, calories are utilized at very high levels, and this accounts for the greater need for calories in infancy, up to 120 Kcal/kg/d. Brown adipose tissue is located in the paracervical, subscapular and perinephric regions. The thermograms (A–C) show changes in skin temperature occurring in an infant exposed to the cold. Thus it was not surprising that premature infants raised in temperature-controlled incubators gained weight at a more rapid rate than those in room air did [5,6]. Furthermore, in obese infants born with a thicker layer of subcutaneous fat, the rates of heat loss are lower, and the subsequent need for calories would be expected to be less (see Fig. 2-9).

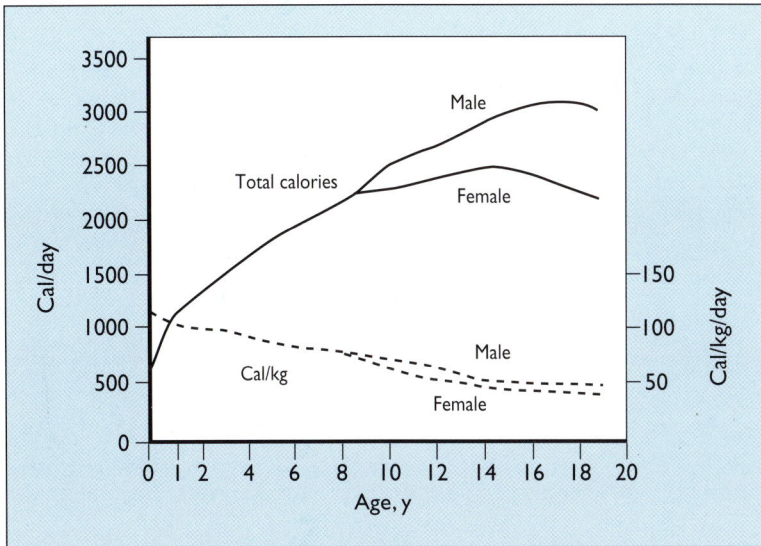

FIGURE 2-4. Infant feeding calorie needs. The caloric requirement is greatest in the neonatal period, often in excess of 120 kcal/kg/24 h, in order to accommodate the caloric requirements for temperature maintenance and growth. The main categories for energy intake are basal metabolic rate, which accounts for 55 kcal/kg/d, and growth, which during the first four months of life utilizes one third of the calories ingested. By the end of the second year the caloric requirements for growth fall to 1% to 2% of calories ingested, energy lost through excretion accounting for 5% to 10% of total calories [7].

BENEFITS OF BREASTFEEDING *VS.* ARTIFICIAL FEEDING

Child
  Fewer gastrointestinal infections
  Less allergies
  Increased jaw muscle usage permits development well-formed jaws and straight teeth
  Increased maternal-child bonding
Maternal benefits
  Oxytocin secretion promotes uterine involution
  Convenience
  Economy
  Decreased risk of breast cancer and postpartum thromboembolism

FIGURE 2-5. Benefits of breast feeding to mother and child. Based on studies of nutrition requirements in infancy, reasonable recommendations for full-term infants include 7% to 16% of calories from protein, 30%-55% from fat, and the remainder from carbohydrate. Both human milk and artificial formulas modeled after human milk provide comparable levels of these macronutrients. There are several benefits to breast feeding that recommend it above formula feeding, without supplementation for the first 6 months of life [8]. Recent studies have shown that infants who were breast-fed have a lower rate of obesity in childhood than did age-matched bottle-fed infants.

SCHEDULE OF SOLID FOODS

An appropriate regimen for introduction of solid foods begins with the grains and fruits. Rice cereal appears to be the least allergenic of the cereals and thus should be offered first. Progression through vegetables, meats, and eggs can be accomplished in the following manner:

5–6 mo:	cereals and fruits
6–7 mo:	meats and vegetables
7–8 mo:	egg yolk
8–9 mo:	egg white

To ensure an adequate amount of protein, fat, and carbohydrate during the sixth through twelfth months, infants should be offered and should consume no more than an average of 28 oz of milk each day in addition to their quota of solids. An example of an infant diet in this age group follows:

Breakfast:	cereal and milk
Midmorning snack::	cup of orange juice
Lunch:	meat, yellow or green vegetables, fruit, milk
Midafternoon snack:	cup of orange juice or milk
Dinner:	cottage cheese or yogurt, egg, vegetable, fruit, and milk
Bedtime:	milk

FIGURE 2-6. Delaying introduction of solid foods. Current practice is aimed at preventing obesity as well as minimizing the risks associated with food allergies. Thus, introduction of solid foods should not usually begin before six months ths of age. The appropriate regimen for introduction of solid foods begins with grains and fruits. Rice cereal appears to be the least allergenic of cereals and thus should be offered first. Progression through vegetables, meat and eggs can be accomplished in the following manner. To ensure an adequate amount of protein, fat, and carbohydrate during the sixth through the twelfth month, infants should be offered 28 oz of milk each day in addition to the solid foods listed [7].

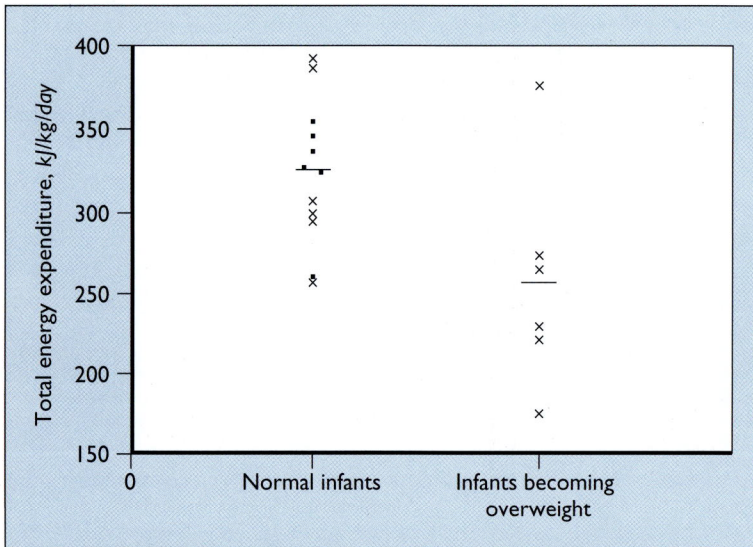

FIGURE 2-7. Decreased energy expenditure. Infants who are likely to gain excess weight in the newborn period, appear to conserve energy more efficiently than those who gain at an abnormal rate do. These infants, identified prospectively as having overweight or diabetic mothers, were monitored for the first year of life. Energy expenditure was determined using deuterium-labeled water. Reduction in energy expenditure could be the result of less thermogenesis occurring because core temperature was more easily maintained [10].

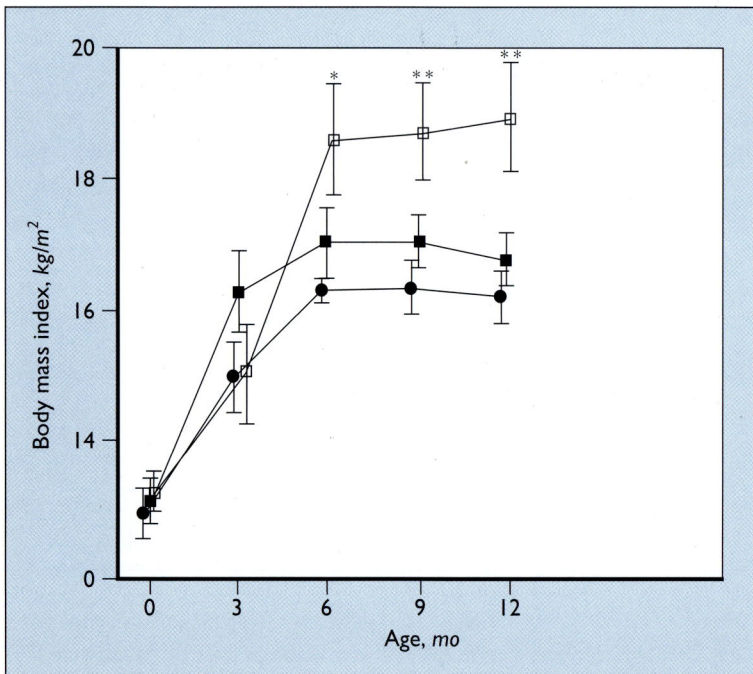

FIGURE 2-8. Increased weight gain in the first year. Infants who exhibited reduced energy expenditure in the first three months of life were then tracked for rate of weight gain during the remainder of the first year. Those infants with the lowest rates of energy expenditure gained the most weight in the first year of life [10].

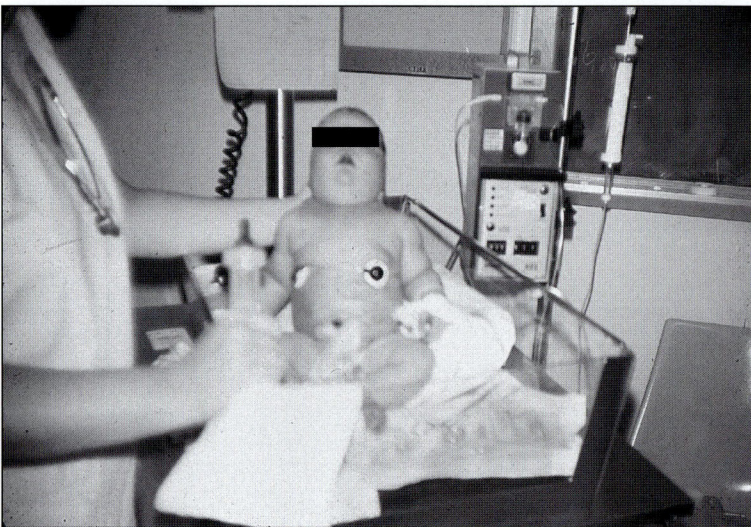

FIGURE 2-9. Twelve-pound infant of a diabetic mother: This is a full-term male infant born to mother with gestational diabetes. Infants of diabetic mothers examined at one year of age were heavier and taller and had larger head circumferences than age-matched control infants. These infants are subsequently at greater risk for developing obesity [11]. (Neufeld personal collection)

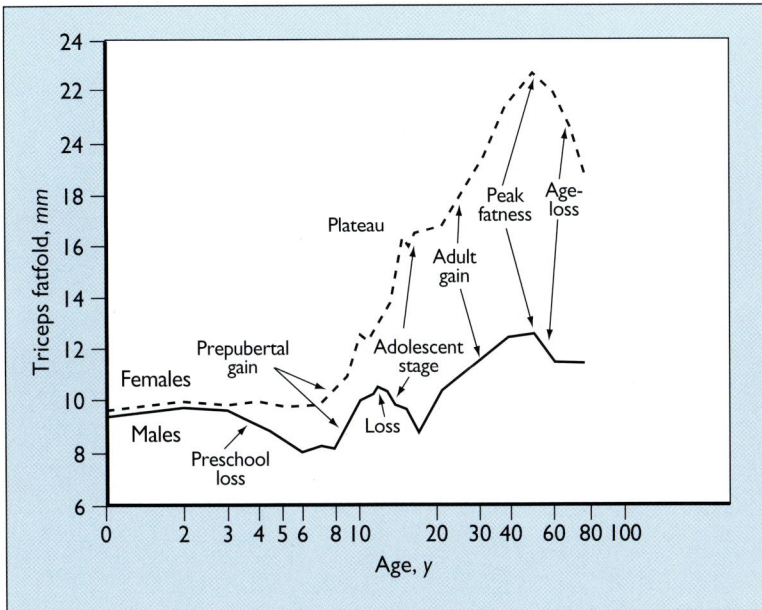

FIGURE 2-10. Fat accumulation with age. Adipose tissue develops according to a predictable timetable during childhood. The first accretion of adipose tissue actually occurs in the fetus during last trimester of pregnancy. The second stage is in mid-childhood, prior to the puberty growth spurt. During adolescence is the third major stage of adipose tissue accumulation. Development of adipose tissue is most strongly related to environmental factors, particularly those that limit or promote nutritional intake. It is during these three stages in particular that the influence of environment as reflected by increased caloric intake and reduced physical activity [12].

Growth and Nutrition in Childhood

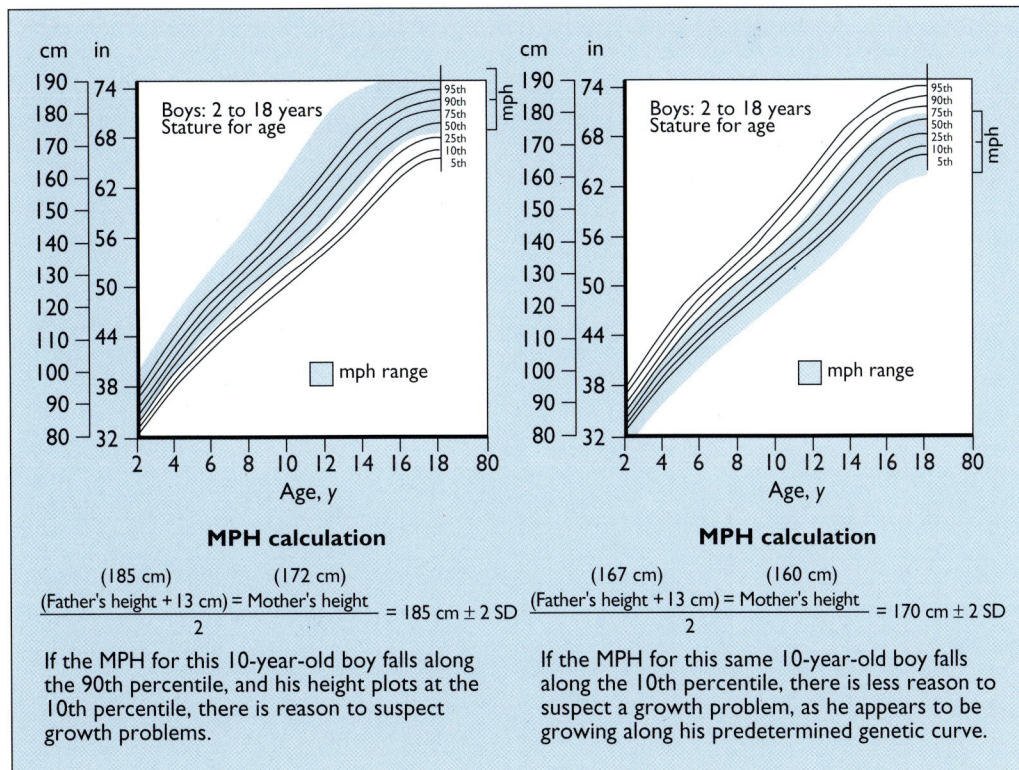

MPH calculation

$$\frac{\text{(Father's height} + 13 \text{ cm)} = \text{Mother's height}}{2} = 185 \text{ cm} \pm 2 \text{ SD}$$
(185 cm) (172 cm)

If the MPH for this 10-year-old boy falls along the 90th percentile, and his height plots at the 10th percentile, there is reason to suspect growth problems.

MPH calculation

$$\frac{\text{(Father's height} + 13 \text{ cm)} = \text{Mother's height}}{2} = 170 \text{ cm} \pm 2 \text{ SD}$$
(167 cm) (160 cm)

If the MPH for this same 10-year-old boy falls along the 10th percentile, there is less reason to suspect a growth problem, as he appears to be growing along his predetermined genetic curve.

FIGURE 2-11. Midparental target height. The calculation of midparental target height allows a means of assessing the genetic potential of a child, based on the heights of his/her biological parents. Using this method, even in the absence of other growth data, permits the physician to assess whether the child is growing appropriately. Excess nutrition and subsequent obesity are often associated with overgrowth, which is characterized by a child's height exceeding the percentile determined by midparental target height. The calculation for midparental target height is as follows: For girls, it is (in inches) the mother's height + (the father's height - 5)/2. For boys, it is (in inches) the father's height + (mother's height + 5)/2.

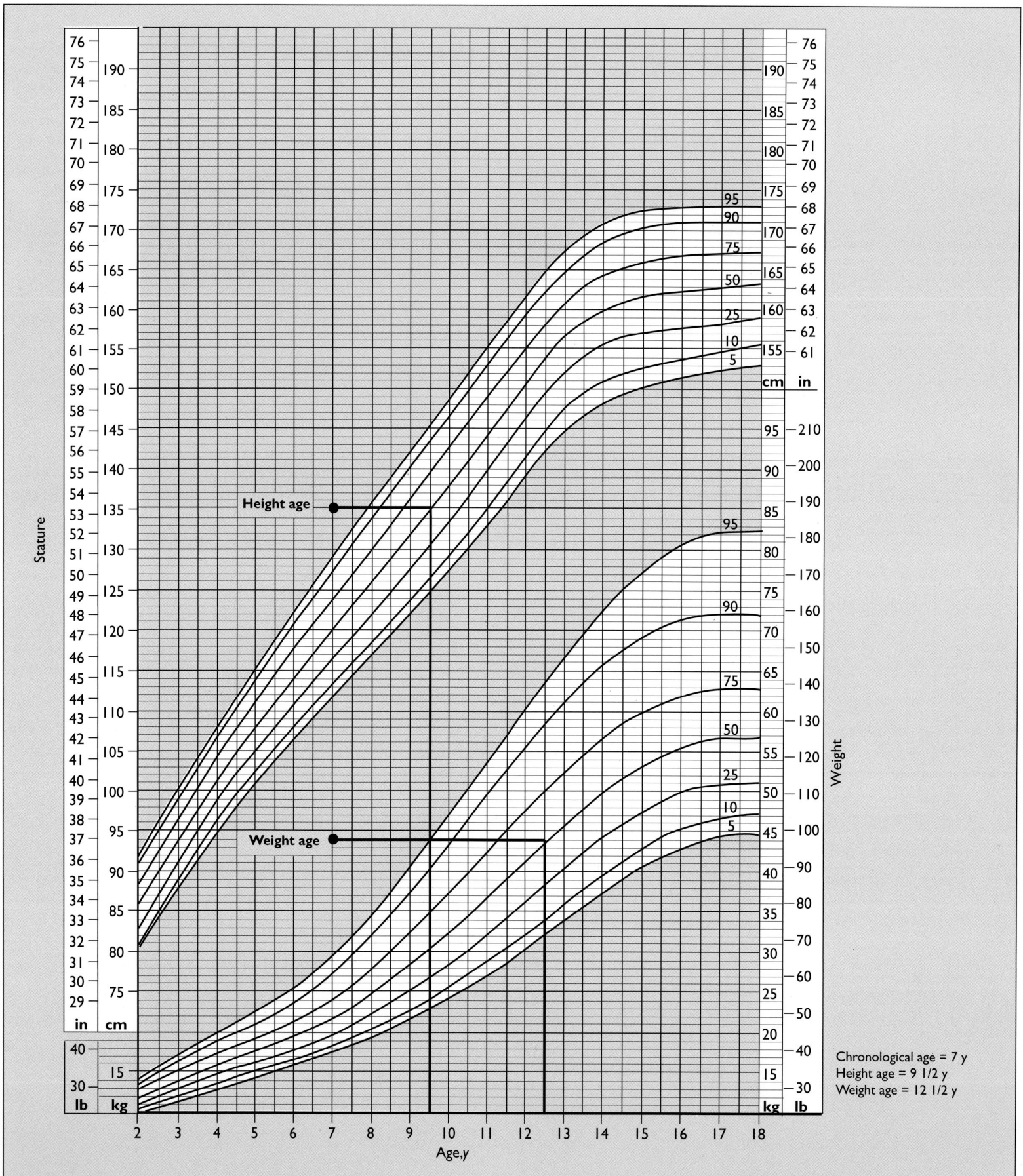

FIGURE 2-12. Assessment of obesity using standard growth curves. Children who are obese demonstrate increases both in weight and in rate of growth. Thus, they are often taller and heavier than their peers are and than might be expected from their midparental target height. These two useful points of information can be determined from the growth curves. The first is height age, ie, the age at which the height of the specific individual intersects the 50th percentile. In children whose growth is overly rapid, the height age often exceeds the chronologic age. The second concept, weight age, is obtained from analysis of the weight curve. Similarly, it is the age at which the individuals weight intersects the 50th percentile. In severely overweight children, the weight age is often considerably higher than the chronologic age [13].

Fats & sweets　　　　　　Eat less

Milk group
2 servings

Meat group
2 servings

Vegetable group
3 servings

Fruit group

Grain group
6 servings

What counts as one serving?

Grain group
1 slice of bread
1/2 cup of cooked rice or pasta
1/2 cup cooked cereal
1 ounce of ready-to-eat cereal

Fruit group
1 piece of fruit or melon wedge
3/4 cup of juice
1/2 cup of canned fruit
1/4 cup of dried fruit

Meat group
2 to 3 ouinces of cooked lean
meat, poultry, or fish
1/2 cup of cooked dry beans,
or 1 egg counts as 1 ounce of
lean meat. 2 tablespoons of
peanut butter count as 1 ounce
of meat

Vegetable group
1/2 cup of chopped raw or
cooked vegetables
1 cup of raw leafy vegetables

Milk group
1 cup of milk or yogurt
2 ounces of cheese

Fats and sweets
Limit calories from these

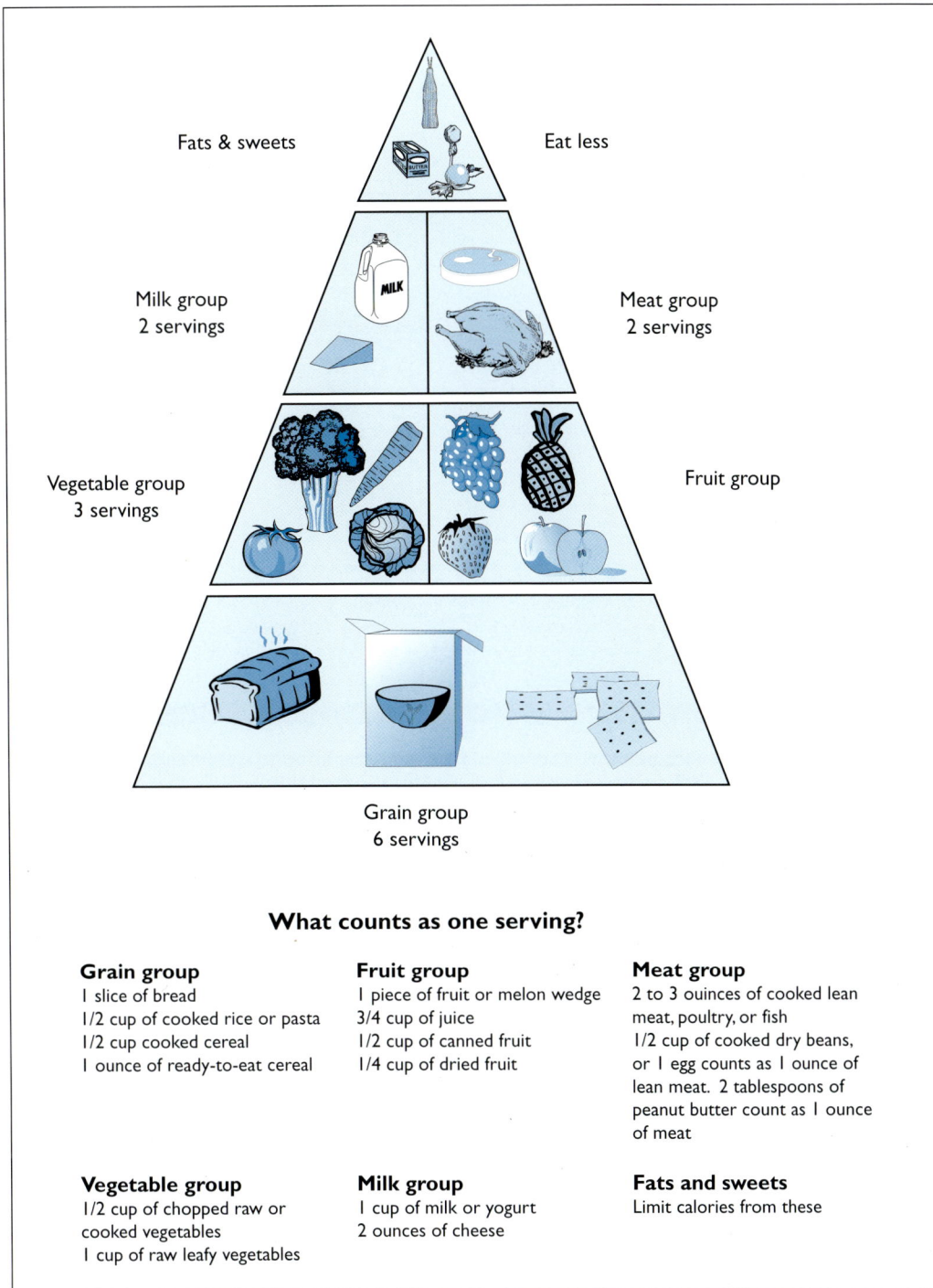

FIGURE 2-13. Food Guide Pyramid for children: prudent diet. The current recommendations of a healthy diet, based on the food Guide pyramid has been modified to clearly address the dietary needs of children, between the ages of two and six. This food guide, emphasizes the need to increase consumption of grain-derived foods, fruits and vegetables, and to reduce the intake of meat, dairy products and foods that are high in fat. The release of this Modified Food Guide Pyramid is prompted by the need to address the growing epidemic of obesity and related disorders seen in children [14].

ADOLESCENT BMI*: 5TH, 15TH, 85TH, AND 95TH PERCENTILES ACCORDING TO SEX AND AGE

Age in Years	Male BMI				Female BMI			
	5th%	15th%	85th %	95th%	5th%	15th%	85th%	95th%
10	14	15	20	23	14	15	20	23
11	15	16	20	24	15	16	21	25
12	15	16	21	25	15	16	22	26
13	16	17	22	26	16	17	23	27
14	16	17	23	27	16	17	24	28
15	17	18	24	28	16	17	24	29
16	17	18	24	29	17	18	25	29
17	17	19	25	29	17	18	25	30
18	18	19	25	30	17	18	26	30
19	18	19	26	30	17	18	26	30
20–21	19	20	27	30	17	19	26	30

The criteria in this table are based on the BMI. BMI is defined as weight (kg) divided by height (m^2). Determine the BMI by translating weight into kg (1lb = 2.2kg) and the height into meters (1 m = 39.37 in). After squaring the meters, divide the kilograms by the square meters. For example, a child weighing 110 pounds is 50 kilograms and standing 60 inches tall is 1.5 meters. After squaring the meters (1.5 x 1.5 = 2.25), divide the kilograms by the meters which, in this example, is 50 divided by 2.25. The BMI for this child is 22.2 and within normal limits.

FIGURE 2-14. Adolescent Body Mass Index (BMI) according to age and sex. The criteria in this table are based on the Body mass index. BMI is defined as weight (kg) divided by height (m^2). The standards of the 5th, 15th, 85th, and 95th percentiles are utilized for establishing normal weight during adolescence. Those children whose BMI exceeds the 95th percentile for age are considered overweight [15].

Assessment of Caloric Requirements

EQUATIONS FOR PREDICTING RESTING ENERGY EXPENDITURE FROM BODY WEIGHT

Sex and Age Range, y	Equation to Derive REE in kcal/d	R*	SD†
Males			
0–3	60.9 × wt†) - 54	0.97	53
3–10	(22.7 × wt) + 495	0.86	62
10–18	(17.5 × wt) + 651	0.90	100
18–30	(15.3 × wt) + 679	0.65	151
30–60	(11.6 × wt) + 879	0.60	164
> 60	(13.5 × wt) + 487	0.79	148
Females			
0–3	(61.0 × wt) - 51	0.97	61
3–10	(22.5 × wt) + 499	0.85	63
10–18	(12.2 × wt) + 746	0.75	117
18–30	(14.7 × wt) + 496	0.72	121
30–60	(8.7 × wt) + 829	0.70	108
> 60	(10.5 × wt) + 596	0.74	108

*Correlation coefficient (R) of reported BMRs and predicted values, and standard deviation (SD) of the differences between actual and computed values.
†Weight of person in kg.

FIGURE 2-15. Equations for predicting resting energy expenditure (REE) from body weight. The equations presented in this table permit a method for estimating the daily calorie requirements of an individual, based on age and weight. They show a decline in resting energy expended with age, reflecting the change in energy required to maintain body temperature and permit other bodily functions. In addition to REE, other needs to be determined include calories for growth and those for activity. In order to promote weight loss in severe childhood obesity, which is characterized not only by excess weight but also by overgrowth and early maturation, it is reasonable to estimate daily calorie requirements using ideal body weight, without adding the obligatory calories for growth and activity [16].

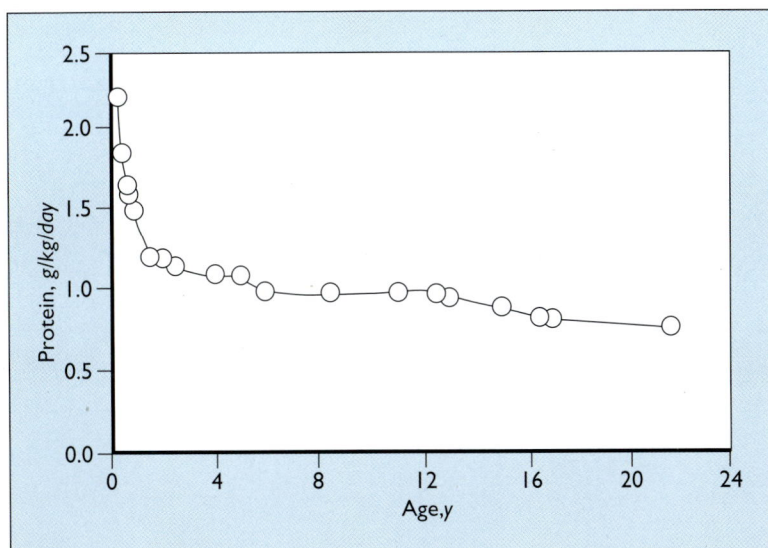

FIGURE 2-16. Estimates of protein requirements as a function of age. Recent surveys show that the average protein intake by Americans is at least twice the estimated requirement [4].

Endocrine Disorders

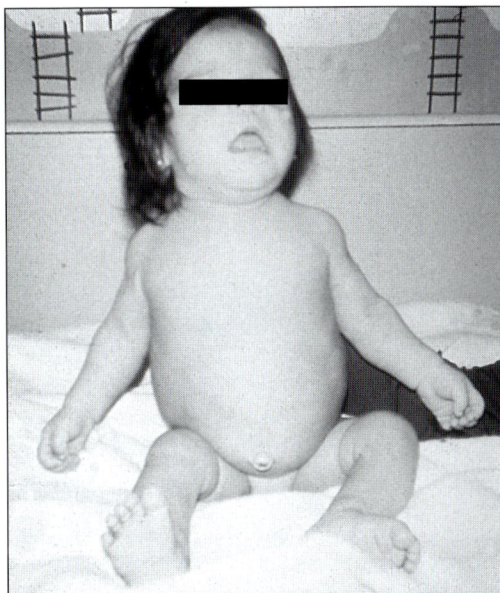

FIGURE 2-17. Role of thyroid hormone in growth in the neonatal period. This child represents a tragic occurrence no longer seen in the United States, namely undiagnosed congenital hypothyroidism. At 16 months of age, despite lacking adequate motor skills, she was of normal weight and length. Growth and weight gains in the first year of life are not dependent on thyroid hormone. It is likely that the reduced availability of thyroid hormone, which is critical to the activation of brown adipose tissue, resulted in sparing of calories that would otherwise be used for thermogenesis (Neufeld, personal collection).

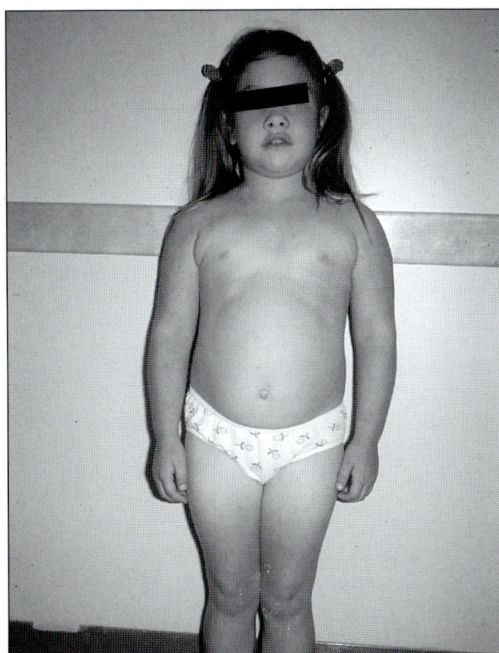

FIGURE 2-18. Hypothyroidism in childhood is associated with short stature, particularly due to lack of growth of the extremities, resulting in upper-to-lower segment disproportion. In addition, as seen in this 7-year-old girl with long-standing unrecognized hypothyroidism, there is evidence of fat accumulation and difference in body proportions. In hypothyroidism, it is not uncommon for the weight to be at a higher percentile than height (*ie*, weight age > height age). (Neufeld, personal collection)

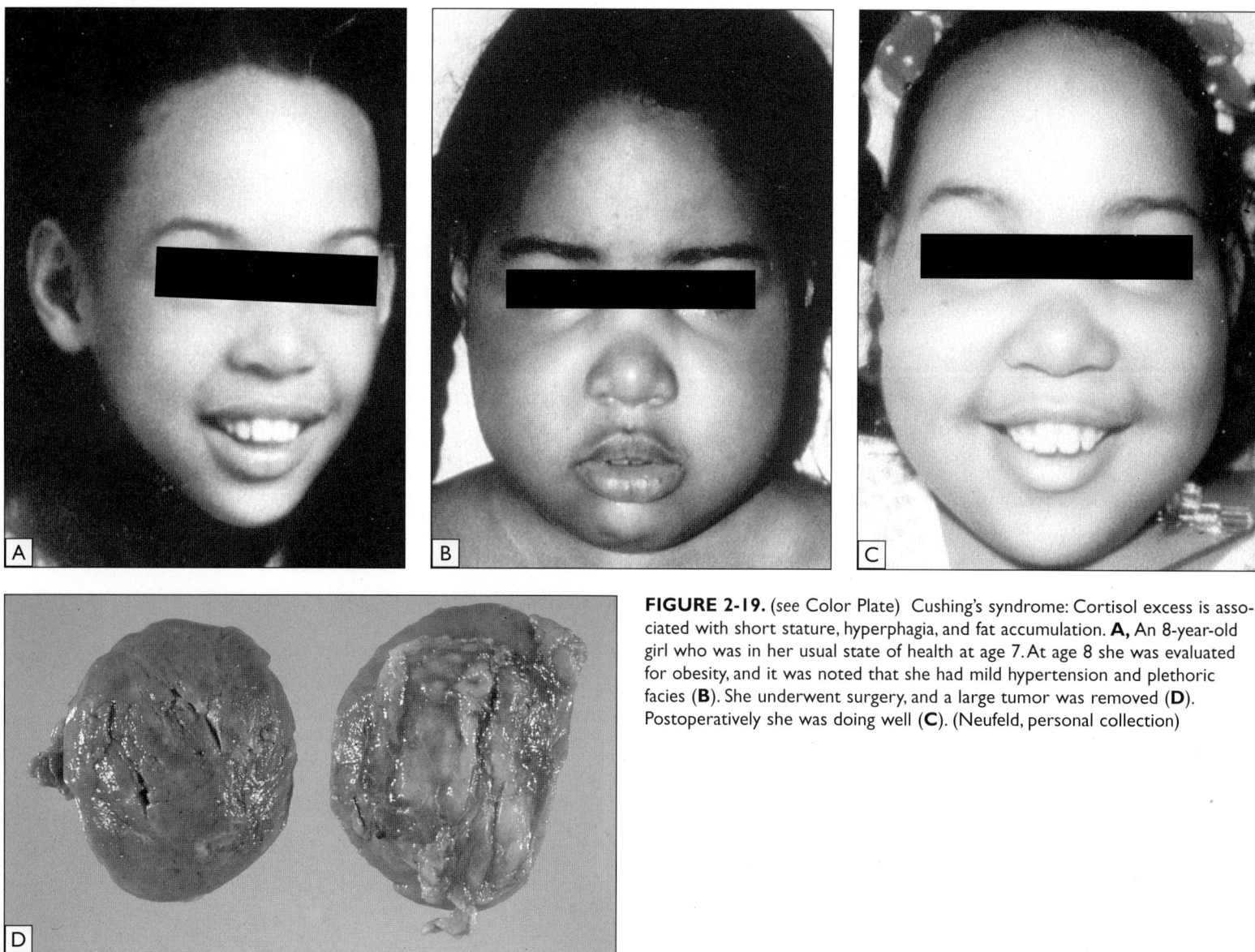

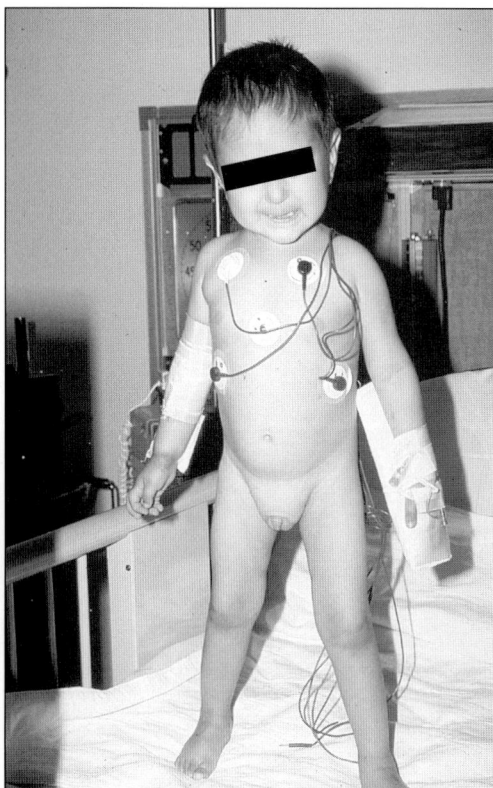

FIGURE 2-19. (*see* Color Plate) Cushing's syndrome: Cortisol excess is associated with short stature, hyperphagia, and fat accumulation. **A,** An 8-year-old girl who was in her usual state of health at age 7. At age 8 she was evaluated for obesity, and it was noted that she had mild hypertension and plethoric facies (**B**). She underwent surgery, and a large tumor was removed (**D**). Postoperatively she was doing well (**C**). (Neufeld, personal collection)

FIGURE 2-20. Human growth hormone deficiency in infancy is associated with normal birthweight and length at birth. At times the only presenting feature may be microphallus (*ie* a phallus < 2.5 cm long) and hypoglycemia. Short stature in children with growth hormone deficiency may not present until after the first year of life. At the time of diagnosis of growth hormone deficiency, chronological age > weight age > height age. (Neufeld, personal collection)

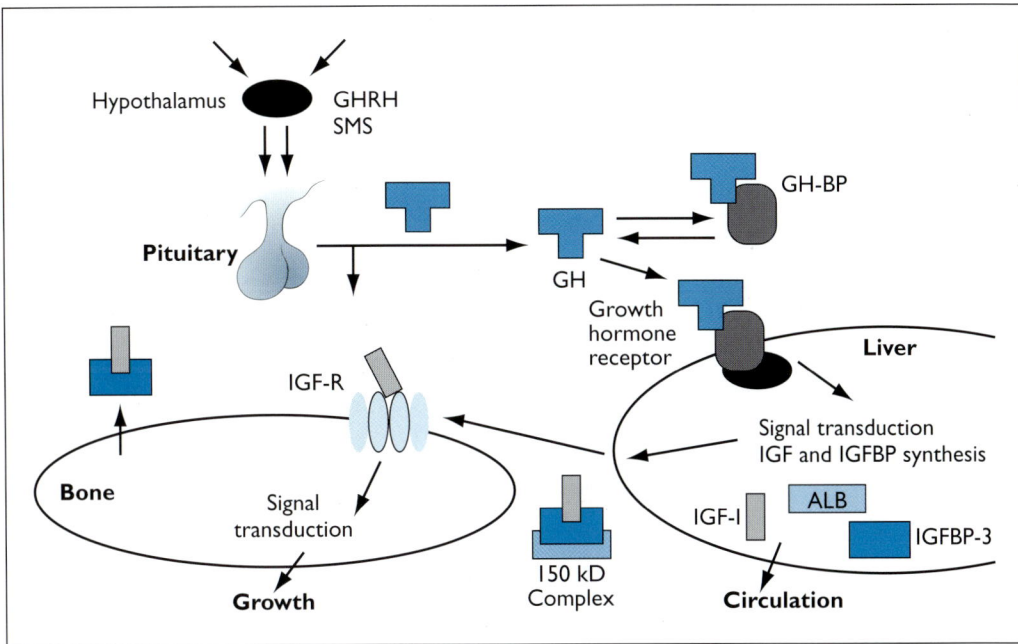

FIGURE 2-21. IGF-GH axis regulation. Growth hormone releasing factor (GHRH) and somatostatin (SMS) regulate pituitary GH secretion. GH binds to the circulating GH binding protein (GHBP), which is the cleaved extracellular domain of the GH receptor, as well as to the receptor itself. Insulin-like growth factor (IGF) binding protein-3 (IGFBP-3) and the acid-labile subunit are produced in response to GH signal transduction. IGF mediates growth by binding to its receptor (IGF-R). In hyperinsulinemic states, serum insulin often interacts with the IGF-R and can further potentiate growth. Such growth has been observed in growth hormone deficient children who have become obese following surgery for craniopharyngioma [17,18].

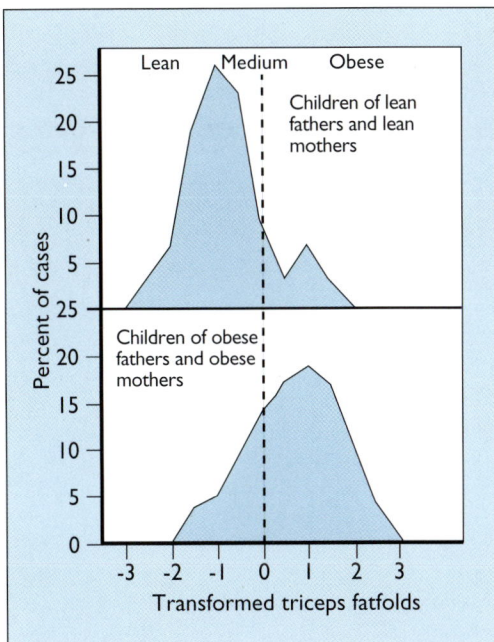

FIGURE 2-22. Genetic influences in the development of obesity. Data from the second NHANES survey were analyzed by examining the offspring of adults who were normal or obese. Children whose parents were thin had triceps skinfold thickness' more often that were less than the norm for age, whereas those whose parents were both obese were more likely to have had triceps skinfold thicknesses that were above normal [12].

MEDICAL PROBLEMS ASSOCIATED WITH CHILDHOOD OBESITY

Endocrine-metabolic
    Growth: increased height, advanced bone age, early menarche, menstrual abnormalities
    Type 2 diabetes (blacks, Mexican-Americans)
    Hypertension
Mechanical
    Respiratory disorders: worsened asthma, sleep apnea
    Orthopedic problems: SCFE, Blount's disease, compression fractures
Emotional
    Psychosocial dysfunction

FIGURE 2-23. Problems in obese children. Children who are overweight have a variety of problems, both physical and emotional as a consequence of their increased body mass. The most commonly observed findings are tall stature and associated early maturation. In some individuals, we also observed hypertension, and some of the most obese children have developed type 2 diabetes. Many children with severe obesity may develop problems in response to the mechanical burdens of the excess weight. These include respiratory problems and orthopedic problems. A significant number of children experience psychosocial problems related to teasing and social exclusion. Sometimes the emotional distress is so great that young people may become severely depressed, socially withdrawn, and suicidal. (Neufeld, personal collection)

SYNDROME X: THE INSULIN RESISTANCE SYNDROME

Known initially as the deadly triad
  Type 2 diabetes
  Hypertension
  Dyslipidemia
In female subjects, insulin resistance is also associated with ovarian
  hyperandrogenism and polycystic ovary disease

FIGURE 2-24. Syndrome X is now seen in children. In 1988 Reaven described the relationship of insulin resistance to the development of three disorders that constitute the deadly triad. These include type 2 diabetes mellitus, hypertension and dyslipidemia. Females suffering from these disorders were also noted to have menstrual disorders and hyperandrogenism. Since 1995, a number of reports of Type 2 diabetes occurring in obese minority children have appeared. More recently, recognition that obesity and insulin resistance are occurring in epidemic proportions has made physicians aware of the long-term impact of obesity in childhood [19].

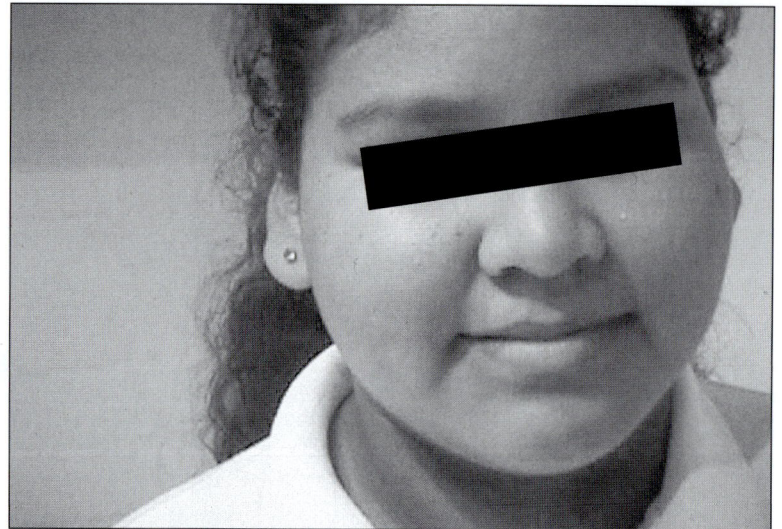

FIGURE 2-25. (see Color Plate) Acanthosis nigricans: Darkening and thickening of skin in the neck creases, the armpits, and the groin are attributable to and associated with hyperinsulinemia. If insulin levels are lowered through calorie restriction, exercise, or medication, the dark pigmentation decreases in intensity. (Neufeld, personal collection)

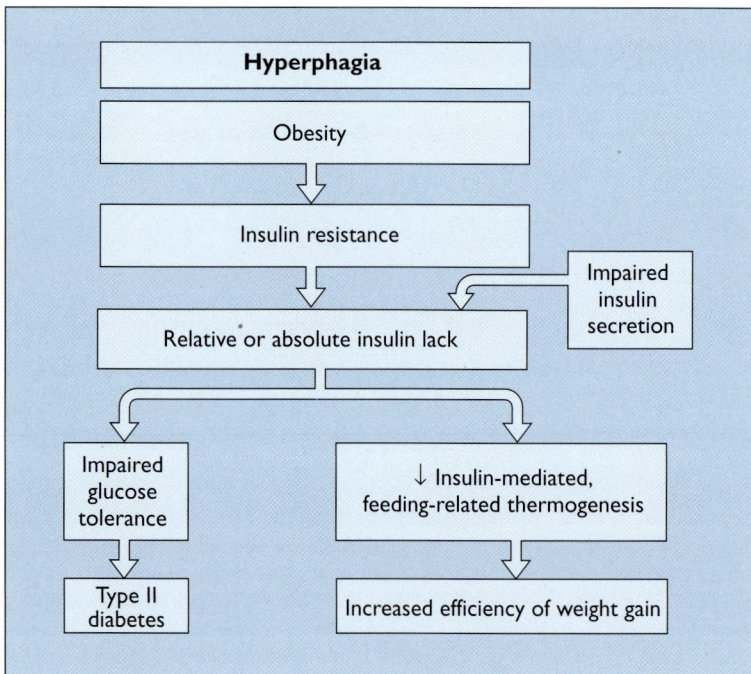

FIGURE 2-26. Hyperinsulinemia and impairment of thermogenesis: proposed interactions among insulin resistance, thermogenesis, and efficiency of weight gain in obesity. The development of relative or absolute lack of insulin results not only in an impairment of glucose tolerance but also in a decrease in feeding-related thermogenesis. As a consequence of the reduced thermogenesis, there is an increase in the efficiency of weight gain, which may accelerate the development or facilitate the maintenance of obesity [20].

References

1. Christoffel KK, Ariza A: The epidemiology of overweight in children: Relevance for clinical care. *Pediatrics* 1998, 101: 103–104.

2. Troiano R, Flegel K: Overweight children and adolescents: Description, epidemiology , and demographics. *Pediatrics* 1998, 101 (suppl): 497–504.

3. Epstein LH, Myers MD, Raynor HA, Saalens BE: Treatment of pediatric obesity. *Pediatrics* 1998, 101 (suppl):554–570.

4. Ogata E: Carbohydrate Metabolism in the Fetus and Neonate and Altered Neonatal Glucoregulation. *Pediatric Clin North Am,* 1986, 33: 25–45.

5. Rylander E , Pribylova H , Lind J: A thermographic study of infants exposed to cold. *Acta Paediatr Scand* 1972, 61(1):42–48.

6. Glass L , Silverman WA , Sinclair JC: Relationship of thermal environment and caloric intake to growth and resting metabolism in the late neonatal period. *Biol Neonat* 1969, 14(5):324–340.

7. Forbes GB: Nutrition 1: Nutritional Requirements. In *Primary Pediatric Care.* Edited by Hoekelman RA. St. Louis: Mosby YearBook; 1992:168–182.

8. Eiger MS: The Feeding of Infants and Children. In *Primary Pediatric Care.* Edited by Hoekelman RA. St. Louis: Mosby YearBook; 1992: 182–194.

9. Von Kries R, Koletzko B, Sauerwald T, *et al.*: Breastfeeding and obesity: Cross-sectional study. *BMJ* 1999, 319:147–150.

10. Roberts SR, Savage J, Coward WA, *et al.*: Energy expenditure and intake in infants born to lean and overweight mothers. *New Eng. J Med* 1988, 319:461–466.

11. Somatic growth of children of diabetic mothers with reference to birth size. *J Pediatr* 1980, 97(2):196–9.

12. Garn SM and Clark DC: Trends in fatness and the origins of obesity. *Pediatrics* 1975, 56:443–456.

13. Hamill PVV, Drizid TA, Johnson CL, *et al.*: Physical growth, National Center for Health Statistics percentiles. *Am J Clin Nutr* 1979, 32:607–629.

14. US Dept. of Agriculture, Center for Nutrition Policy and Prevention, Program Aid 1647, March 1999.

15. California Department of Health Services, Primary Care and Family Health Division, Children's medical Services Branch, Feb 1997, p 310.

16. Recommended Dietary allowances, 10th edition. Copyright 1989 by the National Academy of Sciences, Published by the National Academy Press.

17. Cohen P, Rosenfeld RL: Growth problems in adolescence. In *Textbook of Adolescent Medicine.* 1992.

18. Kaplan SA: Growth and Growth Hormone. In *Clinical Pediatric Endocrinology.* Edited by Kaplan SA. Philadelphia: WB Saunders; 1990: 38.

19. Katsuya T , Horiuchi M , Chen YD, *et al.*: Relations between deletion polymorphism of the angiotensin-converting enzyme gene and insulin resistance, glucose intolerance, hyperinsulinemia, and dyslipidemia. *Arterioscler Thromb Vasc Biol* 1995, 15(6):779–782.

20. Ravussin E, Lillioja S, Knowler WC, *et al.*: Reduced rate of energy expenditure as a risk factor for body-weight gain. *New Engl J Med* 1988, 318(8):467–472.

VITAMINS AND MINERALS

Jeffrey B. Blumberg and Diane L. McKay

3

From antiquity through the turn of the century, the role of nutrition in health promotion and therapeutics has been based on the empiric healing of disease by certain foods and their components. References to the dietary treatment of night blindness with liver date back to ancient Egypt. Examples of the medical use of foods that demonstrate an understanding of the relationship between diet and health can be traced back to the early history of both Hippocratic and Ayurvedic medicine. The first government-endorsed nutrition intervention program can probably be attributed to the 18th century British navy, with its promulgation of official dietary standards to prevent scurvy.

The classic studies by Lunin and Eijkmann 100 years ago demonstrated that such nutrient deficiency diseases as beriberi could be produced in animals. Their work led Hopkins to propose that small amounts of accessory nutrient factors are essential for growth and development, and in 1912 Funk coined the term *vitamin*. Thus began the first phase of the modern era of nutrition with the discovery and isolation of the micronutrient vitamins and minerals, including elucidation of the structure and synthesis of vitamin B_{12} in 1972.

This identification of vitamins and minerals as enzyme cofactors established the central theme of defining the concept for micronutrient requirements. In 1941, the US National Nutrition Conference for Defense directed the National Council to "explore and define our nutrition problems and to map out recommendations for an immediate program of action [to promote] buoyant health [and] ... the building up of our people to a level of health and vigor never before attained or dreamed of." The Food and Nutrition Board, which was established in response to these great expectations, produced in 1943 the first recommended dietary allowances (RDAs) for six vitamins. The scope of nutrients covered by the RDAs as well as the objectives of the recommendations have broadened substantially since then.

The 1989 edition of the RDAs [1] noted that the recommendations were "neither minimal requirements nor necessarily optimal levels of intake" and stated that "it is not possible at this time to establish optima." However, the RDAs being developed today are focused on "the promotion of nutrient function and biologic-physical well-being [and] the consideration of evidence concerning the prevention of disease and developmental disorders in addition to more traditional evidence of sufficient nutrient intake (for example, prevention of deficiency)." This paradigm shift has resulted from the accumulating evidence that micronutrients possess important roles beyond their classically recognized function in preventing deficiency diseases and their biochemical actions as coenzymes. Micronutrients have been shown to function in nonclassical roles as biological regulators and modulators such that they can affect gene expression, maximize physiologic function, delay or prevent the onset of chronic diseases, and serve as adjunctive therapeutic agents.

This chapter reviews the basis for the essentiality of micronutrients and emphasizes the effect of vitamin and mineral status in age-related declines of physiologic function and the development of chronic diseases.

Role of Vitamins and Minerals in Health and Disease

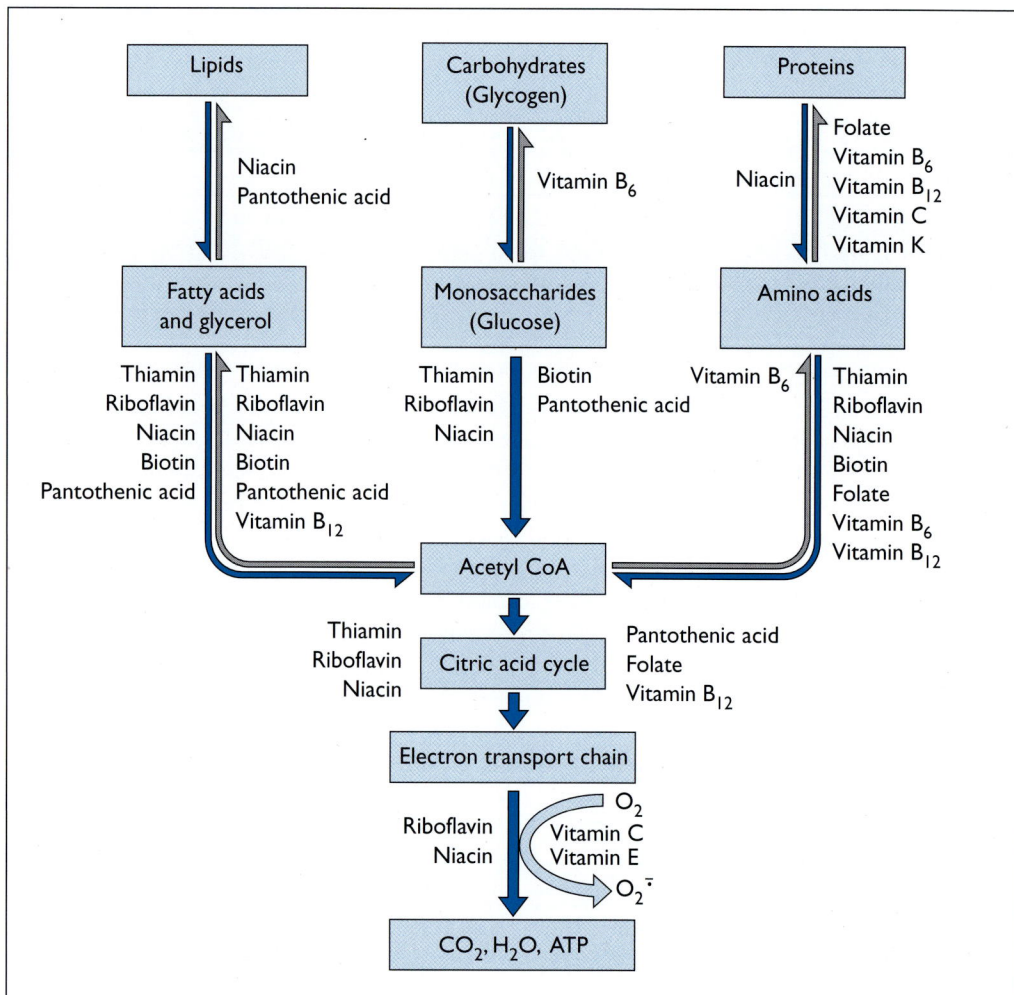

FIGURE 3-1. Integrative vitamin metabolism. Vitamins are essential to both anabolic (*gray arrows*) and catabolic (*blue arrows*) pathways of energy metabolism, usually serving as precursors to or components of coenzymes. Vitamin B_1 as thiamin pyrophosphate is involved in the enzymatic decarboxylation of α-keto acids. Riboflavin and niacin function in oxidation–reduction reactions as flavin adenine dinucleotide (FAD), flavin mononucleotide (FMN), nicotinamide adenine dinucleotide (NAD), and nicotinamide adenine dinucleotide phosphate (NADP), respectively. As pyridoxal phosphate, vitamin B_6 serves as the prosthetic group of enzymes catalyzing the transamination, racemization, and decarboxylation of amino acids. Pantothenic acid is a component of coenzyme A, a transient carrier of acyl groups, and biotin acts similarly with carboxyl groups in carboxylation reactions. As tetrahydrofolic acid, folate functions as an intermediate carrier of one-carbon groups in many enzymatic reactions. As methylcobalamin, vitamin B_{12} participates in enzymatic reactions involving the transfer of methyl groups. Vitamins C and K function as cofactors in hydroxylation and carboxylation reactions, respectively.

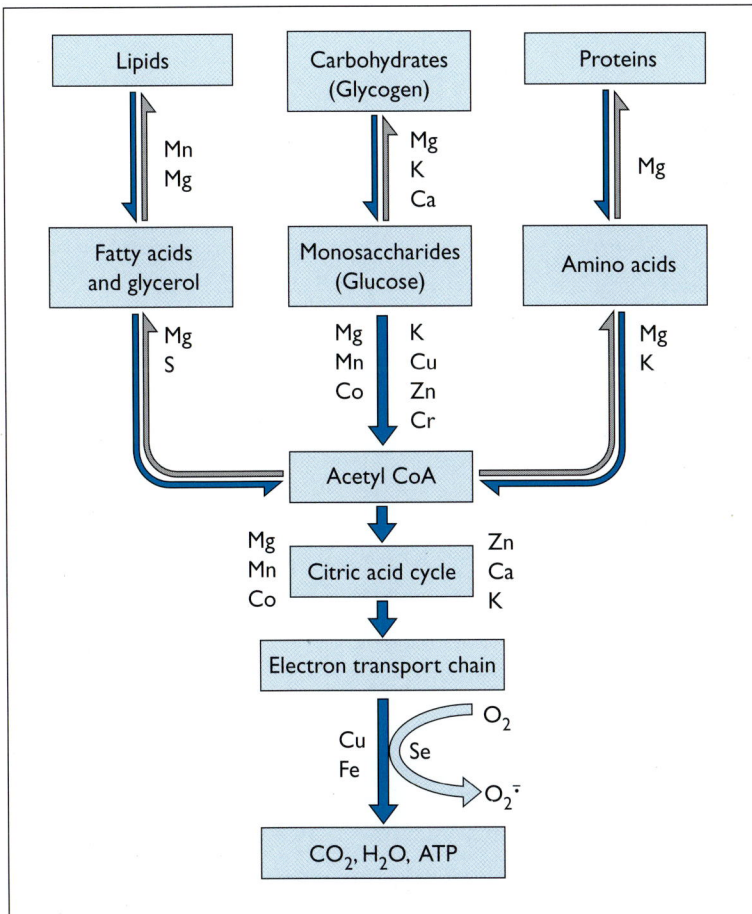

FIGURE 3-2. Integrative mineral metabolism. In both anabolic (*gray arrows*) and catabolic (*blue arrows*) processes, minerals function primarily as either cofactors (eg, manganese for pyruvate carboxylase; zinc for dehydrogenases; molybdenum for xanthine oxidase; manganese, copper, and zinc for superoxide dismutase; and selenium for glutathione peroxidase) or as integral components of macromolecules (eg, cytochromes [copper, iron], hemoglobin [iron], hormones such as thyroxine [iodine] and insulin [chromium], ceruloplasmin [copper], apatite and hydroxyapatite [calcium, phosphorus], fluoroapatite [fluoride], vitamin B_{12} [cobalt], thiamin [sulfur], and ATP [magnesium]), and numerous proteins contain functionally important zinc-finger regions. The ion forms of some minerals (eg, sodium, potassium, calcium, and chloride) function in electrical conduction in neurons and muscle and in the maintenance of cell water balance. Minerals with relatively large recommended dietary intakes (>100 mg) include calcium (1200 mg), phosphorus (1200 mg), and magnesium (350 mg). Minerals required in lesser amounts include iron (15 mg), zinc (15 mg), iodine (150 μg), and selenium (70 μg). CoA—coenzyme A.

ROLE OF VITAMINS IN HEALTH AND DISEASE

Vitamin	Biochemical Function	Deficiency	Prevention/Treatment
Niacin	NAD, NADP component	Pellagra	Hypercholesterolemia
B_6	Transamination cofactor	Convulsions	Carpal tunnel syndrome
B_{12}	Transmethylation cofactor	Anemias	Cognitive dysfunction
Folic acid	Single carbon transport	Megaloblastic anemia	Hyperhomocysteinemia
C	Hydroxylation cofactor	Scurvy	Oxidative stress
D	Calcium transport	Rickets	Osteoporosis
E	Antioxidant	Hemolytic anemia	Relative anergy

FIGURE 3-3. Role of vitamins in health and disease. Several dose-dependent biochemical functions have been identified for most vitamins, only some of which are related to their essentiality in preventing deficiency syndromes. The essentiality of niacin is based on its role in oxidation–reduction (redox) reactions (NAD, NADP), although this mechanism is unrelated to its hypocholesterolemic action at high doses. Pyridoxine is essential to the metabolic transformation of amino acids, which may be related to the epileptiform convulsions of deficiency and its analgesic pharmacology in tenosynovitis. Vitamin C at low intakes supports proline hydroxylation via iron reduction and prevents scurvy, whereas higher consumption provides enough redox capacity for ascorbate to function as an antioxidant. The antioxidant function of vitamin E maintains membrane integrity, but supplemental intake is associated with the inhibition of cyclooxygenase and stimulation of immune function.

ROLE OF MINERALS IN HEALTH AND DISEASE

Mineral	Biochemical Function	Deficiency	Prevention/Treatment
Calcium	Cell signaling	Osteoporosis	Colorectal cancer
Potassium	Cell membrane potential	Muscle weakness	Hypertension
Magnesium	ATPase cofactor	Tetany	Eclamptic convulsions
Iron	Electron transfer	Hypochromic anemia	Cognitive impairment
Zinc	Metalloenzyme cofactor	Growth retardation	Relative anergy
Selenium	Glutathione peroxidase cofactor	Cardiomyopathy	Cancer
Chromium	Insulin cofactor	Impaired glucose tolerance	Diabetes

FIGURE 3-4. Role of minerals in health and disease. Minerals are essential to metalloenzymes, acid–base balance, muscle contraction, and neurotransmission, and function as well in other roles. Consumption of several minerals beyond that necessary for prevention of deficiency symptoms may play a role in health promotion. Generous intakes of calcium, potassium, and magnesium are associated with antihypertensive actions, each via different mechanisms. Iron deficiency anemia in children impairs intellectual ability, but supplemental iron can improve cognitive performance in some children without anemia. Zinc deficiency induces hypogonadism in young men, but increasing zinc status in older adults is associated with improved taste acuity and immune response. Selenium deficiency results in cardiomyopathy, but intakes greater than that needed for glutathione peroxidase activity are associated with chemopreventive actions. Calcium deficiency results in osteomalacia, but high intakes reduce the risk of lead poisoning in children, premenstrual syndrome in women, and colonic neoplasia in older adults.

Recommended Dietary Allowances

PERCENTAGE OF INDIVIDUALS WITH DIETS THAT MEET THE RDA: PROBLEM VITAMINS

Vitamin	Population Meeting RDA, %	Groups at Highest Risk for Not Meeting RDA (years of age)
A	30.4–31.7	Males (20–29), females (12–29)
E	18.9–30.8	Children <5, males (6–11, 60+), females (6–70+)
B_6	33.2–33.8	Females (40–49, 60–69)
Folate	26.0–33.5	Males and females (20+)

FIGURE 3-5. Percentage of individuals with diets that meet the recommended dietary allowances (RDAs): problem vitamins. Assessment of vitamin intakes over a 2-day period reveals that no age/gender group meets 100% of the US RDA for all nutrients [1]. However, low vitamin intake and risk of deficiency can be defined as intake of less than 66% of the RDA over time. Low vitamin A intake, particularly in children and young adults, can result in xerophthalmia; increased susceptibility to infections; and impaired growth, fertility, and embryonic development. The actual requirement for vitamin E depends on the intake of polyunsaturated fatty acids (PUFAs), with recommended ratios ranging from 0.4 to 1.0 mg of vitamin E per gram of PUFA; inverse associations between vitamin E intake and the risk of cancer, cardiovascular disease, and cataract have been reported. Inadequate intake of folate and vitamins B_6 and B_{12} is associated with elevated total plasma homocysteine, an independent risk factor for vascular disease. Poor folate intake/status during the periconceptual period increases the risk for birth of a child with neural tube defects.

PERCENTAGE OF INDIVIDUALS WITH DIETS THAT MEET THE RDA: PROBLEM MINERALS

Mineral	Population Meeting RDA, %	Groups at Highest Risk for Not Meeting RDA
Calcium	13.5–25.3	Females (12–70+)
Phosphorus	33.7	Females (12–19)
Magnesium	17.9–33.5	Males (12–29, 50+), females (12–70+)
Iron	22.1–27.7	Females (12–49)
Zinc	12.4–32.7	Children (1–5), males (40+), females (6+)

FIGURE 3-6. Percentage of individuals with diets that meet the recommended dietary allowances (RDAs): problem minerals. Assessment of mineral intakes over a 2-day period reveals that no age/gender group meets 100% of the US RDA for all nutrients [1a]. However, low mineral intake and risk of deficiency can be defined as intake of less than 66% of the RDA over time. Poor intake of calcium, phosphorus, magnesium, and zinc is associated with lower peak bone mineral density by 35 to 40 years of age and faster loss in postmenopausal women, resulting in an increased risk of osteoporosis; iron is necessary for collagen matrix production, providing a structural framework for bone. Poor iron intake is also associated with anemia and, in children, with cognitive impairment. Poor magnesium intake is also associated with atherosclerosis, diabetes, hypertension, migraine headaches, and stroke.

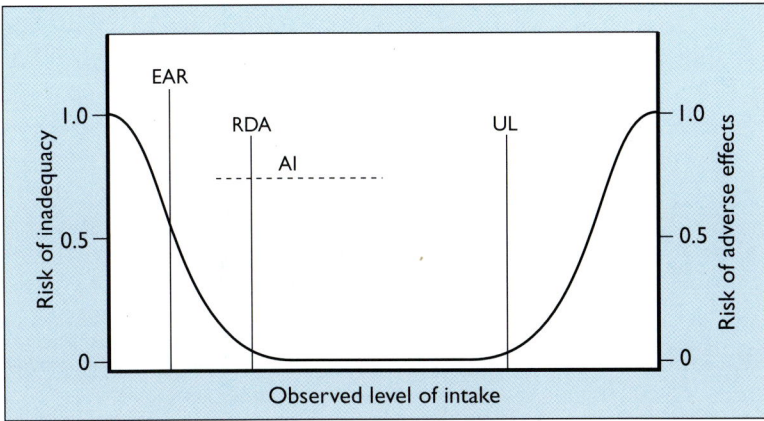

FIGURE 3-7. Redefining the recommended dietary allowances (RDAs): dietary reference intakes (DRIs). The RDAs, which have provided nutrient intake standards since 1941, are being replaced by DRIs [2]. DRIs are quantitative reference estimates of nutrient intakes for planning and assessing the diets of healthy people. DRIs include RDAs and three other reference values: estimated average requirement (EAR), adequate intake (AI), and tolerable upper limit (UL). The RDA is the average daily intake level that is sufficient to meet the nutrient requirements of 97% to 98% of healthy individuals within a specific age and gender group. The EAR is an estimated intake sufficient to meet the requirements of 50% of the individuals in a group. AI is employed when an RDA cannot be determined and represents an approximation of nutrient intake by a group. The UL is the highest level of daily nutrient intake that is likely to pose no risks of adverse health effects to almost all individuals in a group; as intake increases above the UL, the risk of adverse effects increases. (*Adapted from* Institute of Medicine, Food, and Nutrition Board [2].)

Ingredients

Durum wheat semolina, tomato concentrate, spinach powder, niacin, iron (ferrous sulfate), thiamine mononitrate, riboflavin, folic acid.

Nutrition Facts

Serving Size oz (56g 1/8pkg.) Dry.
Servings Per Container 8

Amount Per Serving

Calories 210 Calories from Fat 10

	% Daily Value*
Total Fat 1 g	2%
Saturated Fat 0 g	0%
Cholesterol 0 mg	0%
Sodium 0 mg	0%
Total Carbohydrate 44 g	15%
Dietary Fiber 2 g	8%
Sugars 2 g	
Protein 6 g	

Required by NLEA:
Vitamin A 0% • Vitamin C 0%
Calcium 0% • Iron 10%

Only required when product is fortified:
Thiamine 35% • Riboflavin 15%
Niacin 20% • Folic Acid 30%

*Percent Daily Values are based on a 2,000 calories diet. Your daily values may be higher or lower depending on your caloric needs.

	Calories	2,000	2,500
Total fat	Less than	65 g	80 g
Sat fat	Less than	20 g	25 g
Cholesterol	Less than	300 mg	300 mg
Sodium	less than	2,400 mg	2,400 mg
Total Carbohydrate		300 g	375 g
Dietary Fiber		25 g	30 g

Calories per gram:
Fat 9 • Carbohydrate 4 • Protein 4

Keep in cool dry place.
Pasta is a cholesterol and sodium free product.

FIGURE 3-8. Food labeling requirements for vitamins and minerals. The 1990 Nutrition Labeling and Education Act (NLEA) mandated nutrition labeling of most processed foods and proposed voluntary nutrition labeling of fresh produce, fish, meat, and poultry. For labeling purposes, the % daily value was established to show how the product fits into an overall healthy diet. The daily value is derived from the recommended dietary intakes (RDIs) for micronutrients and the daily recommended value (DRV) for protein, fat, and carbohydrates. The RDI represents the highest 1968 recommended dietary allowance (RDA) value except those for pregnant and lactating women. Among the 14 nutrients required on nutritional labeling, the only micronutrients included are vitamins A and C, calcium, and iron because they reflect current health concerns. Listing other vitamins and minerals is required only when the product is fortified, the product is a dietary supplement, or a health claim is made on the label.

Heart Disease

Antioxidants

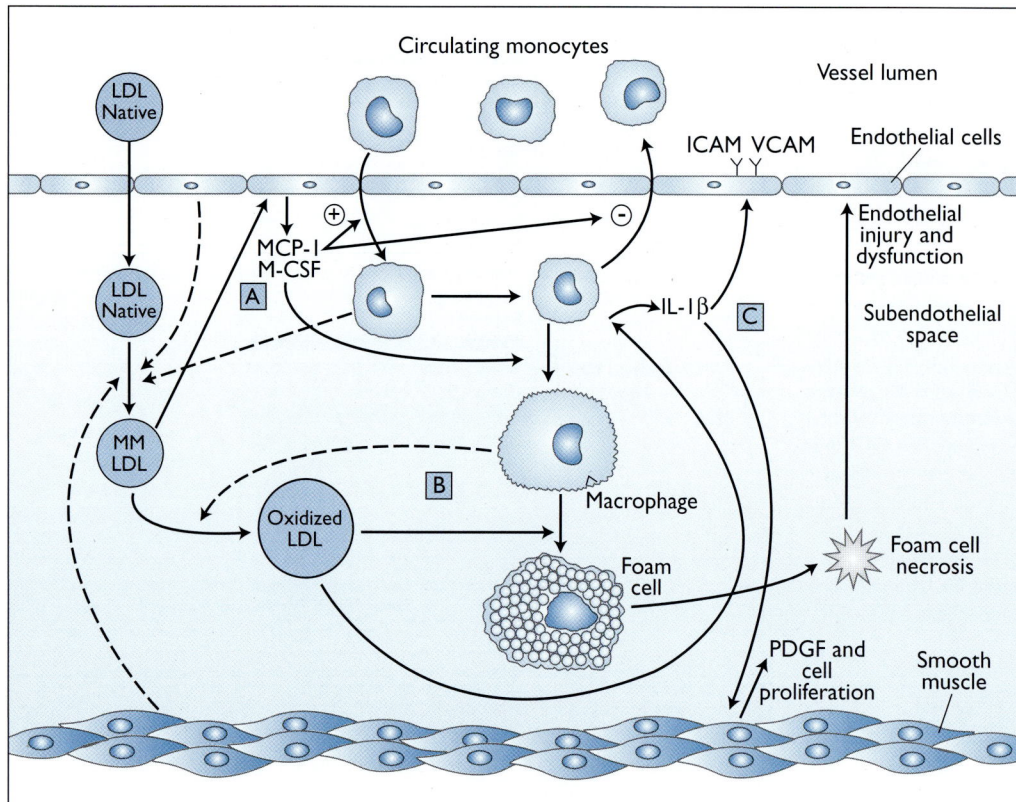

FIGURE 3-9. Low-density lipoprotein (LDL) oxidation as an early event in atherogenesis. The oxidative modification of LDL represents a critical early step in atherogenesis. Native LDL trapped in the subendothelial space can be minimally modified (MM-LDL) by smooth muscle cells (SMCs), endothelial cells, and monocytes/macrophages (*dashed lines*). MM-LDLs stimulate (+) monocyte chemotaxis via endothelial secretion of monocyte chemotactic protein-1 (MCP-1), inhibit (-) monocyte egress, and promote their differentiation with macrophage colony-stimulating factor (M-CSF) (*A*). Mature macrophages further oxidize MM-LDL into a ligand internalized via the scavenger receptor, resulting in foam-cell formation, necrosis, and subsequent release of lysosomes and necrotic debris (*B*). Oxidized LDL stimulates monocyte secretion of interleukin-1 (IL-1), which induces expression of endothelial (intracellular [ICAM] and vascular [VCAM]) cell adhesion molecules and stimulates SMC proliferation via platelet-derived growth factor (PDGF) secretion (*C*). Oxidized LDL also promotes endothelial dysfunction and injury, resulting in the formation of fatty streaks. Dietary antioxidants have been demonstrated to have an effect at multiple points in this process.

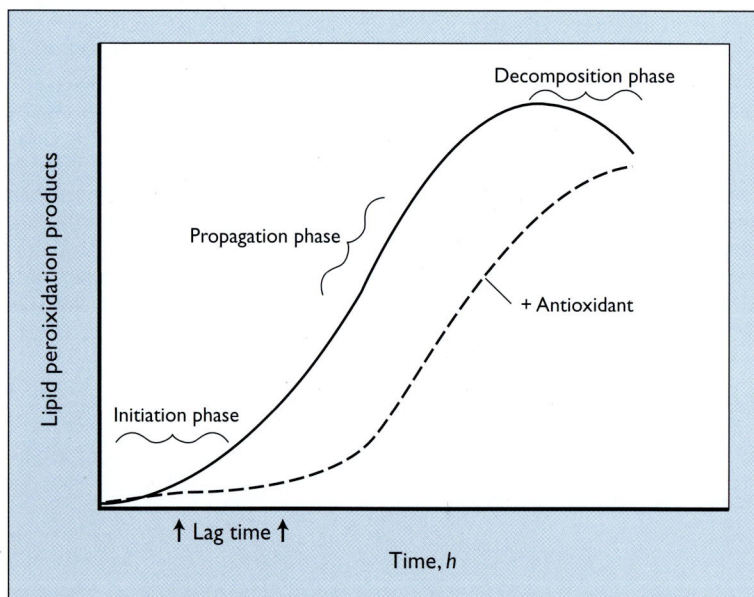

FIGURE 3-10. Role of antioxidants in the pathogenesis of atherogenesis. Incorporation of antioxidants (including vitamins C and E, coenzyme Q10, and possibly carotenoids) into lipoproteins and vascular tissue decreases the susceptibility of low-density lipoprotein (LDL) to oxidation by slowing the rate of the initiation and/or progression of LDL oxidation. LDL oxidation is determined by the production of lipid peroxidation products such as conjugated dienes and malondialdehyde. Increasing the antioxidant concentration of vascular cells may improve their function and reduce the clinical expression of heart disease by reducing monocyte adhesion, foam-cell formation, and cytotoxic reactions leading to the formation and activation of atherosclerotic lesions.

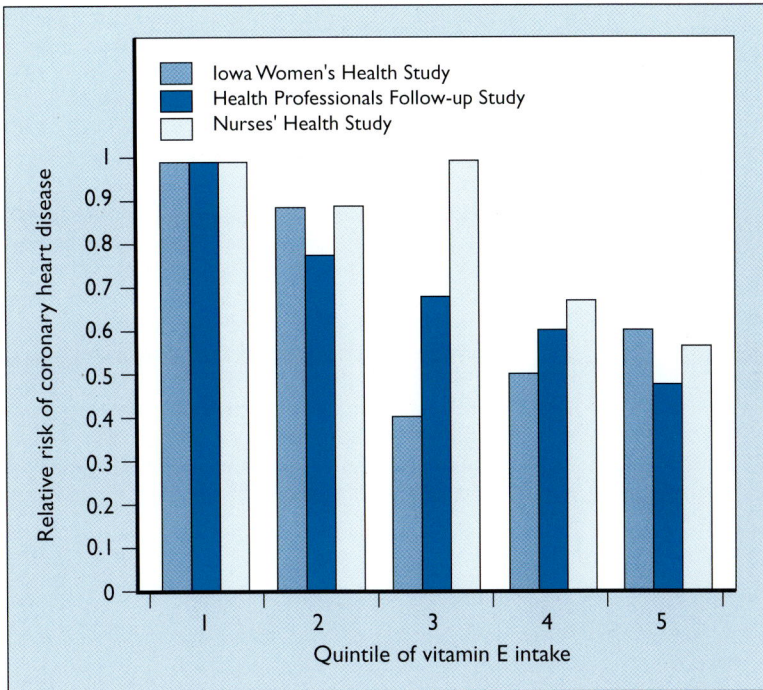

FIGURE 3-11. Vitamin E intake and relative risk of coronary heart disease (CHD). Several epidemiologic observations indicate an inverse association between vitamin E intake and CHD. For example, the Iowa Women's Health Study (n = 34,486) [3], Nurses' Health Study (n = 87,245) [4], and Health Professionals Follow-Up Study (men only; n = 39,910) [5] revealed that subjects in the highest quintile of vitamin E consumption from food (36,208 IU) and supplements (419 IU) had relative CHD risks of 0.78, 0.59, and 0.59, respectively, after adjustment for confounding variables such as age. Regular supplementation for at least 2 years appears important to the observation of such a benefit.

B Vitamins

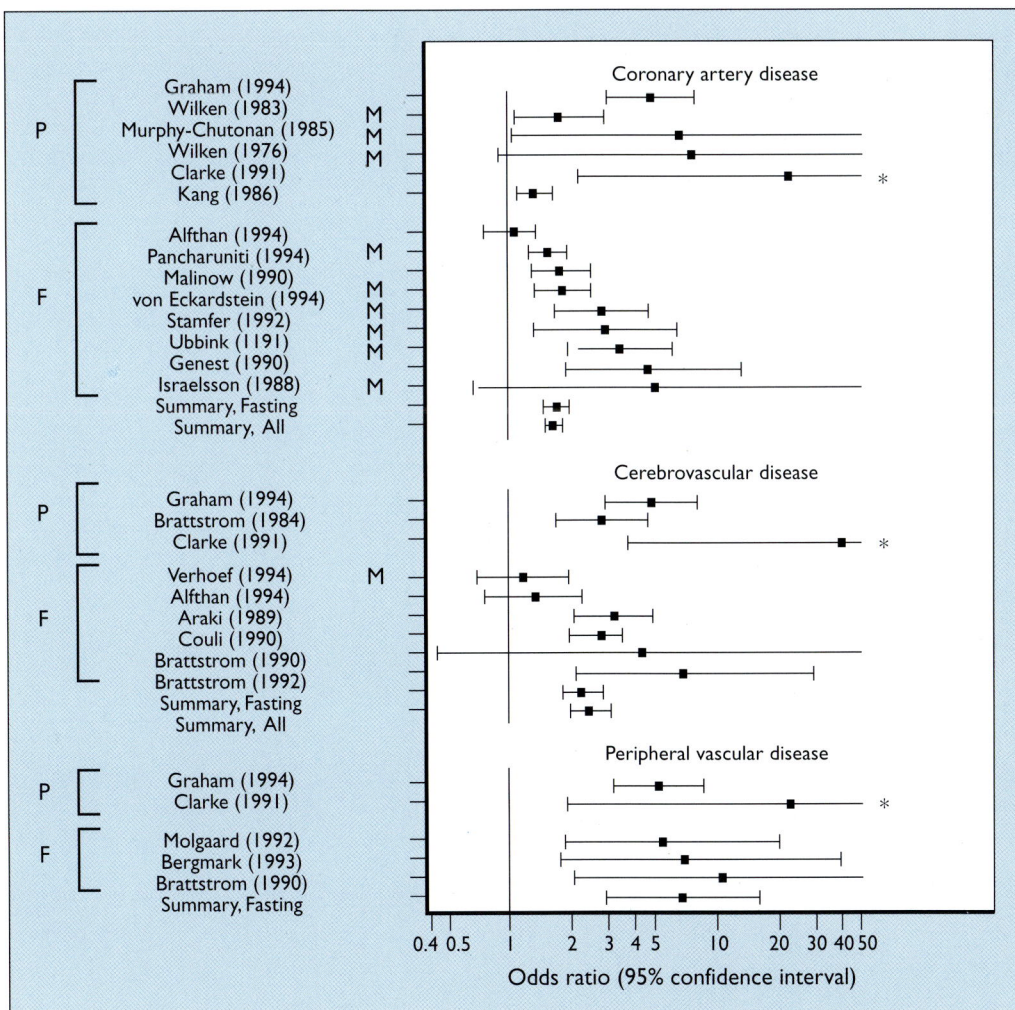

FIGURE 3-12. Homocysteine and risk of vascular disease. Hyperhomocysteinemia is an independent risk factor for vascular disease. Premature thrombotic and arteriosclerotic complications in children with hyperhomocysteinuria first suggested that elevated total plasma homocysteine may increase the risk of vascular disease. Moderate elevations of homocysteine are observed in many patients with arteriosclerosis of coronary, cerebral, and peripheral arteries. Data from relevant selected studies [6] are presented as odds ratios with 95% confidence intervals (CI) on a log scale. Unless indicated, odds ratios are for both men (M) and women. Asterisks indicate the infinite upper bound of risk estimate, P indicates homocysteine measured by the postmethionine load test, and F indicates fasting total homocysteine. (Adapted from Boushey et al. [6].)

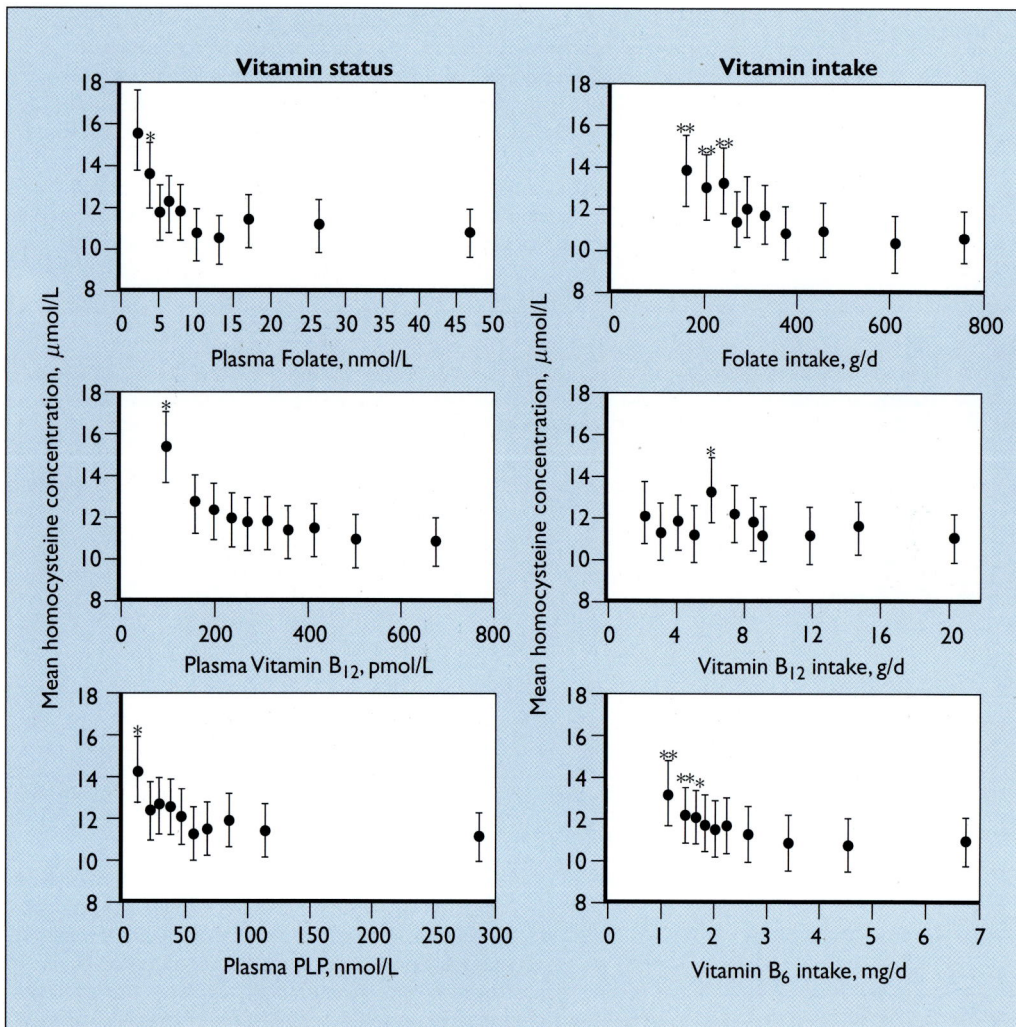

FIGURE 3-13. Relationship between homocysteine concentration, B vitamin status, and age. After adjustment for age, sex, and plasma vitamins, mean (±95% confidence intervals) total plasma homocysteine was found to increase with age and low intake and status of B vitamins (by deciles) in the oldest cohort (n = 1160) of the Framingham Heart Study [7]. Adequate levels of vitamins B$_6$, B$_{12}$, and folate appear necessary to maintain relatively low levels of homocysteine. The absence of a dose–response relationship between vitamin B$_{12}$ intake and plasma homocysteine reflects the lack of correlation between vitamin B$_{12}$ intake and status, possibly due to hypochlorhydria. A substantial portion of the elderly population may be at risk for elevated homocysteine, although the impact of a 1998 federal mandate for the fortification of flour with folic acid has not been evaluated. PLP—pyridoxal phosphate. (Adapted from Selhub et al. [7].)

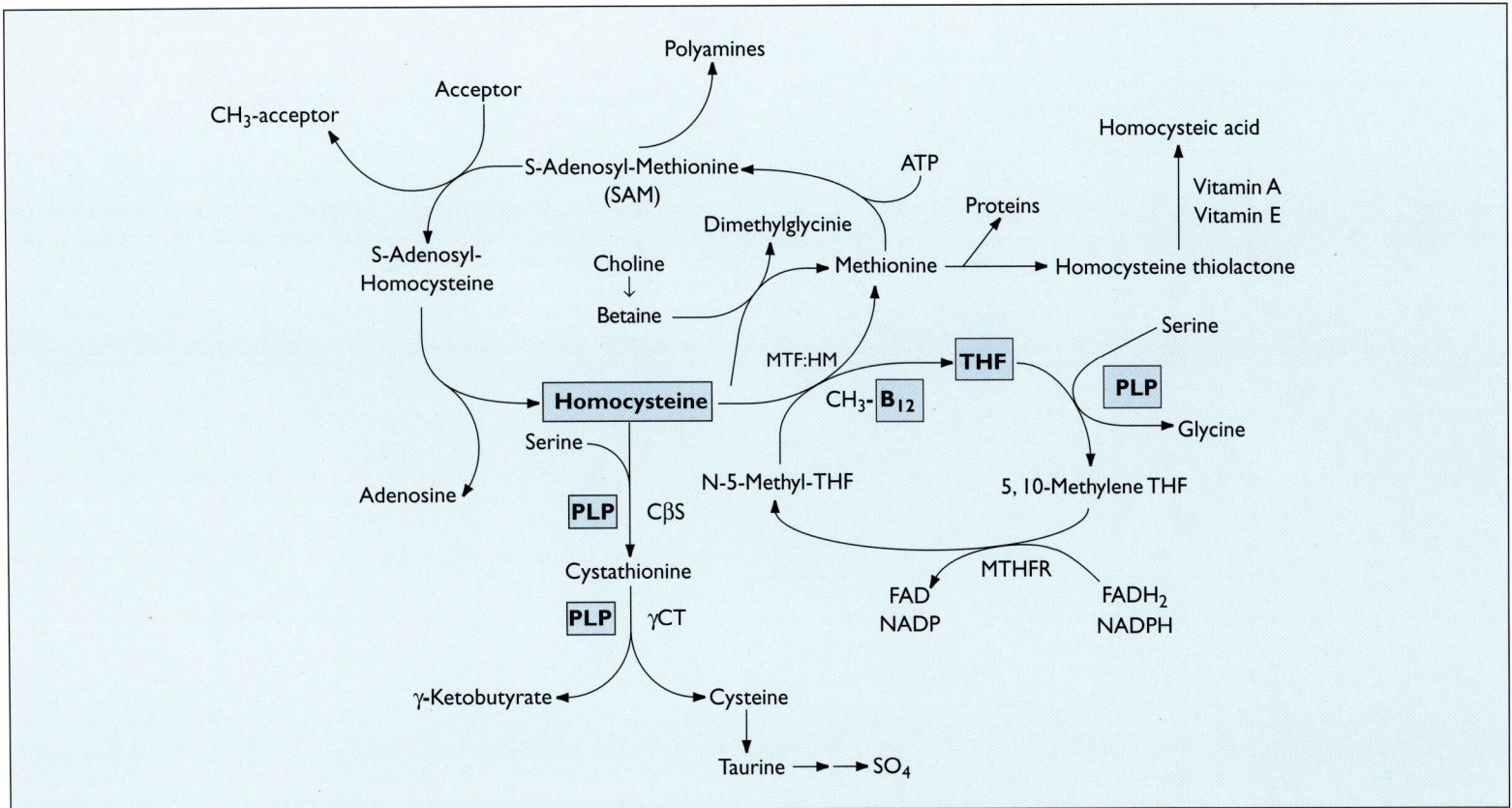

FIGURE 3-14. Homocysteine metabolism. The status of homocysteine, a sulfur-containing amino acid, depends on its rate of remethylation and transsulfuration. Homocysteine is methylated by N-5-methyltetrahydrofolate (MTHF; ultimately derived from dietary folate) or betaine to form methionine in a reaction catalyzed by the vitamin B_{12}-containing enzyme, N-5-MTHF:homocysteine methyltransferase (MTHF:HM, EC 2.1.1.13). Methionine then forms S-adenosyl-methionine (SAM) in an ATP-dependent process, and SAM serves as a methyl donor to a variety of acceptors, including guanidinoacetate, nucleic acids, neurotransmitters, phospholipids, and hormones. Homocysteine condenses with serine to form cystathionine in an irreversible transsulfuration reaction catalyzed by the pyridoxal-5'-phosphate (PLP)– containing enzyme, cystathionine β-synthase (CβS, EC 4.2.1.22). Cystathionine is hydrolyzed by a second PLP-containing enzyme, γ-cystathionase (γCT, EC 4.4.1.1). The de novo synthesis of methionine methyl groups requires both vitamin B_{12} and folate coenzymes, whereas the synthesis of cystathionine requires PLP. Nutritional inadequacy of vitamins B_6, B_{12}, and/or folate is a determinant of homocysteinemia. FAD—flavin adenine dinucleotide; $FADH_2$—reduced form of FAD; MTHFR—methyl tetrahydrofolate reductase.

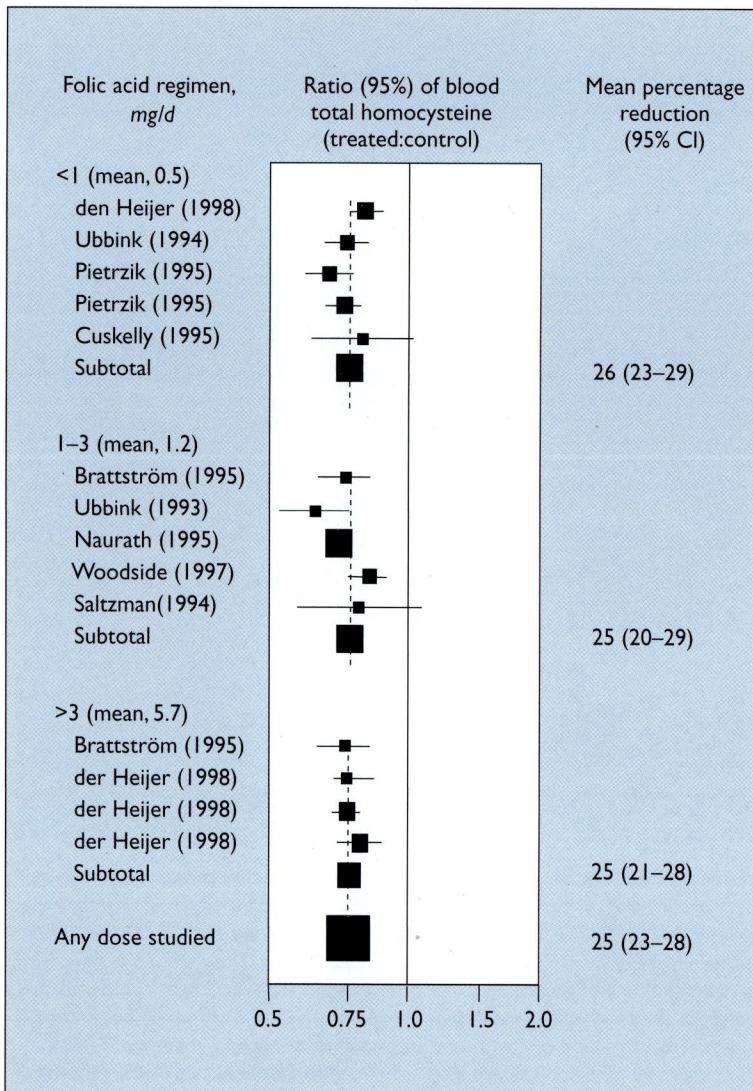

FIGURE 3-15. Effect of B vitamins on homocysteine metabolism. Randomized, controlled trials of folic acid supplementation with and without vitamins B_6 and B_{12} indicate that 0.5 to 5 mg/d of folic acid significantly reduces total homocysteine concentrations, especially among patients initially presenting with median plasma homocysteine concentrations of 12 mmol/L or higher and/or folate levels of 12 nmol/L or lower [8]. The addition of 0.2 to 1 mg/d of vitamin B_{12} induces a further reduction in homocysteine. Vitamin B_6 has little impact on fasting homocysteine concentrations but appears effective in lowering homocysteine following a methionine loading test. *Squares* indicate the ratios of posttreatment blood homocysteine among subjects allocated folic acid supplements to those of controls (the size of the squares is proportional to the number of subjects), and *horizontal* lines indicate 95% confidence intervals (CIs). (*Adapted from* the Homocysteine Lowering Trialists' Collaboration [8].)

Minerals and Hypertension

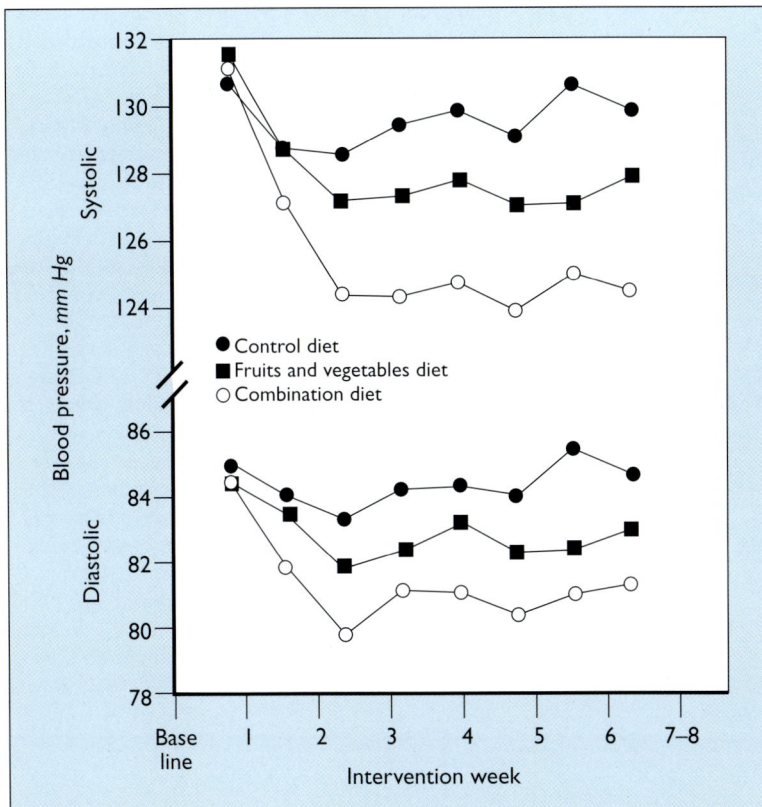

FIGURE 3-16. Role of minerals in hypertension. Dietary modification in patients with moderate hypertension is an effective alternative or adjunct to antihypertensive drug therapy. Arterial pressure is decreased by salt depletion in about half of hypertensive patients. Mechanisms underlying the salt sensitivity of blood pressure may include decreased renal capacity for sodium excretion, increased sympathetic nervous system activity and baroflex function alterations, and alterations of ion transport in vascular smooth muscle. Potassium has a natriuretic action and may also inhibit renin release, antagonize the pressor response to angiotensin II, induce vasodilation, decrease thromboxane production, and increase kallidin synthesis. High calcium intake induces diuresis, stabilizes membranes, and elevates plasma calcitonin-gene—related peptide (CGRP). Magnesium decreases vascular tone and contractility, possibly through decreasing cellular uptake and cytosolic concentrations. The Dietary Approaches to Stop Hypertension (DASH) clinical trial [9] demonstrated that a diet low in sodium and rich in calcium (from low-fat dairy products), magnesium, and potassium (at levels close to the 75th percentile of US consumption) in moderately hypertensive (mean, 132/85 mm Hg) adults (n = 459) lowered systolic (-5.5%) and diastolic (-3.0%) blood pressures more than did a control diet poor in these minerals (at levels close to 25th percentile of US consumption). A fruit-and-vegetable diet rich only in magnesium and potassium also lowered systolic (-2.8%) and diastolic (-1.1%) blood pressures more than did the control diet. (*Adapted from* Appel *et al.* [9].)

Cancer Prevention

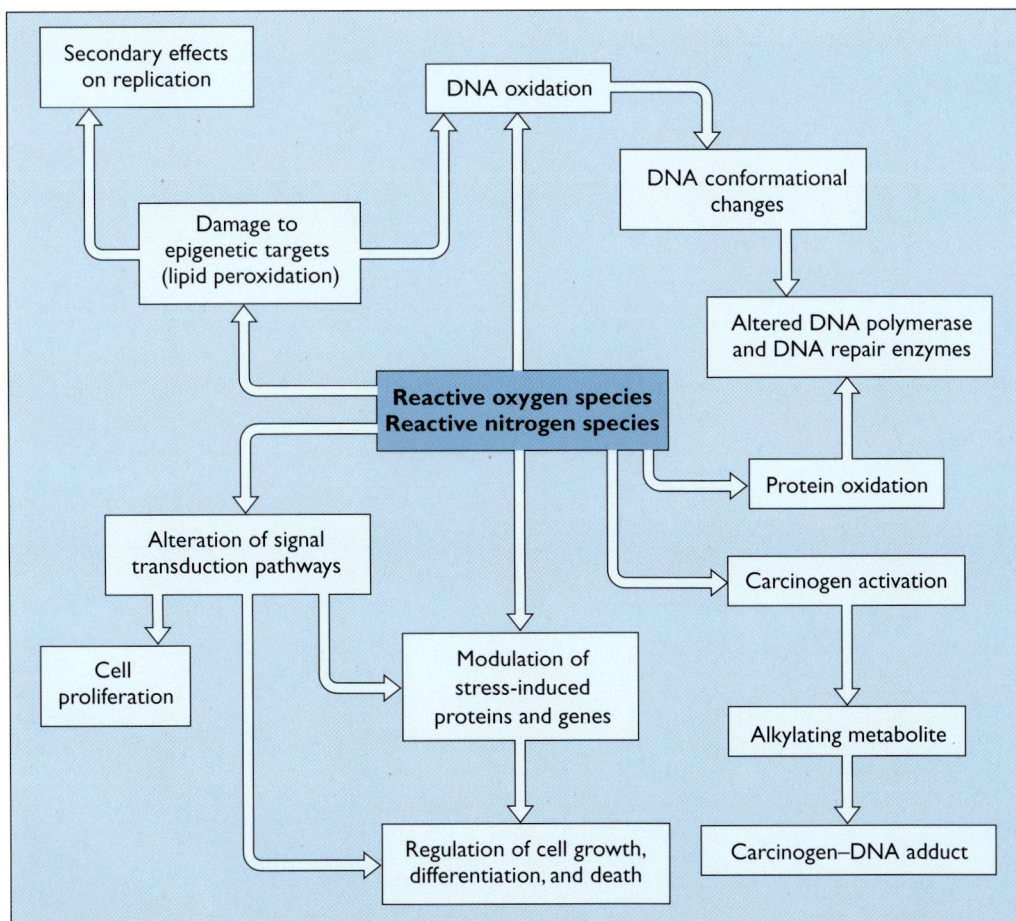

FIGURE 3-17. Relationship between free radicals and carcinogenesis. Reactive oxygen and nitrogen species, including superoxide anion, hydroxyl radical, hydrogen peroxide, nitric oxide, and peroxynitrite, appear to play a major role in carcinogenesis. These free radicals may act directly to oxidize DNA and cause mutations or indirectly via damage to lipids and proteins or alteration of signal transduction pathways for cell growth and apoptosis. Poor intake and status of antioxidants, including vitamins C and E, carotenoids, and retinol, are associated with an increased risk of several forms of cancer. Low serum concentrations of mineral cofactors in antioxidant enzymes, including copper, selenium, and zinc, are also associated with an increased cancer risk.

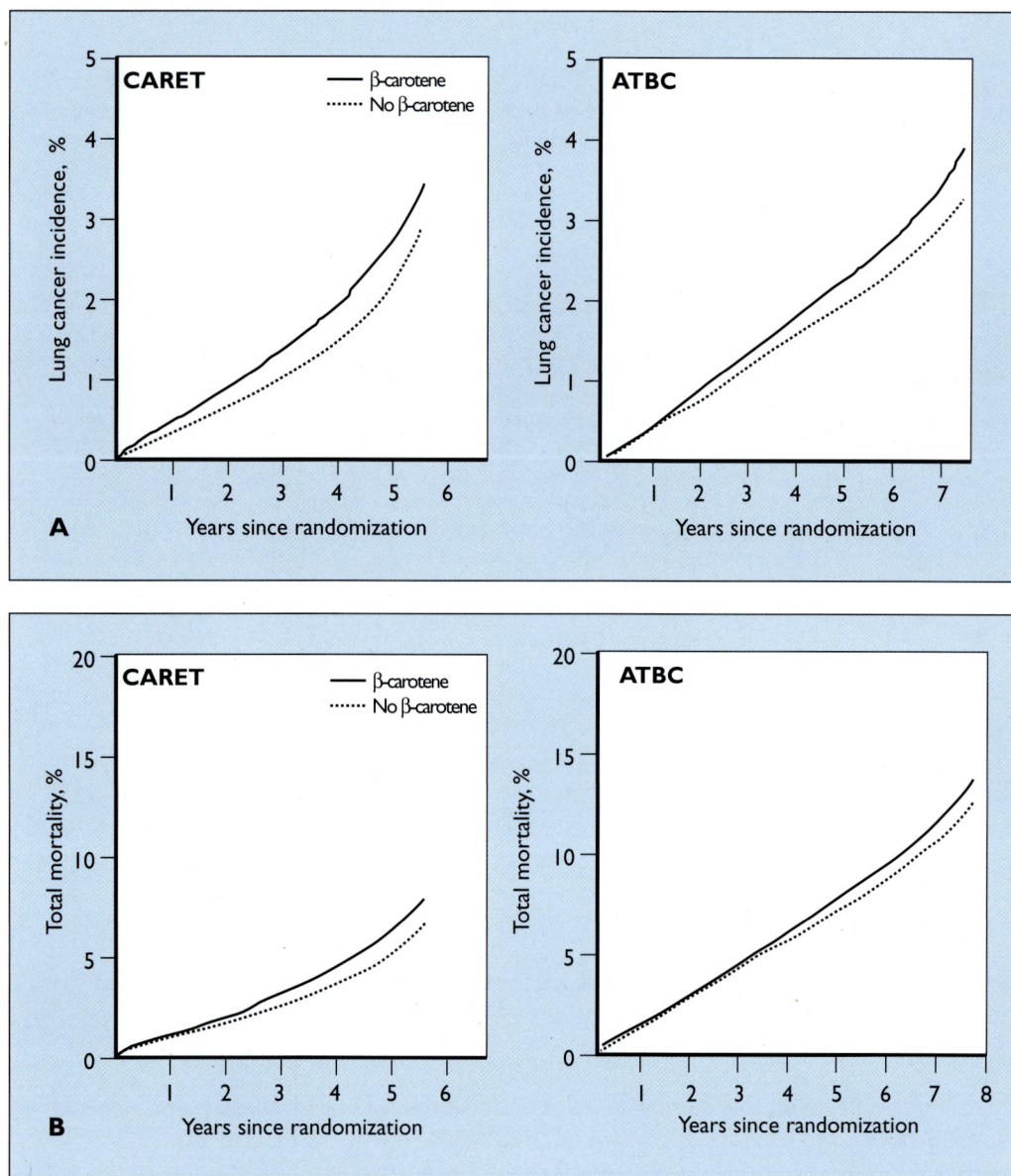

FIGURE 3-18. Beta-carotene supplementation and lung cancer. Most epidemiologic studies generally show an inverse correlation between low dietary intake (0.5 to 2.9 mg/d) and status (≤0.23 μmol/L) of beta-carotene and several forms of cancer, particularly lung cancer. The controlled Alpha-Tocopherol, Beta-Carotene Lung Cancer Prevention Study (ATBC; *n* = 29,133) [10] and the Carotene and Retinol Efficacy Trial (CARET; *n* = 18,314) [11] administered 20- and 30-mg supplements of beta-carotene daily (with 25,000 IU vitamin A in CARET), respectively, to subjects at high risk of lung cancer owing to lifelong smoking and/or occupational exposure to asbestos. The treatment increased plasma beta-carotene levels 18-fold (to 3.0 μmol/L) and 12-fold (to 2.1 μmol/L) in ATBC and CARET, respectively. Lung cancer incidence (18%, 28%; **A**) and mortality (8%, 17%; **B**) were significantly greater in the supplemented groups in ATBC and CARET, respectively. Consistent with epidemiologic observations, the incidence of lung cancer in the placebo groups was significantly higher among the subjects in the lowest quartile of baseline serum beta-carotene. The Physicians Health Study (*n* = 22,071) [12] reported no effect of 50-mg beta-carotene supplements administered every other day on cancer incidence or mortality in a population comprised principally of nonsmokers.

A. CARCINOGENIC MECHANISMS FOR FOLATE-RELATED ENHANCEMENT OF CARCINOGENESIS

Induction of DNA hypomethylation
Increased chromosomal fragility and/or diminished DNA repair
Secondary choline deficiency
Diminution in natural killer cell surveillance
Misincorporation of uridylate for thymidylate in DNA synthesis
Facilitation of tumorigenic virus metabolism

FIGURE 3-19. Folate and cancer. **A,** Several candidate mechanisms have been proposed to explain the association between poor folate status and a high risk of some forms of cancer, particularly colorectal cancer [13]. **B,** Increasing folate intake reduces DNA hypomethylation, a putative biomarker of early neoplastic lesions in the colorectum. Intrinsic DNA methylation evaluated in normal-appearing and lesion sites from the rectal mucosa of patients with colonic carcinomas or adenomas and healthy controls revealed significantly greater hypomethylation in carcinomas based on *in vitro* incorporation of ^{3}H-methyl-*S*-adenosylmethionine, an assay in which the radioisotope accumulates in inverse proportion to the content of methylated DNA [14]. (Part A *adapted from* Mason and Levesque [13]; part B *adapted from* Gravo et al. [14].)

B. [^{3}H-METHYL] INCORPORATION INTO DNA FROM SPECIMENS (MEAN ±SEM)

Group	[^{3}H-methyl] Incorporation Into DNA, *dpm* x 10^3	
	Neoplastic lesions	**Normal-Appearing Rectal Mucosa**
Carcinomas	383 ± 52	245 ± 27
Adenomas	209 ± 21	156 ± 20
Controls	—	109 ± 12
P value	0.004	0.002

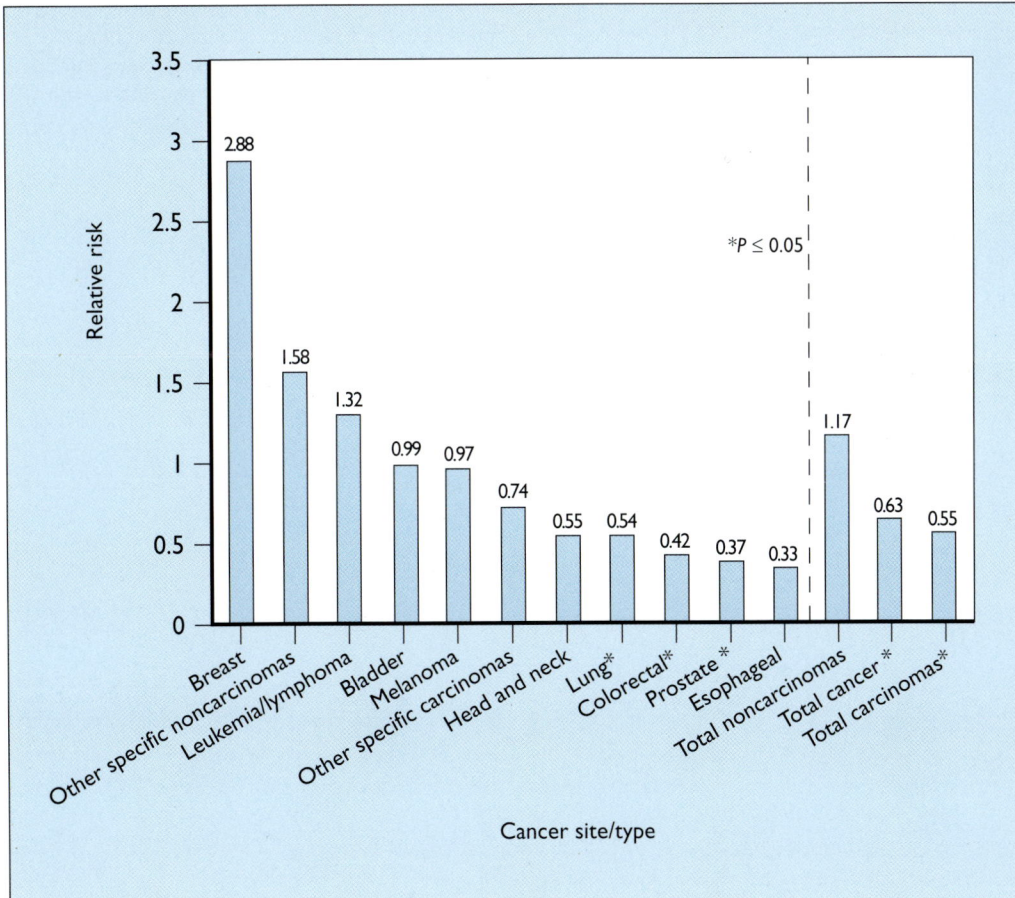

FIGURE 3-20. Selenium in chemoprevention. Epidemiologic investigations reveal an inverse correlation between selenium status and cancer incidence in both industrialized and less developed countries. Animal studies suggest an antitumorigenic effect of high-dose selenium intake. Proposed chemopreventive mechanisms of selenium include enhanced antioxidant protection by selenium-dependent glutathione peroxidase; alterations in carcinogen metabolism to decrease mutagenicity; endocrine-mediated alterations in carcinogen metabolism to less potent compounds; stimulation of immune responses; production of cytotoxic selenium metabolites; inhibition of protein synthesis and cell proliferation; and/or stimulation of apoptosis. Secondary endpoint analyses of a multiclinic trial of patients at high risk for skin cancer ($n = 1312$) employing a selenium supplement of 200 µg/d for 4.5 ± 2.8 years revealed significant reductions ($P \leq 0.05$) in the relative risk of several forms of cancer after 6.4 ± 2.0 years of follow-up [15].

Bone Health

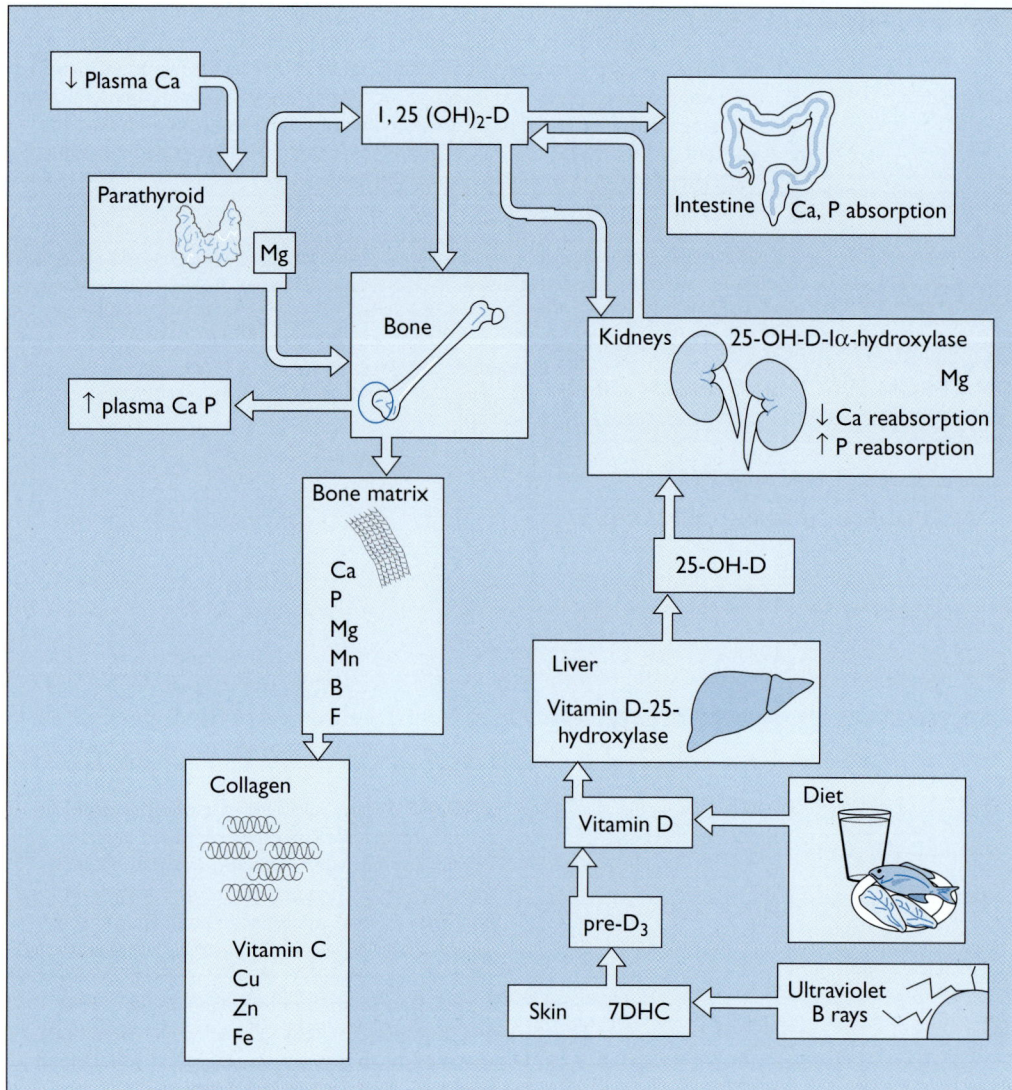

FIGURE 3-21. Nutrients required for bone remodeling. A significant amount of the body's mineral content is found within bone and teeth (eg, calcium [99%], phosphorus [90%], magnesium [60%], and manganese [25%]). Although mineralization during bone calcification principally involves the incorporation of apatite (calcium phosphate) and/or hydroxyapatite (calcium hydroxide) into the bone structure, magnesium, boron, and fluoride are also important components of this process. In addition to promoting the absorption of calcium, phosphorus, and magnesium, vitamin D is necessary to bone remodeling through activating osteoclasts, facilitating parathyroid hormone (PTH) action, and maintaining calcium and phosphorus homeostasis. Magnesium is required for PTH release, bioactivation of vitamin D, and, together with ATP, formation of hydroxyapatite. Manganese is a cofactor of glycosyl transferase and is necessary for the synthesis of the chondroitin sulfate side chains in proteoglycans. Zinc is essential to metalloenzymes such as carbonic anhydrase and collagenase that are involved in bone resorption and remodeling and to the synthesis of growth factors and chondro-osseous matrix. Copper is bound by cartilage matrix glycoprotein and required by lysyl oxidase for cross-linking elastin and collagen. Fluoride replaces hydroxyl groups in hydroxyapatite to form fluoroapatite and is employed therapeutically to reduce fracture risk. Vitamin C is a cofactor for bone hydroxylases and promotes the formation of connective tissue matrices (collagen, elastin, proteoglycans) and bone mineral through its metabolic interactions with calcium, copper, fluoride, and phosphorus. 7-DHC—7-dehydrocholesterol.

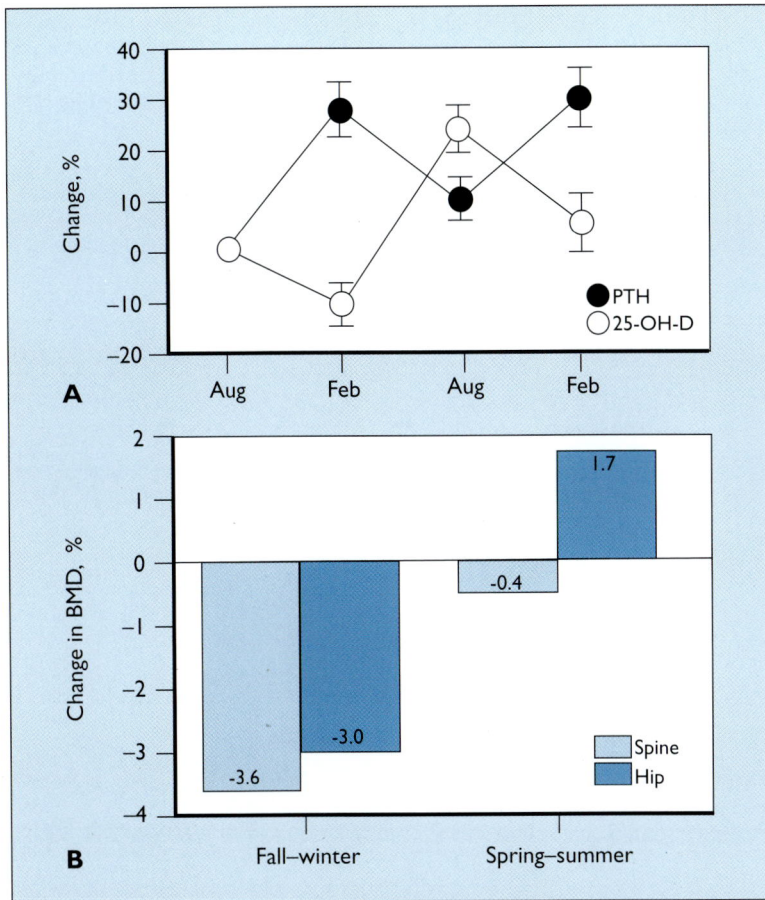

FIGURE 3-22. Interactions between age, vitamin D status, and bone mineral density (BMD) (**A** and **B**). The decline in vitamin D status with advancing age is the result of several factors, including less sun exposure, decreased dietary intake, lower skin 7-DHC concentrations, loss of intestinal vitamin D receptors, and decreased responsiveness of gastrointestinal mucosa to 1,25-$(OH)_2$-vitamin D and renal 1α-hydroxylase to parathyroid hormone (PTH). Further, several drugs commonly taken by older adults impair vitamin D status and/or action, including cholestyramine, isoniazid, phenolphthalein, and phenytoin. Increases in circulating ionized calcium resulting from postmenopausal estrogen loss can suppress PTH secretion and reduce 1,25 $(OH)_2D$ status as well. Weak ultraviolet light irradiation during winter in northern latitudes results in a seasonal increase in PTH, a decrease in 25-OH vitamin D production, and a related loss of BMD in the hip and spine as noted in 15 women living in New England (mean age, 77 years) [16]. Increasing vitamin D intake can compensate for several of these changes as well as age-related declines in the absorption efficiency of calcium. (*Adapted from* Holick [16].)

A. NUMBER OF FIRST NONVERTEBRAL FRACTURES

Site of Fracture	Placebo (n = 202)	Calcium–Vitamin D (n = 187)
Face	1	1
Shoulder, humerus, or clavicle	4	3
Radius or ulna	5	1
Hand	1	1
Ribs	2	2
Pelvis	2	0
Hip	1	0
Tibia or fibula	1	1
Ankle or foot	7	2
Multiple Sites	2	0
Total	26	11

FIGURE 3-23. Effect of calcium and vitamin D supplementation on fracture incidence. Inadequate intake of calcium and vitamin D reduces calcium absorption, increases serum parathyroid hormone (PTH), and promotes loss of bone density. Low bone mass is a significant determinant of fracture. Randomized clinical trials have demonstrated that supplemental calcium reduces bone loss in middle-aged postmenopausal women and lowers the rate of vertebral fracture in those with previous vertebral fractures. Women with the lowest dietary calcium intake appear to benefit most from supplementation, but adequate vitamin D is necessary to achieve the full benefit of calcium.

(Continued on next page)

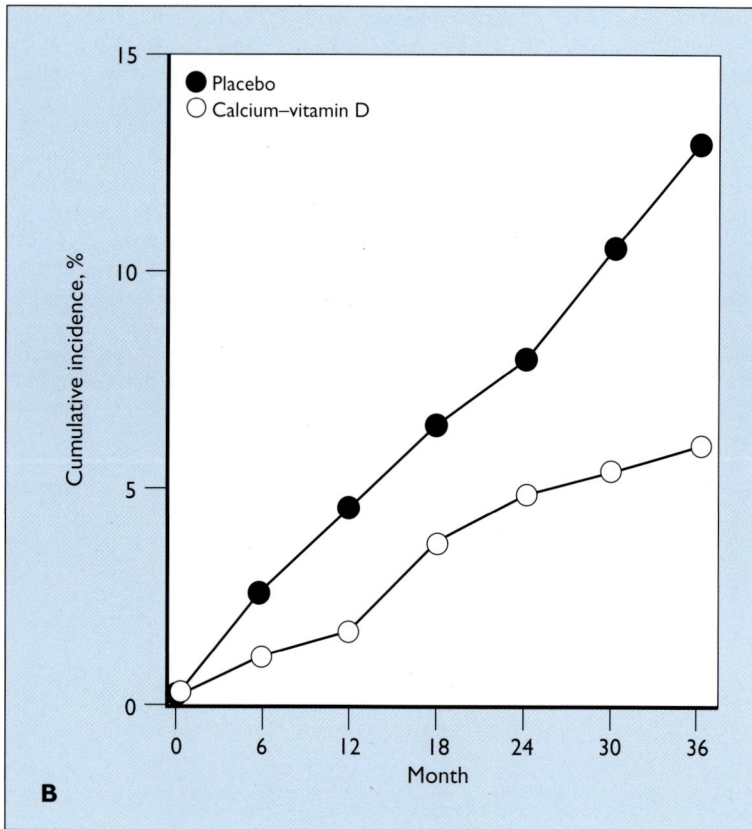

FIGURE 3-23. (*Continued*) **A** and **B,** Daily supplementation with 500 mg of calcium and 700 IU of vitamin D significantly reduced bone loss and the incidence of nonverterbral fractures among 187 men and women older than 65 years of age over a 36-month period compared with 202 placebo-treated control subjects [17]. (*Adapted from* Dawson-Hughes, *et al.* [17].)

Cognitive Function

NEUROLOGIC AND BEHAVIORAL EFFECTS OF VITAMIN DEFICIENCIES

Vitamin	Presentation
Thiamin	Beriberi, Wernicke-Korsakoff psychosis
Niacin	Pellagra, dementia
Pantothenic acid	Myelin degeneration
Pyridoxine (B$_6$)	Peripheral neuropathy, convulsions
Folate	Irritability, depression (?), paranoia (?)
Cobalamin (B$_{12}$)	Peripheral neuropthy, subacute combined system degeneration, dementia
Vitamin E	Spinocerebellar degeneration, peripheral axonopathy

FIGURE 3-24. Micronutrients and cognitive function. Overt clinical deficiencies of B vitamins have been implicated in many central nervous system disorders, including dementia (vitamin B$_{12}$), depression (folate), convulsions (vitamin B$_{12}$), and Wernicke-Korsakoff syndrome (thiamin) [18]. Studies also suggest that subclinical vitamin deficiencies play a role in the pathogenesis of declining neurocognitive function with age. Low blood levels of folate, vitamin B$_{12}$, vitamin C, and riboflavin in healthy elderly individuals are associated with poor performance on tests of memory and nonverbal abstract thinking. Poor folate and vitamin B$_{12}$ status, along with elevated total plasma homocysteine, are associated with the incidence and progression of Alzheimer's disease. Vitamin E supplementation may slow the progression of Alzheimer's disease in patients with moderately severe impairment. (*Adapted from* Rosenberg and Miller [18].)

Vision

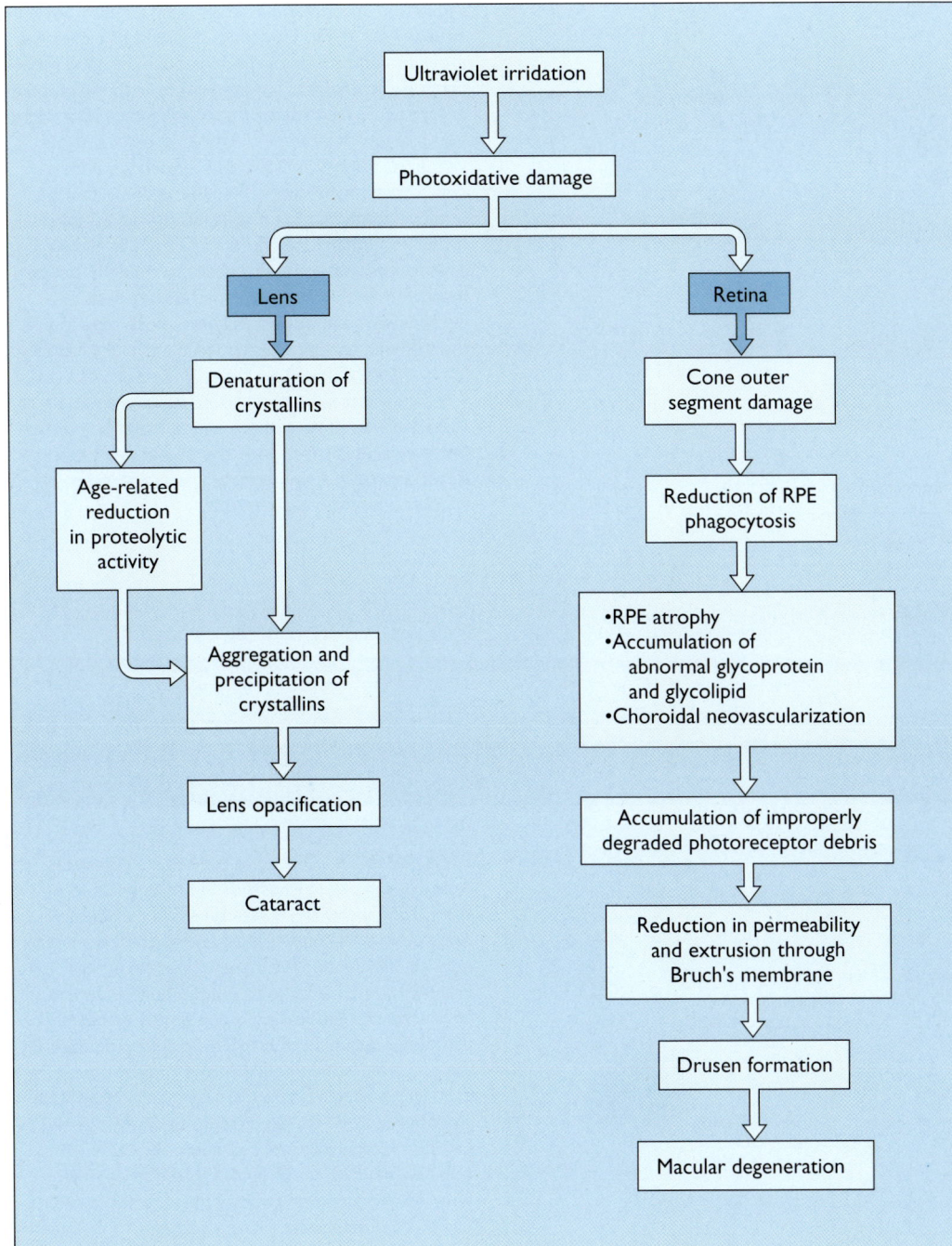

FIGURE 3-25. Oxidative pathogenesis of age-related cataract formation and macular degeneration. Photooxidative damage mediated via reactive oxygen species appears to play an important role in the pathogenesis of age-related cataract formation and macular degeneration. Although each event and its proposed sequence in the pathogenesis of these diseases has not been established, most of the components in the pathway are identified here. The lens and retina contain many molecules that absorb visible or near-ultraviolet light and therefore act as photosensitizers. The sensitizer molecule is excited to a singlet state (^1S), which can dissipate its energy through a radiationless transition to a less excited triplet state (^3S) with a high quantum yield. The ^3S molecules can initiate either direct photochemical oxidation–reduction reactions not involving oxygen to produce radicals or photodynamic reactions with molecular oxygen to produce singlet oxygen or superoxide anion. The net result of either type of reaction is the production of oxyradicals with the potential for damage to lens and retinal tissue. Antioxidants such as vitamins C and E in the lens can serve to quench the ^3S state and reactive oxygen species. Such carotenoids as lutein and zeaxanthin in the retinal macula can protect as well through the physical absorption of blue light, thereby preventing light from reaching the sensitizing molecules. RPE—retinal pigment epithelium.

Diet
  Jacques and Chylack (1991)
  Leske et al. (1991)
  Leske et al. (1991)
  Leske et al. (1991)
  Leske et al. (1991)
  Hankinson et al. (1992)
  Mares-Perlman et al. (1995)
    Women
    Men
Supplements
  Robertson et al. (1989)
  Hankinson et al. (1992)
  Jacques et al. (1997)
    Early
    More advanced
  Jacques and Chylack (1997)
Blood
  Mohan et al. (1989)
  Jacques and Chylack (1991)
  Vitale et al. (1993)
  Vitale et al. (1993)

Cataract type
■ Any
● Nuclear
▲ Cortical
□ Posterior
   subcapsular
○ Mixed
△ Extraction

Risk ratio (95% CI)

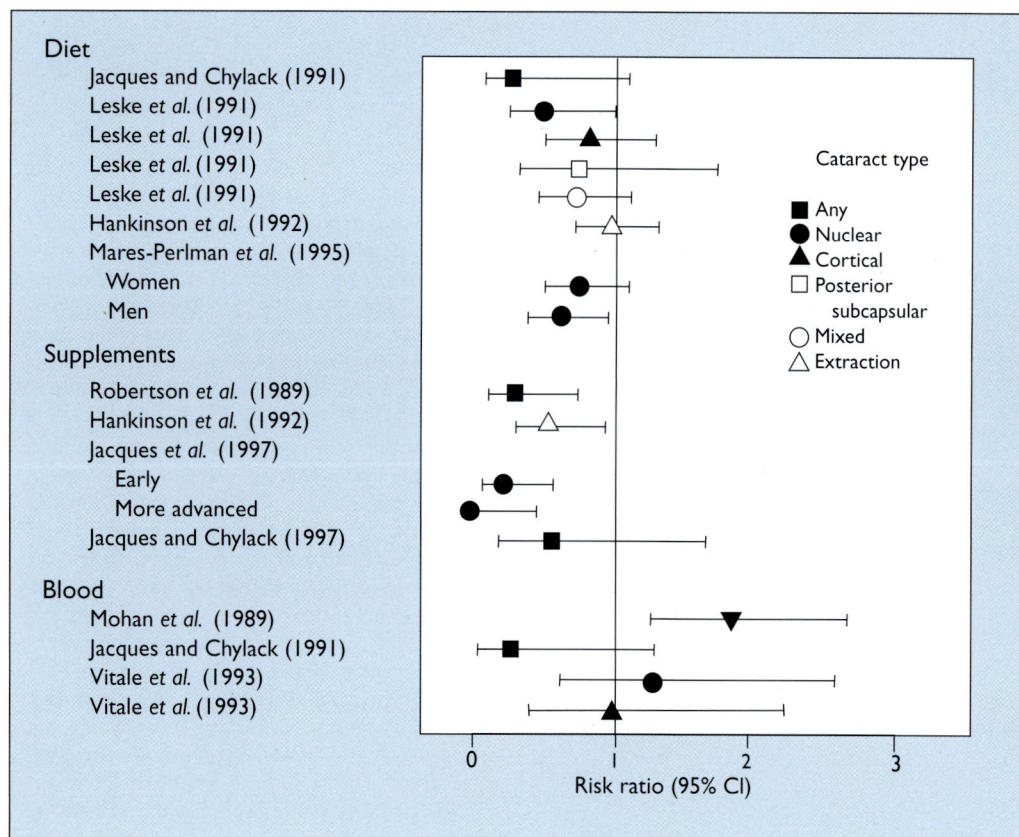

FIGURE 3-26. Vitamin C and the risk of cataract. Epidemiologic studies suggest a protective role of dietary antioxidants, particularly vitamins C and E and the carotenoids, in the prevention of age-related cataract formation and macular degeneration. Several studies have demonstrated a reduced risk of some types of cataract or of the lens opacities that may progress to cataract among people with high intake of vitamin C from diet or supplements and/or high blood levels of vitamin C. The long-term use of vitamin C supplements is also associated with a significantly lower rate of lens extraction. Vitamin C is actively concentrated to levels 20- to 60-fold higher in human lens and macula than in plasma. The concentration of ascorbate in the lens can be increased further via supplementation, even in persons who habitually consume more than 120 mg/d (twice the recommended dietary allowance for vitamin C). This figure shows the results of studies in which the risk ratios and 95% confidence intervals (CIs) for vitamin C and age-related cataract were determined [19]. Although the protective capacity is not as marked, similar data are available for vitamin E and the carotenoids.

Diabetes

Glucose

Enolization

Protein

Free radical attack

Enediol anions

Schiff base

Cu^{2+}, Fe^{3+}
Cu^{+}, Fe^{2+}

Nonenzymatic reaction with O_2

O_2

$H_2O_2 + \cdot OH \xleftarrow{Fe} O_2^{-}$

Semidione radical $+ O_2^{-}$

Amadori product

Decay reaction

Dicarbonyl

Hydroxylalkyl radical $+ H_2O_2$

Advanced glycation end-products

Protein damage via reaction with $^{-}NH_2$

Increased vascular permeability Inelastic vessel wall

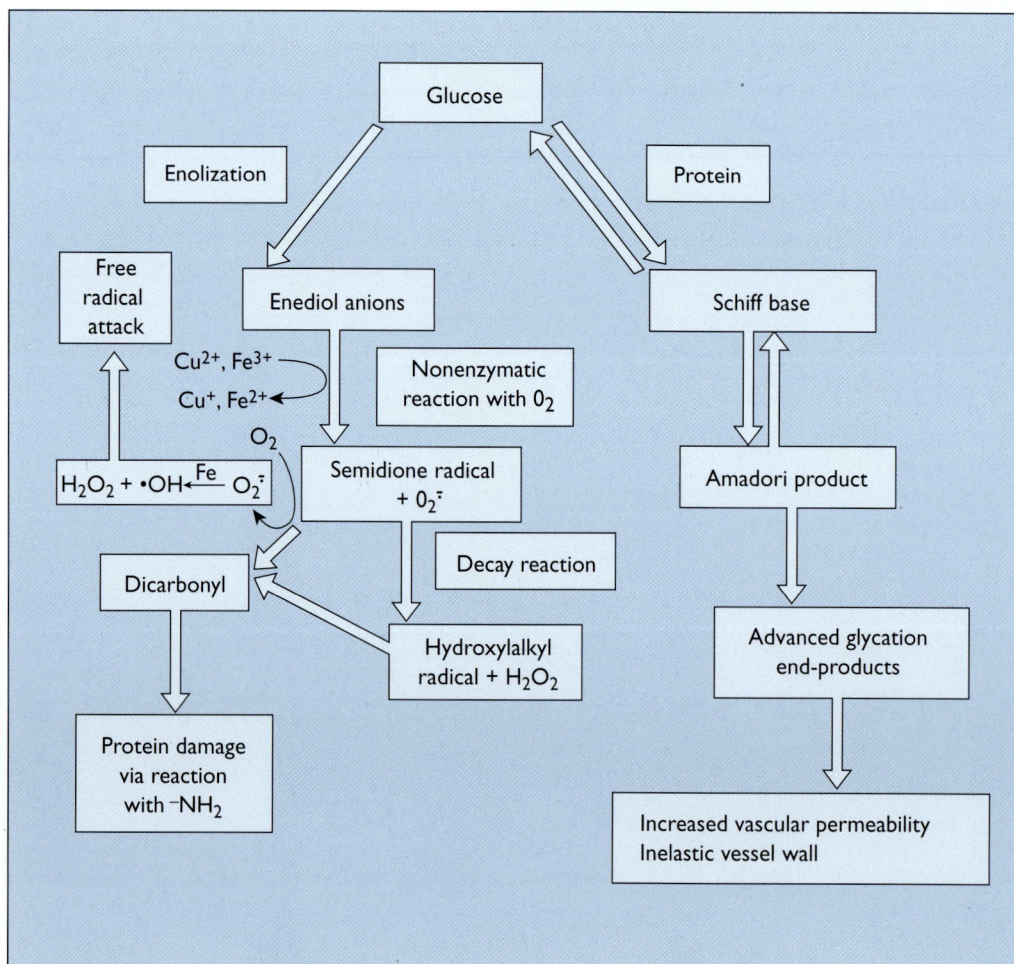

FIGURE 3-27. Oxidative pathways in diabetes. Reactive oxygen species (ROS) are implicated in the pathogenesis of insulin-dependent diabetes mellitus (type 1) and complications associated with non–insulin-dependent diabetes mellitus (type 2). Free radicals contribute to autoimmune destruction of pancreatic islet beta cells and type 1 diabetes. The pathologic sequelae of diabetes, including damage to the eye lens, kidney, neurons, and microvasculature involves, in part, oxidative changes associated with glucose metabolism. Glucose in its straight-chain form is an aldehyde and can react very slowly in a nonenzymatic glycation with DNA and proteins with a slow turnover such as those in the eye lens. Glycation is detectable in many proteins from diabetic patients, and glycated hemoglobin serves as an index of blood glucose control. Monosaccharide oxidation can lead to protein damage by ROS (eg, superoxide $[O_2 \cdot -]$, hydrogen peroxide $[H_2O_2]$ and hydroxyl radicals $[\cdot OH]$) and by the covalent binding of the carbon products of the process. Diabetics present with increased lipid peroxides and dehydroascorbate: ascorbate ratios in plasma; decreased glutathione and copper/zinc superoxide dismutase in erythrocytes; and loss of vitamin E in platelets.

ROLE OF MICRONUTRIENTS IN DIABETES

Nutrient	Role in Diabetes
Retinol	Protects islet beta cells
Vitamin C	Reduces glycation of hemoglobin, reduces erythrocyte sorbitol
Vitamin D	Required for insulin secretion and glucose tolerance
Vitamin E	Reduces glycation, improves glycemia
Niacin	Delays onset in high-risk individuals (type 1 or 2), delays increase in islet cell antibody titer (type 1 or 2)
Chromium	Enhances insulin action
Vanadium	Insulin-mimetic

FIGURE 3-28. Role of micronutrients in diabetes. Several micronutrients enhance insulin action and/or are associated with potential benefit in reducing the onset or progression of diabetes mellitus, and they may play an adjunctive role with established therapies. Dietary antioxidants such as vitamins C and E can beneficially affect those adverse processes mediated by reactive oxygen species (ROS), including glycation and lipid peroxidation. ROS-mediated damage to DNA and mitochondria can also deprive cells of niacin (NAD). Cellular NAD is consumed as a source of ADP–ribose in DNA repair, resulting in a sharp fall in intracellular NAD and ATP levels and a subsequent reduction in insulin release. In vitro studies have shown that the combination of nicotinic acid, glutathione, and trivalent chromium—known as glucose tolerance factor (GTF)—potentiates insulin action better than does chromium alone. The regulatory role of chromium in glucose and insulin metabolism, however, appears to be more of a nutritional rather than a pharmacologic effect (ie, chromium is most effective if at least a marginal deficiency state exists). Normal intakes of the ultra–trace mineral vanadium are well above marginal; therefore, its effects on improving glucose tolerance and alleviating insulin insensitivity are pharmacologic in nature. A postreceptor mechanism for the in vivo action of oxovanadium compounds has been suggested.

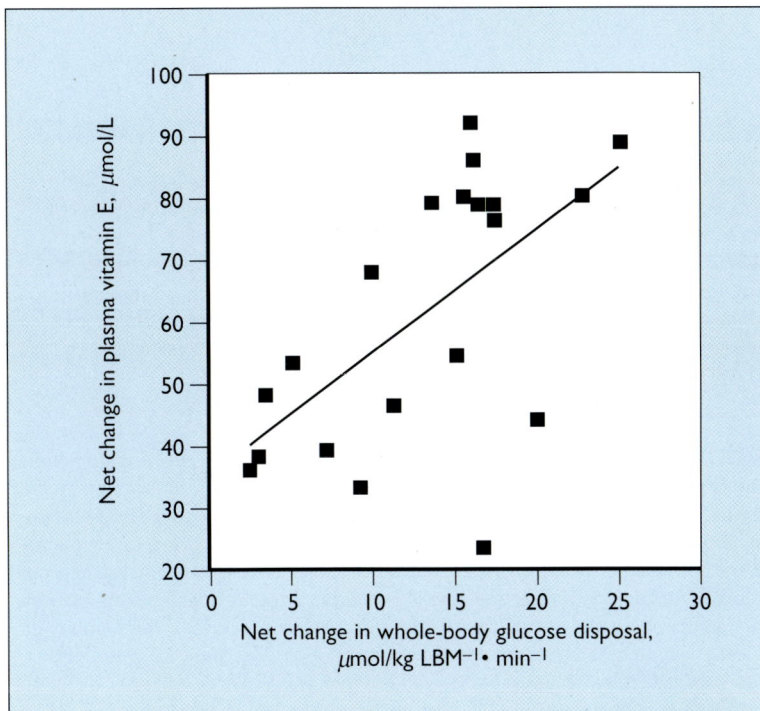

FIGURE 3-29. Improved glucose tolerance with vitamin E. Epidemiologic observations indicate that low vitamin E status is associated with an elevated risk of type 2 diabetes. Insulin-mediated stimulation of whole-body glucose disposal (following a euglycemic glucose clamp) was significantly potentiated in 20 nonobese subjects (age, 77 ± 0.4 years) with normal glucose tolerance after daily supplementation with 900 mg of vitamin E for 3 months compared with placebo controls [20]. Net changes in plasma vitamin E concentration correlated with net changes in insulin-stimulated whole-body glucose disposal [20]. Supplementation with vitamin E reduces measures of oxidative stress status and protein glycation in diabetics. Vitamin E supplementation reduces insulin resistance and improves metabolic control of glucose in patients with type 2 diabetes. LBM—lean body mass. (Adapted from Paolisso, et al. [20].)

Immunity

MICRONUTRIENT DEFICIENCIES IMPAIR IMMUNITY

Nutrient	Antibody Response	Lymphocyte Proliferation	Phagocytic Function	Delayed-type Hypersensitivity	Neutrophil Production	Natural Killer Cell Activity
Vitamin A	✓	✓		✓		✓
Vitamin C	✓	✓	✓	✓	✓	
Vitamin E	✓	✓	✓		✓	
Vitamin B$_6$	✓	✓		✓		
Vitamin B$_{12}$		✓			✓	
Folate	✓	✓	✓	✓	✓	
Copper	✓	✓	✓		✓	
Iron	✓	✓	✓	✓	✓	
Manganese	✓	✓			✓	
Zinc	✓	✓	✓	✓	✓	✓

FIGURE 3-30. Micronutrient deficiencies impair immunity. Micronutrients are essential to the support of immune function. Studies of peripheral blood, lymph nodes, spleen, thymus, tonsils, bone marrow, and other immune system tissues suggest that each may be differentially responsive to specific nutrients. Vitamins A, B$_6$, B$_{12}$, C, E, and folate and the minerals copper and zinc have been established to play critical roles in nonspecific immunity, particularly in the maintenance of skin, mucous membranes, and phagocyte activity. These and other micronutrients are necessary in specific cell-mediated and humoral immune responses such as mitogen-stimulated lymphocyte production and antibody production. The impact of vitamin deficiency on immunocompetence is recognized, and it appears that recommended dietary intakes are generally sufficient to prevent significant impairments in function such as anergy. It is not clear that these intakes are optimized, however, for levels of immune function associated with a reduced risk of infectious diseases, noninfectious inflammatory conditions, cancer, or mortality, particularly in populations such as the elderly.

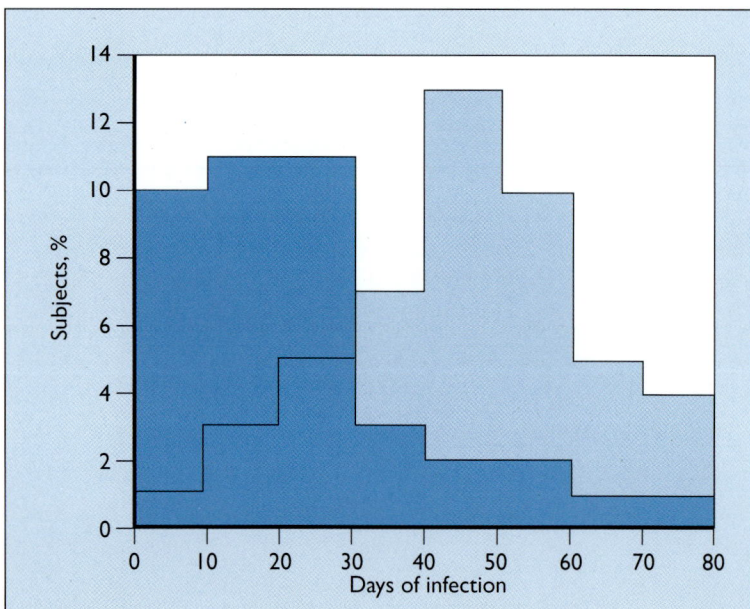

FIGURE 3-31. Effects of multivitamin–mineral supplementation on immune function. Age-related functional declines in cell-mediated and humoral immunity are modulated by nutritional status. This loss of immune responsiveness contributes significantly to increased morbidity and mortality in the elderly. Increasing micronutrient status, particularly in older adults with poor dietary patterns, may improve immune function and affect the risk of infectious diseases. Supplementation with a multivitamin–multimineral preparation for one year increased the number of T cells, lymphocyte response to phytohemagglutinin, interleukin-2 production and receptor release, natural killer cell number and activity, and antibody response to influenza vaccine in 48 free-living subjects 66 to 86 years of age compared with 48 subjects receiving a placebo [21]. Infection-related illness was significantly less frequent in the supplemented group (23 ± 5 days/y; *dark blue area*) than in the placebo group (48 ± 7 d/y; *light blue area*).

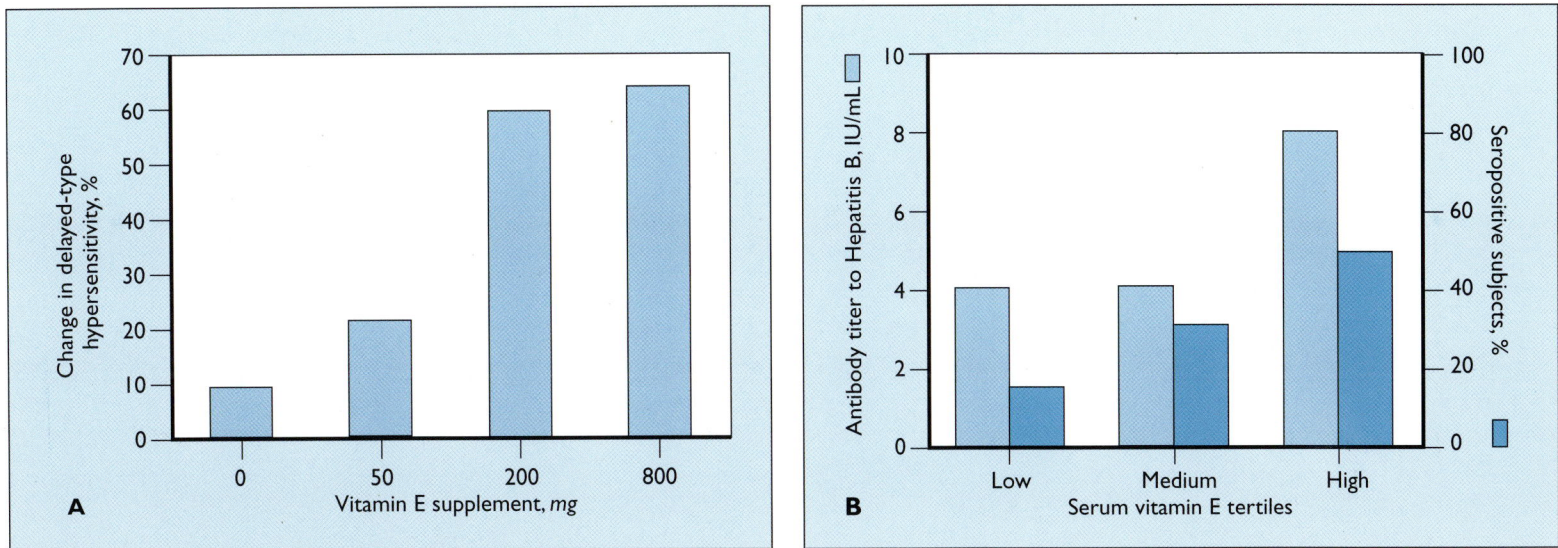

FIGURE 3-32. Effects of vitamin E supplementation on immune function. Supplementation with vitamin E enhances indices of cell-mediated and humoral immunity in the elderly without any apparent adverse effects. **A,** Supplementation with daily doses of vitamin E for 4 months improved delayed-type hypersensitivity responses in skin to seven recall antigens in healthy subjects older than 65 years of age (*n* = 19 or 20/group) [22]. **B,** Increasing levels of vitamin E in serum achieved by supplementation (expressed by tertile) induced greater antibody titers to hepatitis B vaccination and seropositive conversion [22]. Vitamin E supplementation has also been shown to improve mitogen-stimulated lymphocyte proliferation and interleukin-2 production in healthy older subjects. (*Adapted from* Meydani, et al. [22].)

References

1. National Research Council (U.S.) Subcommittee on the Tenth Edition of the RDAs, Food and Nutrition Board, Commission on Life Sciences. Recommended Dietary Allowances. National Academy Press, Washington, DC, 1989.

1a. U.S. Department of Agriculture, Agricultural Research Service: 1997 Data tables: results from USDA's 1994-96 Continuing Survey of Good Intakes by Individuals and 1994-96 Diet and Health Knowledge Survey. ARS Food Surveys Research Group. Available online under "Releases" at: http://www.barc.usda.gov/bhnrc/foodsurvey/home.htm.

2. Institute of Medicine, Food and Nutrition Board: *Dietary Reference Intakes for Thiamin, Riboflavin, Niacin, Vitamin B6, Folate, Vitamin B12, Pantothenic Acid, Biotin, and Choline.* Washington, DC: National Academy Press; 1998.

3. Kushi LH, Folsom AR, Prineas RJ, et al.: Dietary antioxidant vitamins and death from coronary heart disease in postmenopausal women. *N Engl J Med* 1996, 334:1156–1162.

4. Stampfer MJ, Hennekens C, Manson JE, et al.: Vitamin E consumption and risk of coronary disease in women. *N Engl J Med* 1993, 328:1444–1449.

5. Rimm EB, Stampfer MJ, Ascherio A, et al.: Vitamin E consumption and the risk of coronary heart disease in men. *N Engl J Med* 1993, 328:1450–1456.

6. Boushey CJ, Beresford SA, Omenn GS, Motulsky AG: A quantitative assessment of plasma homocysteine as a risk factor for vascular disease: probable benefits of increasing folic acid intake. *JAMA* 1995, 274:1049–1057.

7. Selhub J, Jacques P, Wilson P, et al.: Vitamin status and intake as primary determinants of homocysteinemia in an elderly population. *JAMA* 1993, 270:2693–2698.

8. Homocysteine Lowering Trialists' Collaboration: Lowering blood homocysteine with folic acid based-supplements: meta-analysis of randomized trials. *BMJ* 1998, 316:894–898.

9. Appel LJ, Moore TJ, Obarzanek E, et al.: A clinical trial of the effects of dietary patterns on blood pressure. *N Engl J Med* 1997, 336:1117–1124.

10. The Alpha-Tocopherol, Beta Carotene Cancer Prevention Study Group: The effect of vitamin E and beta carotene on the incidence of lung cancer and other cancers in male smokers. *N Engl J Med* 1994, 330:1029–1035.

11. Ommen GS, Goodman GE, Thornquist MD, et al.: Effects of a combination of beta-carotene and vitamin A on lung cancer and cardiovascular disease. *N Engl J Med* 1996, 334:1150–1155.

12. Hennekens CH, Buring JE, Manson JE, et al.: Lack of effect of long-term supplementation with beta-carotene on the incidence of malignant neoplasms and cardiovascular disease. *N Engl J Med* 1996, 334:1145–1149.

13. Mason J, Levesque T: Folate: effects on carcinogenesis and the potential for cancer chemoprevention. *Oncology* 1996, 10:1727–1743.

14. Cravo M, Fidalgo P, Pereira A, et al.: DNA methylation as an intermediate biomarker in colorectal cancer: modulation by folic acid supplementation. *Eur J Cancer Prev* 1994, 3:473–479.

15. Clark L, Combs G, Turnbull B, et al.: Effects of selenium supplementation for cancer prevention in patients with carcinoma of the skin: a randomized controlled trial. *JAMA* 1996, 276:1957–1963.

16. Holick M: Vitamin D and bone health. *J Nutr* 1996, 126 (suppl):1159S–1164S.

17. Dawson-Hughes B, Harris S, Krall E, Dallal G: Effect of calcium and vitamin D supplementation on bone density in men and women 65 years of age or older. *N Engl J Med* 1997, 337:670–676.

18. Rosenberg I, Miller J: Nutritional factors in physical and cognitive functions of elderly people. *Am J Clin Nutr* 1992, 55 (suppl):1237S–1243S.

19. Jacques P: Nutritional antioxidants and prevention of age-related eye disease. In *Antioxidants and Disease Prevention.* Edited by Garewal HS. New York: CRC Press; 1997:149–177.

20. Paolisso G, Di Maro G, Galzerano D, et al.: Pharmacological doses of vitamin E and insulin action in elderly subjects. *Am J Clin Nutr* 1994, 59:1291–1296.

21. Chandra RK: Effect of vitamin and trace-element supplementation on immune responses and infection in elderly subjects. *Lancet* 1992, 340:1124–1127.

22. Meydani SN, Meydani M, Blumberg JB, et al.: Vitamin E supplementation and in vivo immune response in healthy elderly subjects: a randomized controlled trial. *JAMA* 1997, 277:1380–1386.

4

IMMUNE FUNCTION AND THE ADAPTATION TO STARVATION

Benjamin Bonavida

It is widely recognized that nutrition and immune function are tightly linked. Impaired immune function was originally observed in children with protein–energy malnutrition. The most common cause of death in an epidemic of starvation is typically simple bacterial pneumonia caused by acquired nutrition immunodeficiency. The negative impact of starvation on immune function accounts for the lethal effects of starvation.

A complex series of biochemical and physiologic adaptations are geared toward conserving protein during starvation, with concomitant maintenance of immune function. This requires a shift from the "fed" state, in which glucose and amino acids are consumed readily, into an adapted fasted state called a *fat-fuel economy* because fat stores are mobilized for energy with the result that protein stores are spared. Plasma amino acids measured in venous blood give nonspecific indications of the adaptations taking place in protein metabolism during the course of starvation.

The impact of the adaptation to a fat-fuel economy is reflected in the rapid changes in urinary nitrogen excretion during starvation reflecting net protein sparing through two processes. Overall nitrogen is conserved so that nitrogen excretion decreases from 12 g/d in the postabsorptive state to 5 g/d 7 to 10 days later. This translates into a decrease from 75 to 20 mg/d in muscle protein breakdown. Based on theoretic calculations of the time necessary to reach the critical 50% of body cell mass, survival is extended through these adaptations from approximately 60 to over 260 days provided adequate fluid and electrolytes are administered.

The beneficial effects of individual nutrients on immune function, including vitamins and minerals, have also been examined. Deficiencies of vitamins A, E, B_6, and folate are associated with reduced immunocompetence. Conversely, overnutrition can also be deleterious to the immune system. For example, excess fat intake, particularly such polyunsaturated fats as linoleic acid, can lead to impaired immune function. Continued research on immune function in aging and disease promises to elucidate new strategies for maintaining immune function. There are a number of clinical implications of this extensive body of basic research. Preoperative assessment of immunocompetence is predictive of the risk of postoperative infection. Response to immunization is improved when malnutrition or vitamin deficiencies are corrected. Research is being conducted on the use of immunomodulators as interventions for malnutrition-associated infection.

Metabolic Functions

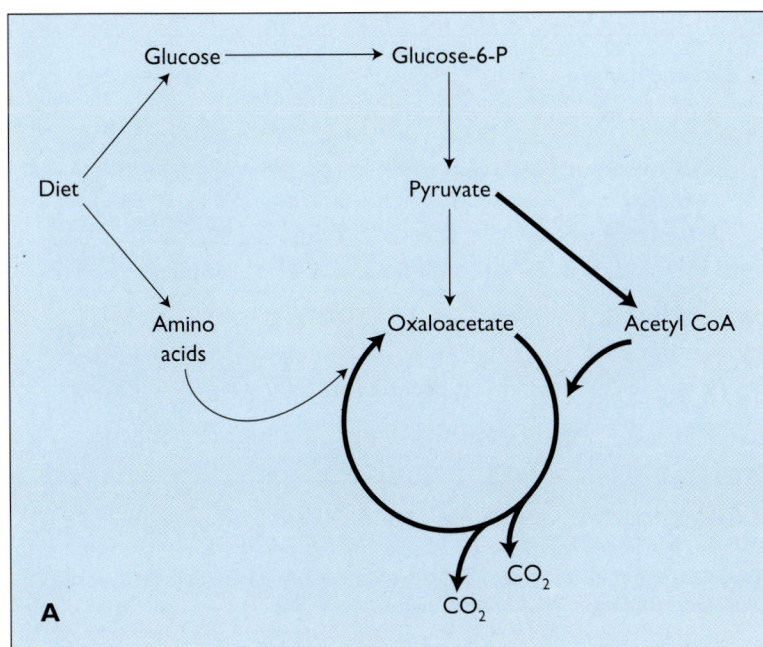

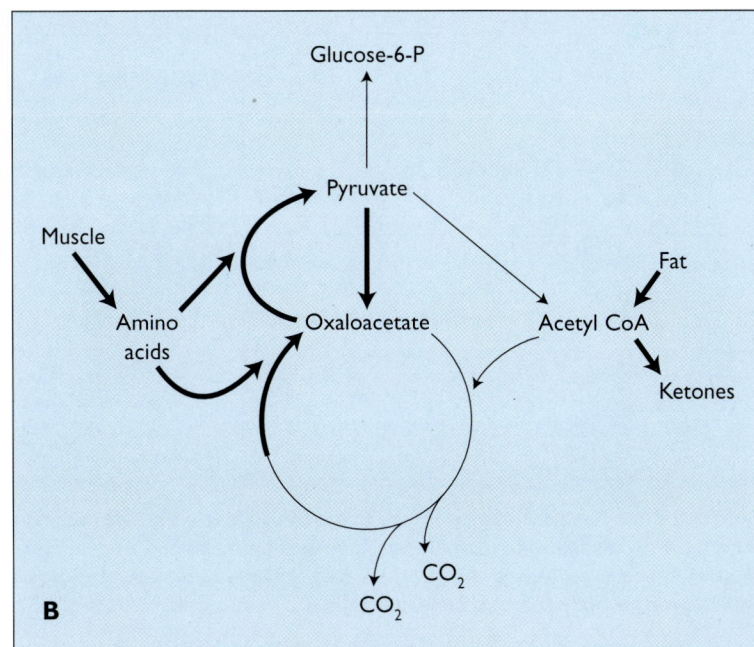

FIGURE 4-1. Fed versus fasting metabolism. The basic metabolism of the body shifts from a fed (**A**) to a fasted (**B**) state with the shift to a fat-fuel economy. Although amino acids must be broken down for energy as shown here, the body adapts to reduced protein needs as it uses fat rather than glucose for energy. CoA—coenzyme A. (*Adapted from Heber [1].*)

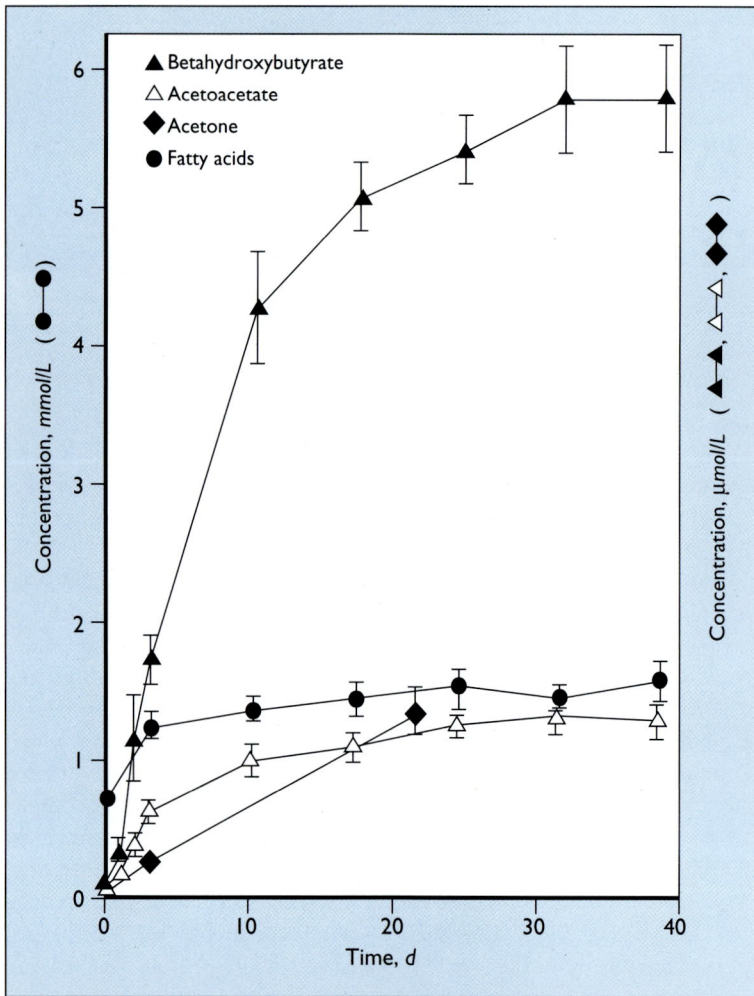

FIGURE 4-2. Blood ketones and fatty acids during starvation. The concentrations of ketone bodies (betahydroxybutyrate, acetoacetate, and acetone) and fatty acids in the bloodstream rise as fats are mobilized from adipose tissue during the adaptation to starvation. (*Adapted from* Heber [1].)

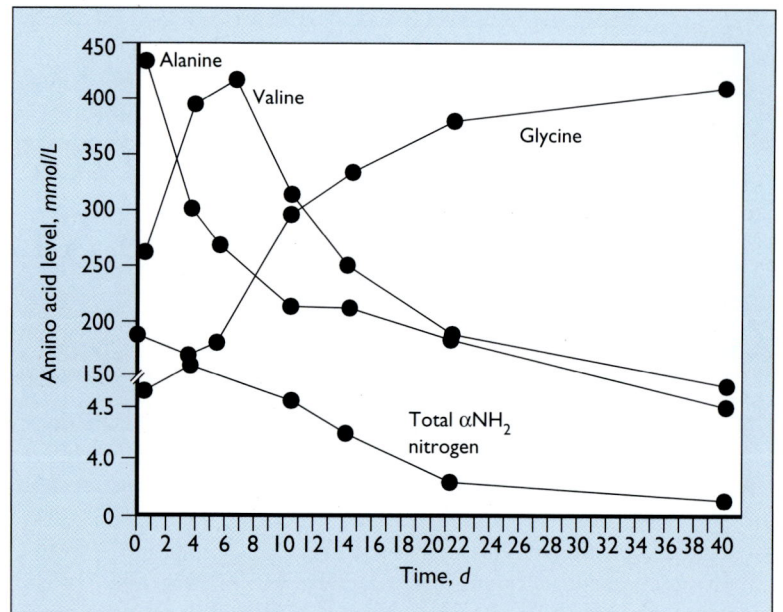

FIGURE 4-3. Amino acid levels during starvation. The levels of amino acids change dramatically over the course of starvation, illustrating the different roles of various amino acids in intermediary metabolism. Alanine excretion parallels that of nitrogen because it is the primary amino acid used for glucose production during early, acute starvation. As alanine levels decrease, the shift to a fat-fuel economy is occurring and net nitrogen output in the urine is reduced. (*Adapted from* Heber [1].)

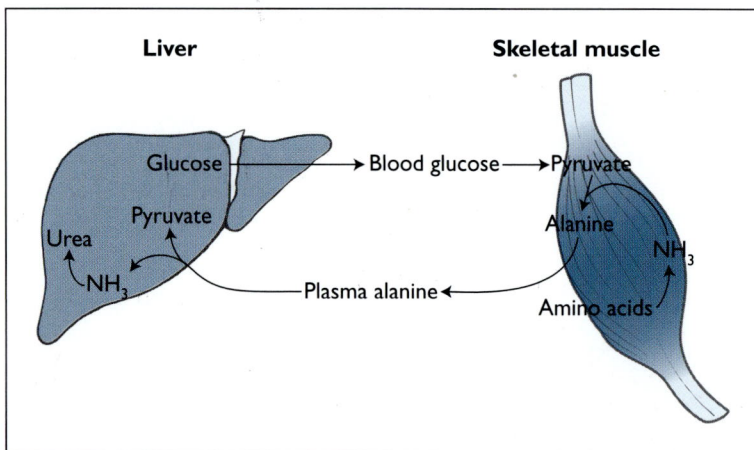

FIGURE 4-4. The alanine cycle. The alanine cycle illustrates the interrelationships between alanine and glucose production. Carbon chains and ammonia are shuttled from skeletal muscle to liver where they are used to synthesize glucose and urea, respectively. (*Adapted from* Heber [1].)

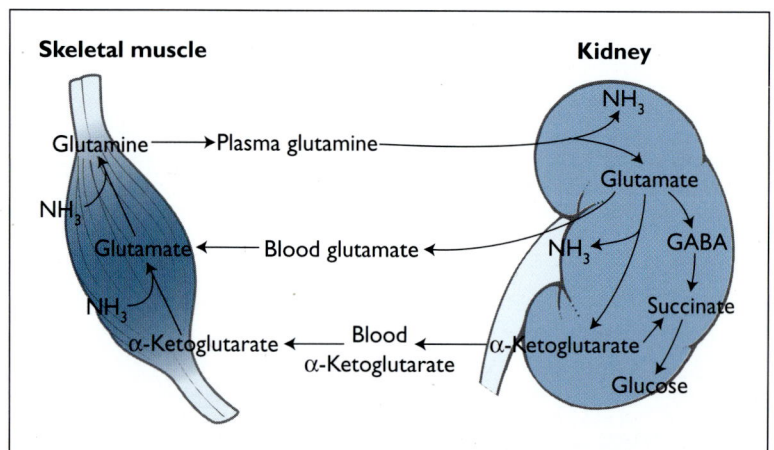

FIGURE 4-5. The glutamine cycle. The glutamine cycle is analogous to the alanine cycle and is shuttled from skeletal muscle and the kidneys. It assumes importance in the later stages of starvation. GABA—γ-aminobutyric acid. (*Adapted from* Heber [1].)

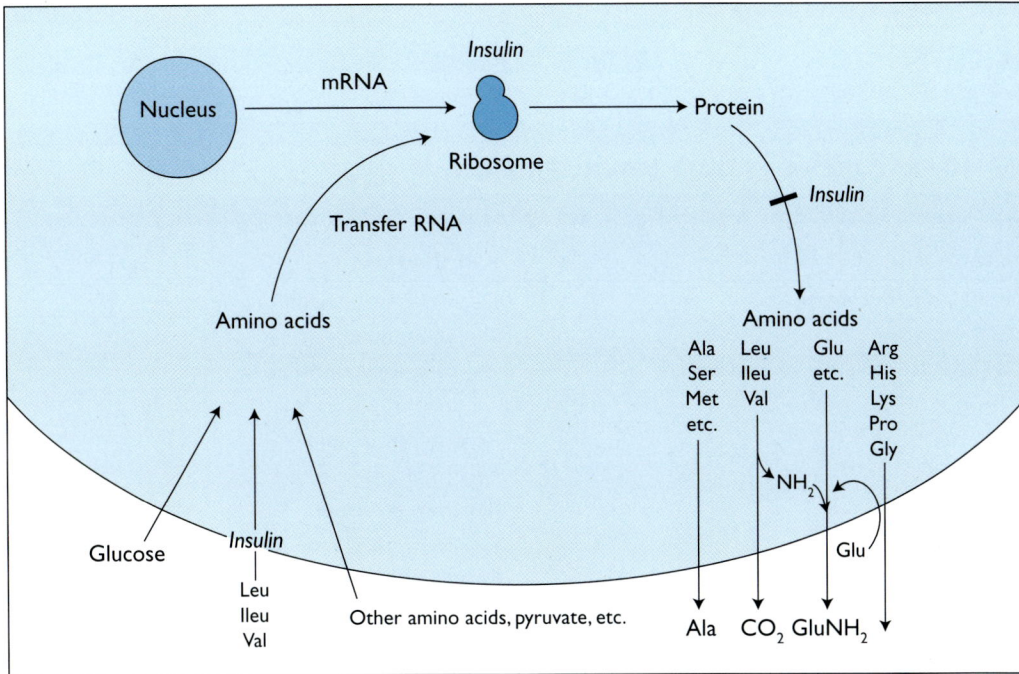

FIGURE 4-6. Intracellular actions of insulin in promoting glucose uptake and inhibiting proteolysis. Insulin is also important in modulating immune function. There are insulin receptors on lymphocytes and other cells of the immune system. Ala—alanine; Arg—arginine; Glu—glutamic acid; Gly—glycine; His—histidine; Ileu—XXX; Leu—leucine; Lys—lysine; Met—methionine; Pro—proline; Ser—serine; Val—valine. (*Adapted from* Heber [1].)

CHANGES IN SERUM LEVELS OF HORMONES IN OBESE SUBJECTS AFTER 12 HOURS AND AFTER 7 DAYS OF FASTING*

Parameter	12-Hour Fast	7-Day Fast
Triiodothyronine, ng/dL	130±15	59±5[†]
Free triiodothyronine, pg/dL	322±32	159±13[†]
r triiodothyronine, ng/dL	35±3	57±5[†]
Thyroxine μg/dL	9.1±0.7	9.3±0.8
Free thyroxine ng/dL	4.7±0.2	3.0±0.3
Insulin, μU/mL	34±6	15±2[†]
Morning cortisol, mg/dL	19.1±2.1	26.4±3.4[†]
Urinary free cortisol, μg/dL	27.1±3.2	41.8±6.3[†]

*Data are expressed as the mean ± SEM for nine subjects.
[†]$p <0.05$

FIGURE 4-7. Serum hormone level changes in obese subjects after 12 hours and after 7 days of fasting. In addition to insulin, other hormones that potentially affect the immune system, such as thyroid hormone and cortisol, change dramatically during starvation [1]. Such changes result in immunosuppression. (*Adapted from* Heber[1].)

Immunologic Manifestations

DIAGNOSTIC FEATURES OF ADULT MALNUTRITION

Parameter	Marasmus	Kwashiorkor
Clinical setting	Decreased caloric intake	Decreased protein intake plus stress
Time course to develop	Months to years	Weeks to months
Physical examination	Cachectic, fat depletion, muscle wasting	May look well nourished
Anthropometrics		
Triceps skinfold	Depressed	Relatively preserved
Arm muscle circumference	Depressed	Relatively preserved
Weight for height	Depressed	Relatively preserved
Creatinine–height index	Depressed	Relatively preserved
Skin test responses	Normal or depressed	Relatively preserved
Visceral proteins		
Albumin	Relatively normal	Low
Transferrin	Relatively normal	Low
Lymphocyte cell	Relatively normal	Low

FIGURE 4-8. Diagnostic features of adult malnutrition. Marasmus represents a slower adaptation to malnutrition with intact immune function. Kwashiorkor represents rapid or unadapted malnutrition in which the immune system is impaired [1]. Stress induces impairment of both innate and adaptive immunity. Decrease in lymphocyte count may result in impaired humoral antibody response and cell-mediated immunity to environmental infections (Adapted from Heber [1].)

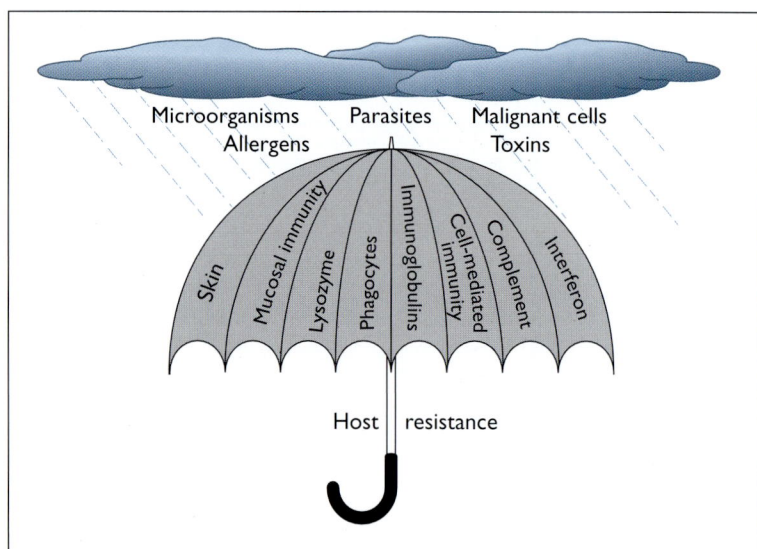

FIGURE 4-9. The protective umbrella of host defenses. A number of host protective systems come under the rubric of the immune system. These systems work together to protect the host but are affected by nutrition status. A simple view of host defense is presented as a protective umbrella, consisting of physical barriers (skin and mucous membranes), nonspecific mechanisms (complement, interferon, lysozymes, and phagocytes), and antigen-specific processes (antibodies and cell-mediated immunity). (*Adapted from* Chandra [2].)

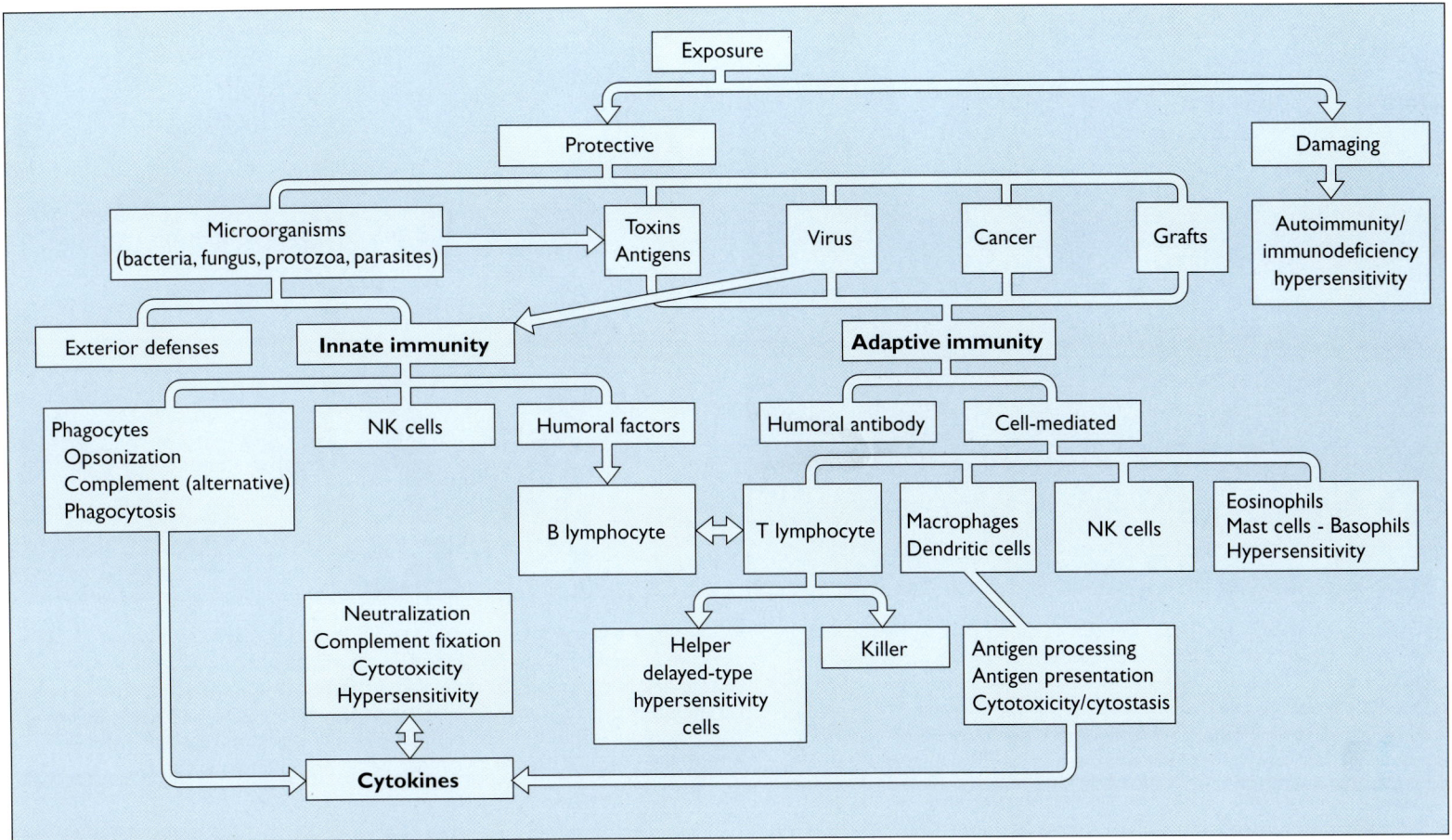

FIGURE 4-10. Journey into the immune system. Cellular interactions in the immune response illustrate components of both humoral and cellular immunity. The innate immune response is differentiated from the adaptive immune response. The early phases of the host response to infection depend on innate immunity, in which a variety of innate resistance mechanisms recognize and respond to the presence of a pathogen. Innate immunity is present in all individuals at all times, does not increase with repeated exposure to a given pathogen, and does not discriminate between pathogens. It is followed by adaptive immunity, which is mediated by clonal selection of specific lymphocytes and leads to both immediate and long-term protection from diseases. Adaptive immunity is the response of antigen-specific lymphocytes to antigen, including the development of immunologic memory.

Immune responses are mediated by leukocytes, which are derived from stem cells in the bone marrow. These cells give rise to the polymorphonuclear leukocytes, the macrophages of the innate immune system, and the lymphocytes of the adaptive immune system. There are two major types of lymphocytes: B lymphocytes mature in the bone marrow and are responsible for antibody production, whereas T lymphocytes mature in the thymus and are responsible for cell-mediated immunity. Lymphocytes recirculate continuously from the bloodstream through the peripheral lymphoid organs, where the antigen is trapped, returning to the bloodstream through the lymphocytic vessel. The three major types of peripheral lymphoid tissues are the spleen, which collects antigens from the blood; the lymph nodes, which collect antigens from sites of infections in the tissues; and gut-associated lymphoid tissue, which collects antigens from the gut. NK—natural killer. (*Adapted from* Heber [1].)

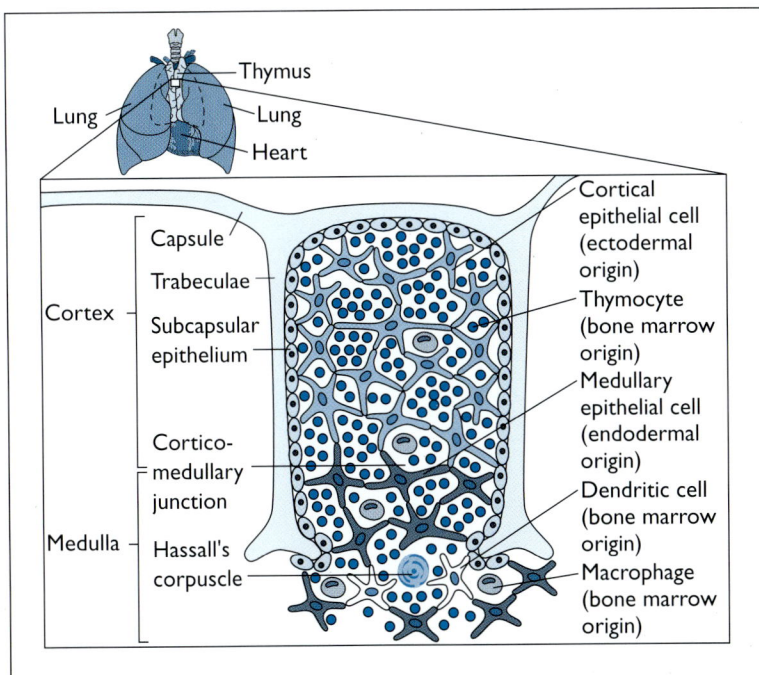

FIGURE 4-11. Development of T cells in the thymus. Like B cells, T cells derive from bone marrow stem cells and undergo gene rearrangements in a specialized microenvironment to produce a unique antigen receptor on each cell. T cells migrate at a very early stage to the thymus, a central lymphoid organ that provides the specialized microenvironment where receptor gene rearrangement and T-cell maturation occur. T cells recognize antigens in the form of peptide fragments bound to molecules encoded by the major histocompatibility complex (MHC). Because T cells are MHC restricted, only those able to recognize the body's own MHC molecules bearing foreign peptides will be capable of contributing to adaptive immune responses. (*Adapted from* Janeway and Travers [3].)

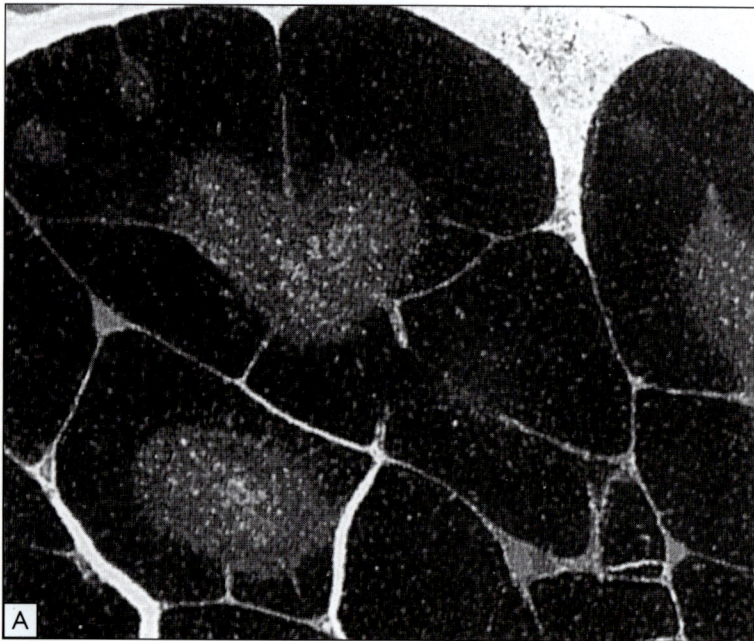

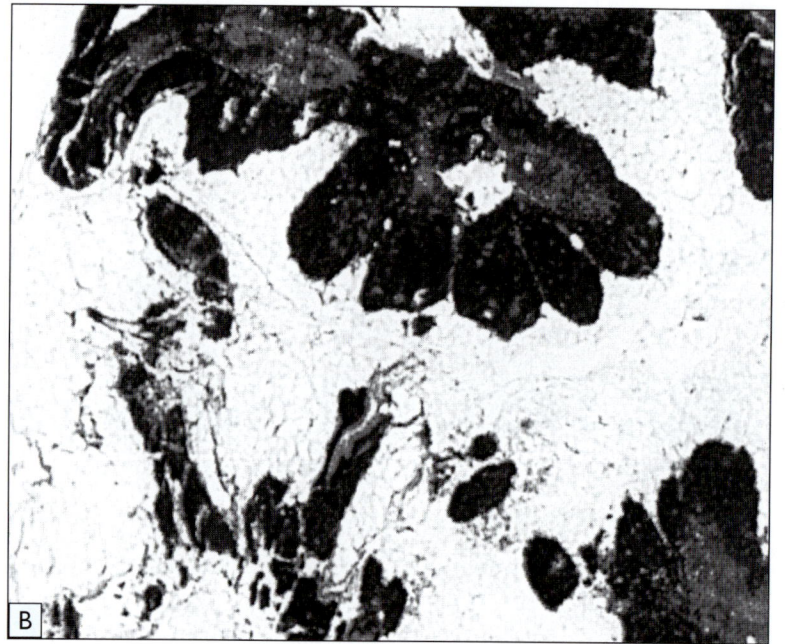

FIGURE 4-12. (*see* Color Plate) The size of the thymus decreases with age. Until about 20 years of age, more than 80% of the thymus is composed of lymphoid tissue. That proportion declines continuously with age until, from about 40 years of age and older, only about 5% of the thymus is morphologically lymphoid. Loss of lymphoid tissue—called *thymic involution*—seems to occur at the level of the thymic epithelium because, in mice, a young thymus can thrive when grafted into an old host, indicating that T-cell progenitors are active in aged bone marrow. Histologic examples of thymus sections from a child (**A**) and an adult (**B**) show dense thymic tissue in the young thymus only. The older thymus is massively infiltrated by nonthymic tissue, mostly fat, but still harbors islands of lymphoid tissue, including both cortical and medullary histologic regions. (*Adapted from* Rodewald [4]; with permission.)

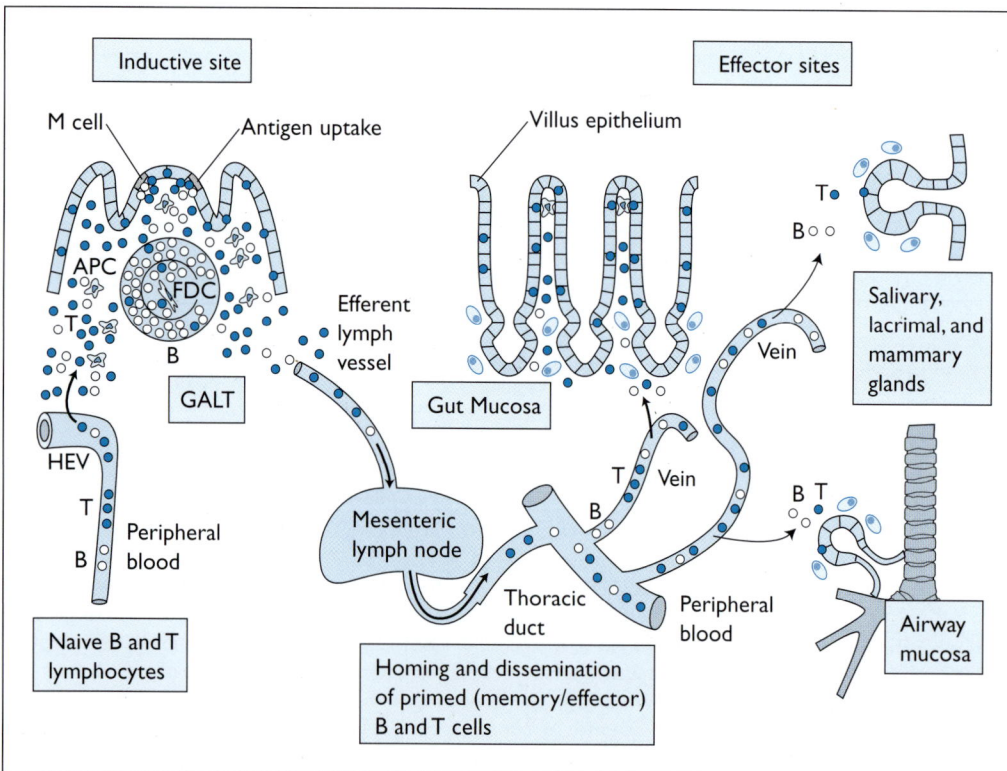

FIGURE 4-13. Schematic depiction of the integrated ("common") human mucosal immune system. Naive B and T lymphocytes are recruited to organized gut-associated lymphoid tissue (GALT) via high endothelial venules (HEVs) in the parafollicular T-cell zone. Such lymphoepithelial inductive sites contain activated B-cell follicles with follicular dendritic cells (FDCs), and the domes are covered with a specialized epithelium where "membrane" (M) cells transport luminal antigens inward. Antigen-primed B and T lymphocytes migrate through lymph and reach peripheral blood for subsequent homing to mucosal effector sites. Their extravasation is particularly efficient in the gut lamina propria (*thick arrows*), but dissemination also takes place from GALT to more distant effector sites in an integrated manner as indicated (*thin arrows*). APC—antigen-presenting cell. (*Adapted from* Brandtzaeg *et al.* [5].)

A. INFLUENCE OF PEM ON IMMUNE RESPONSE IN THE ELDERLY

Parameter	Apparently Healthy Elderly*	Mildly Undernourished Elderly*	Profoundly Undernourished Elderly*
CD2/MM^3	1655±410	1540±440	[†]1295±360[‡]
CD3/mm^3	1395±240	[§]1240±380	920±22.5[‡]
CD2+CD3-/mm^3	260±230	300±270	375±220
CD4/mm^3	850±290	620±305[‡]	390±240[‡]
48-hr lymphocyte proliferation	—	—	—
PHA 1 μg/10^6 cells in 10^3 cpm	52±37	41±37	19±17[‡]
24-hr PHA lymphocyte	—	—	—
Culture IL-2 release, *ng/ml*	1.1±0.4	0.9±0.70	0.65±0.5[‡]
24-hr PHA lymphocyte	—	—	—
Culture IL-6 release, *ng/ml*	1.2±0.4	1.0±0.4[§]	0.7±0.3[‡]
24-hr LPS monocyte	—	—	—
Culture IL-1 release, *ng/ml*	1.8±2.1	1.4±1.1	0.8±0.7[†]

*Apparently healthy elderly (n = 46) were 78.4 ±6.8 year of age; mildly undernourished elderly (n = 42) were 83.4±5.9 years of age with serum albumin levels ranging from 30 to 35g/l; profoundly undernourished elderly (n = 35) were 86.2 ±4.7 years of age with serum albumin levels ranging from 25 to 30 g/L.

[†] $P < 0.01$.

[‡] $P < 0.001$.

[§] $P < 0.05$.

IL—interleukin; LPS—lipopolysaccharide; PHA—phytohemogglutinin.

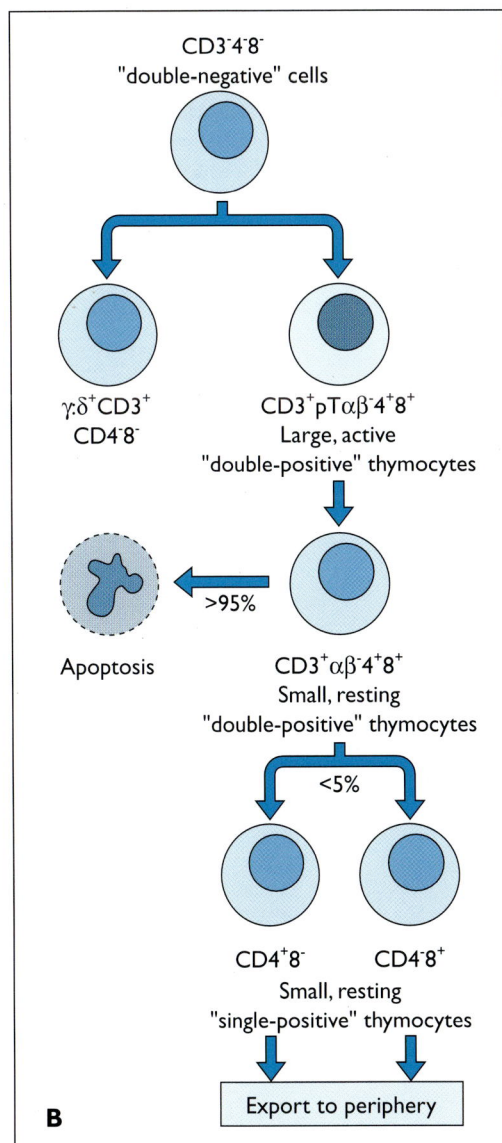

B

FIGURE 4-14. **A,** Influence of protein–energy malnutrition (PEM) on immune response in undernourished elderly (albumin <35 g/L) without important acute phase responses (C-reactive protein [CRP] <20 mg/L, α1-glycoprotein acid <1 g/L) compared with apparently healthy elderly. All immune parameters were simultaneously tested for each individual, but subjects from the different groups were quantified on separate days. Statistical differences between the undernourished and the apparently healthy subjects are presented on the right side of each column and between the two undernourished groups on the left side of each column. These findings demonstrate that undernourished elderly have a compromised immune system and are at risk for infection [6].

B, T-cell maturation in the thymus and selection and exit to the periphery. T cells in the thymus go through a series of stages that can be detected by the differential expression of surface markers and the expression of the CD3:T-cell receptor complex proteins and the coreceptor proteins CD4 and CD8. The CD4$^+$ T lymphocytes are subdivided into two subsets of T-helper cells: T-helper 1 (Th1) cells mediate inflammatory responses, and T-helper 2 (Th2) cells mediate help for antibody production by B cells. The CD8$^+$ T cells are responsible for cell-mediated cytotoxicity against infected cells and tumor cells. (Part A *adapted from* LeSourd, et al. [6]; part B *adapted from* Janeway and Travers [3].)

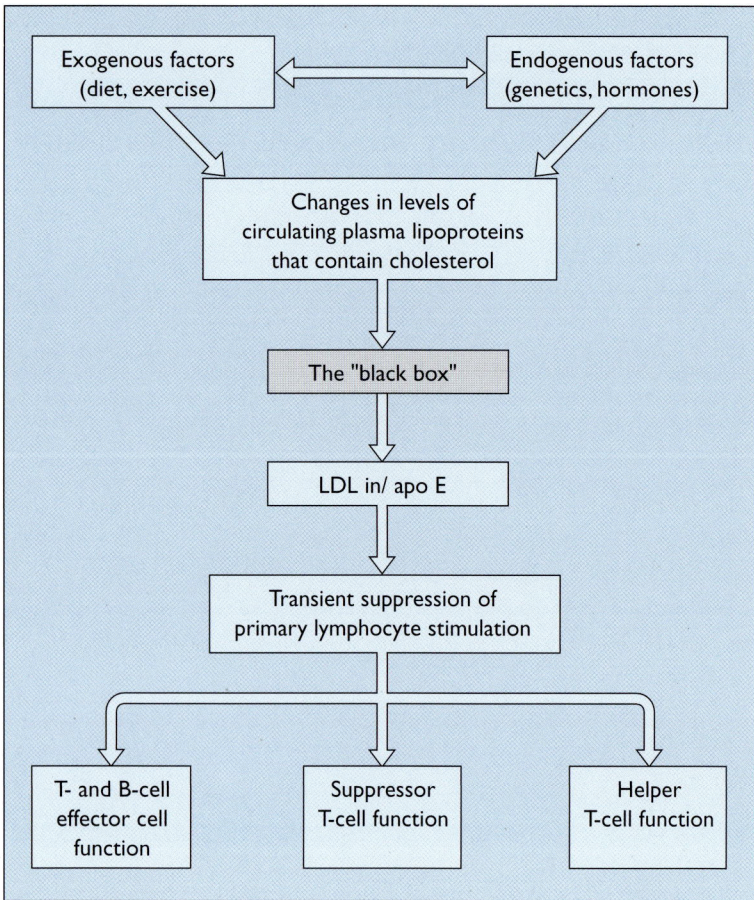

FIGURE 4-15. The impact of dietary fats on immune cell function through low-density lipoprotein (LDL) and apoprotein E (apo E). Changes in levels of circulating plasma lypoprotein that contain cholesterol undergo biochemical change by yet unknown mechanisms and sites "the black box." The specific immune response initiated by T and B cells, responsible for cell-mediated immune and antibody response, respectively, is compromised. Therefore, the response to infection is not optimal [7]. (*Adapted from* Curtiss [7].)

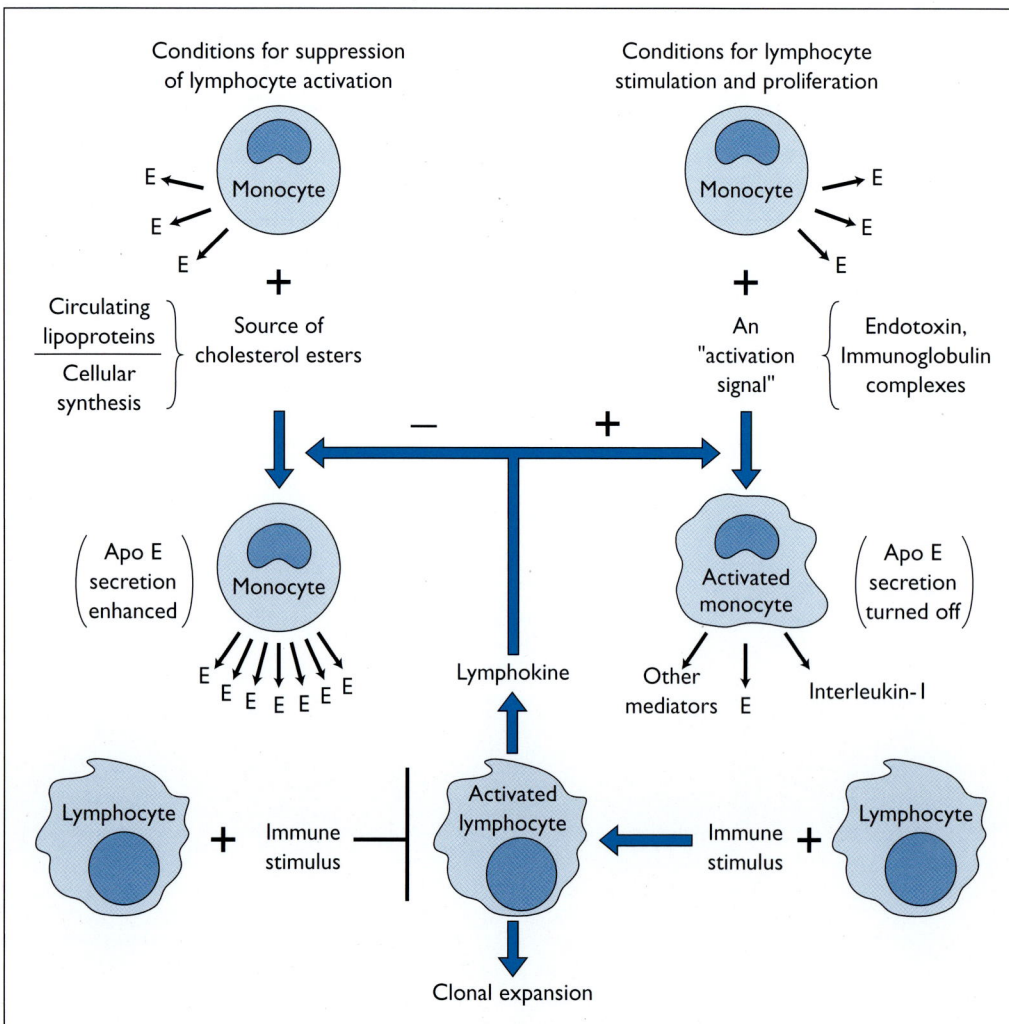

FIGURE 4-16. The immunoregulatory network. The exact impact of dietary fats and cholesterol on the immune system is shown here in the regulation of apoprotein E (apo E) in monocytes and macrophages, which participate in atherosclerosis and some forms of dementia. Dietary fats and cholesterol activate the monocyte for augmenteed secretion of apo E. This results in the inhibition of lymphocytes to be activated, which is necessary for the immune response to take place against infection [7]. (*Adapted from* Curtiss [7].)

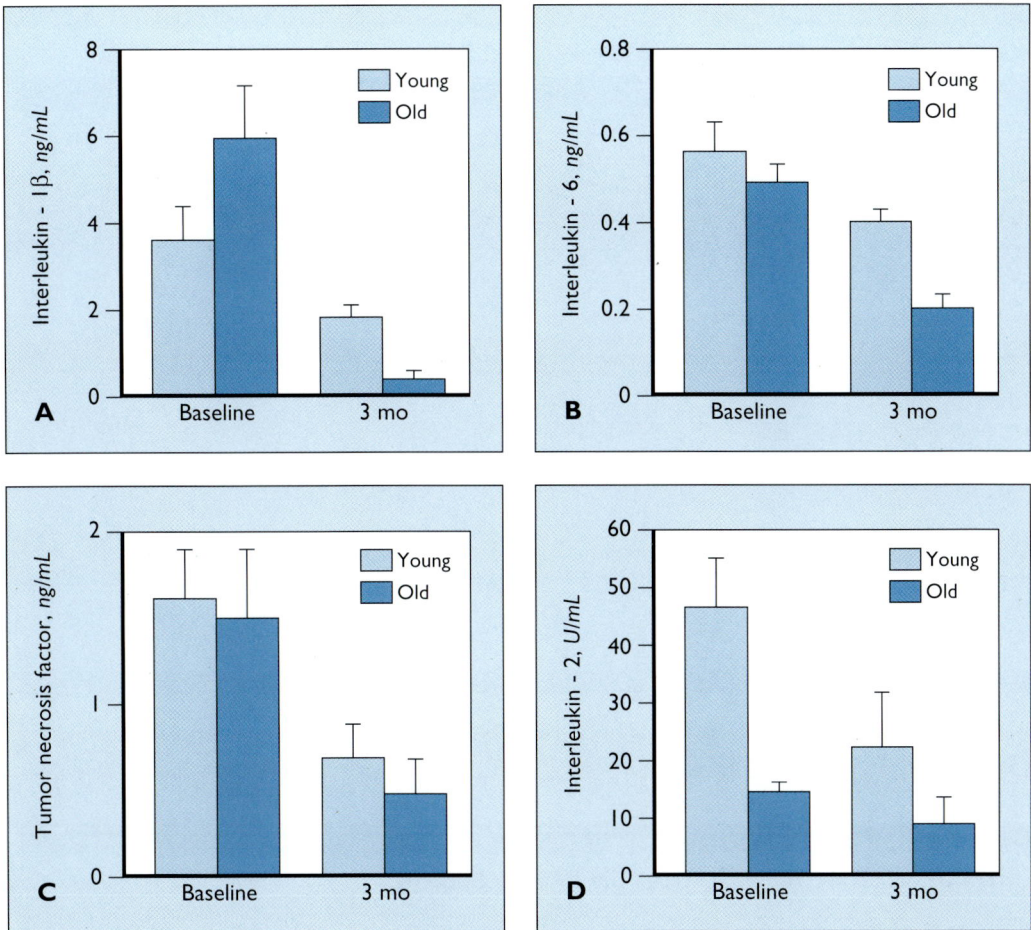

FIGURE 4-17. The effect of dietary supplementation with omega-3 polyunsaturated fatty acids (PUFAs) on cytokine production by peripheral blood mononuclear cells from healthy individuals. The omega-3 PUFAs, eicosapentaenoic and docosahexaenoic acid, competitively inhibit the oxygenation of arachidonic acid by cyclooxygenase and elicit a concomitant decrease in the synthesis of eicosanoids from arachidonic acid. Thus, omega-3 PUFAs can modulate immune and inflammatory cell functions by eicosanoid-mediated effects. Clearly, all cytokines that mediate immune function are inhibited both in the young and in adults. The levels of interleukin-1β (**A**), interleukin 6 (**B**), tumor necrosis factor-α (**C**), and interleukin-2 (**D**) are significantly reduced after 3 months of dietary supplementation. For certain cytokines like Il-1β and Il-6, more depression is seen in the old versus the young. (*Adapted from* Calder [8].)

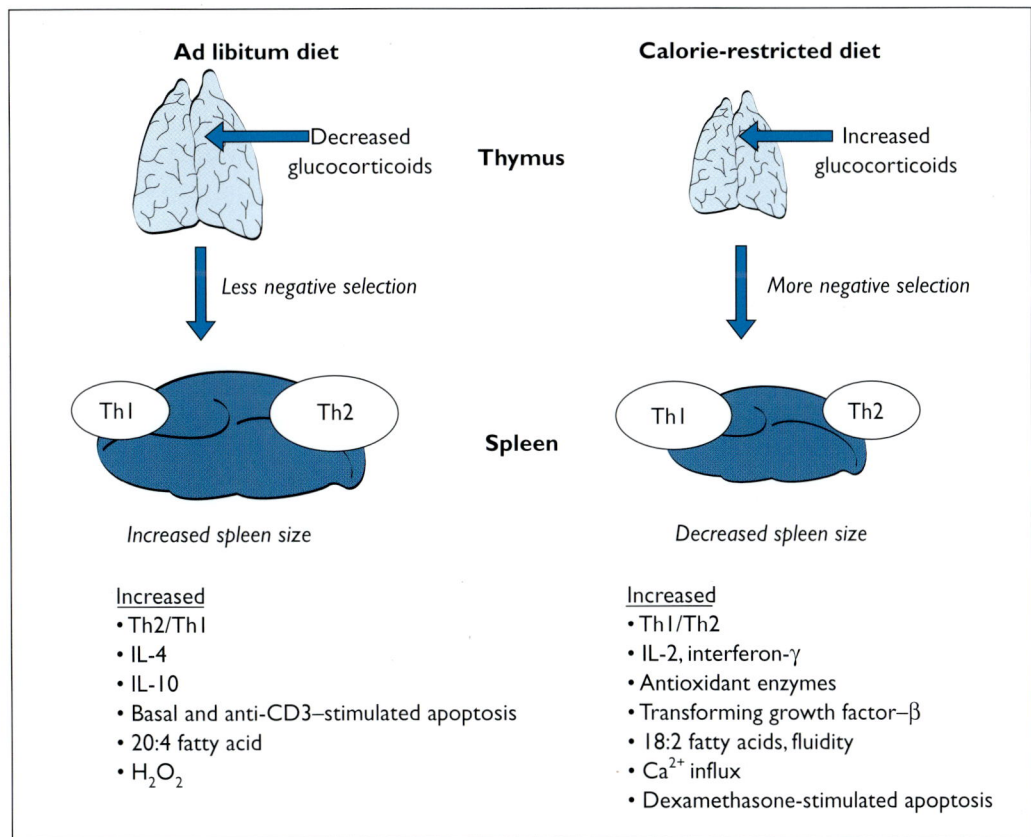

FIGURE 4-18. Influence of ad libitum diets and calorie restriction on modulation of T-helper 1 (Th1) and T-helper 2 (Th2) cells. IL—interleukin. In the ad libitum diet, there is less negative selection of unwanted thomocytes and their exit in the periphery results in horning in the spleen. There is a shift in the ratio of TH_2/TH_1 with inhibition of cell-mediated immunity and a shift towards antibody production. In contrast, in the calorie-restricted diet, the ratio TH_1/TH_2 increases with augmented cell-mediated immunity and protection against infections. (*Adapted from* Fernandez and Jolly [9].)

THYMUS WEIGHT IN MALNOURISHED AFRICAN CHILDREN

Age and Nutrition Status	Patients, n	Age*	Weight* kg	Thymus Weight* Reference, g	Patients, g	Thymus:Body Ratio, g/kg
Neonates	23	5 d	3.0	10.9(6.5–17.5)†	12.1	3.96
1–12 mo						
Kwashiorkor	7	10 mo	6.4	19.5(5.5–38.5)	2.9	0.45
Marasmus	11	5 mo	4.0		3.7	0.91
Adequate	20	6 mo	6.3		8.7	1.37
13 mo to 5 yr						
Kwashiorkor	25	21 mo	8.5	28.0(16.5–38.5)	2.7	0.32
Marasmus	15	21 mo	7.4		2.7	0.36
Adequate	55	30 mo	10.8		21.9	2.03
Sudden death	9	36 mo	11.7		38.6	3.30

*Mean value
†Range

FIGURE 4-19. Effect of malnutrition on thymus weight in African children. Thymus weight is a biomarker of cell-mediated immunity. Decreased thymus weight correlated with immune deficiencies, morbidity, and mortality associated with malnutrition in African children [10]. (*Adapted from* Keusch [10].)

RECIPROCAL INFLUENCES OF AGING AND PEM IN THE ELDERLY

Parameter	Healthy Adults (n = 50)	Healthy Elderly (n = 40)	Elderly with PEM (n = 50)
Age, yr	34.3±13.7	78.7±7.4	78.4±9.3
Serum albumin g/L	43.3±2.7	42.1±2.8	31.4±3.7
T-lymphocyte subsets, X 10^9/L			
Total count	2.190±0.330	1.940±0.510	1.450±0.560
CD3+	1.855±0.305	1.470±0.325	0.980±0.425
CD2$^+$CD3$^-$	0.105±0.085	0.285±0.140	0.410±0.270
CD57+	0.155±0.105	0.350±0.250	0.520±0.220
CD4+	1.190±0.220	1.085±0.285	0.680±0.270
CD8+	0.610±0.180	0.515±0.250	0.425±0.280
CD45RA+	0.895±0.530	0.425±0.430	0.540±0.380
CD45RO+	0.785±0.380	1.095±0.280	0.650±0.310
Cytokine release			
From lymphocytes (IL-2), μg/L	1.6±0.25	1.5±0.35	0.84±0.23
From lymphocytes (IL-6), μg/L	1.3±0.15	1.9±0.30	0.74±0.28
From monocytes (IL-1), 10^3 U/L*	18.4±10.1	13.1±11.4	4.2±4.8
T-cell proliferation			
With phytohemagglutinin (1 μg/10^6 cells)	104±25	98±31	54±27
With purified protein-derivated antigen (IL-1), (10 μg/10^6 cells)	30±14	25±15	12±12

*1 U = 10 g/L.

FIGURE 4-20. Immunosuppression in the elderly with protein–energy malnutrition (PEM). Reciprocal influences of aging and PEM in the elderly: comparison of healthy adults, healthy elderly selected with the Senieur protocol, and mildly undernourished elderly [11]. Elderly patients with PEM suffer from severe effects on their global immune system with a significant decrease in total T-lymphocyte counts and a decrease in response to antigens as manifested by cell proliferation and cytokine release. IL—interleukin. (*Adapted from* LeSourd [11].)

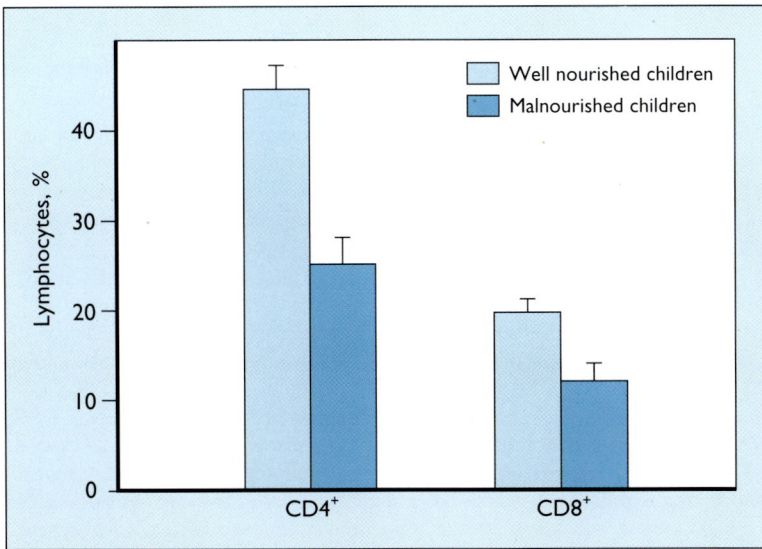

FIGURE 4-21. Decrease in both CD4+ T helper and CD8+ T cytotoxic lymphocytes in undernourished children. CD4+ and CD8+ are significantly reduced in malnourished children. This reduction in the number of lymphocytes results in a marked reduction of the cell-mediated and humoral antibody responses to infection. Therefore, malnourished children are immune compromised. (*Adapted from* Chandra [12].)

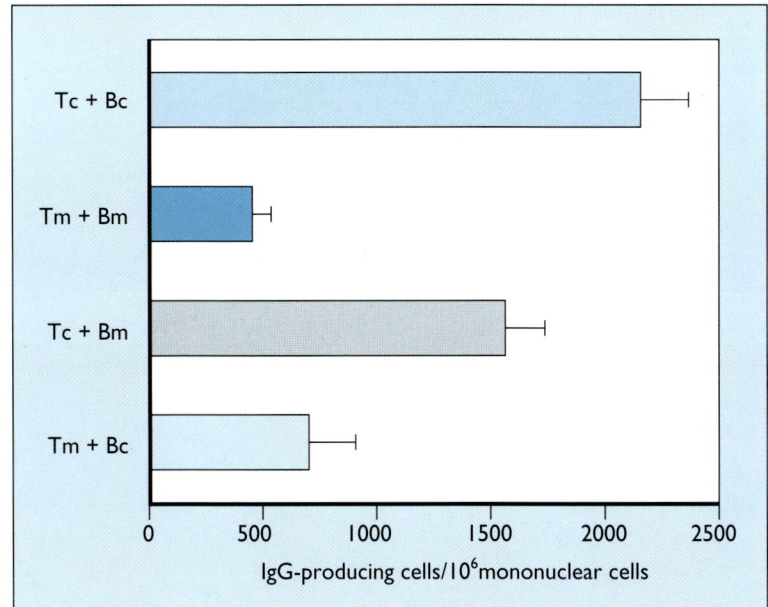

FIGURE 4-22. The reduction in malnourished children of CD4+ T cells, which are primarily responsible for providing T-helper cells for antibody production by B cells, is accompanied by a significant reduction in the frequency of IgG-producing plasma cells. Tc—T cells from control; Tm—T cells from malnourished; Bc—B cells from control; Bm—B cells from malnourished (*Adapted from* Chandra [12].)

A. LYMPHOCYTE COUNTS IN COLOMBIAN CHILDREN WITH PEM

Parameter	Normal	Marasmus	Marasmus-Kwashiorkor	Kwashiorkor
Number studied	25	11	11	21
Mean age (range), mo	44.2 (27–60)	33.7 (24–41)	35.4 (18–51)	44.2 (32–60)
Total lymphocytes on admission	4007±329	5291±793	4316±772	3952±58
Total lymphocytes on discharge	—	5952±699	5533±912	4422±469

B. LYMPHOCYTE SUBPOPULATIONS IN PEM

	Cells Reactive with Monoclonal Antibodies %							
	T3+		T4+		T8+		T4:T8	
Subjects	Before*	After*	Before*	After*	Before*	After*	Before*	After*
Malnourished (n = 6)	26±2.5	65±2.7	15±6.5	41±1.2	18±0.1	22±0.8	0.87±.11	1.86±0.07
Controls (n = 10)	67±4.3		41±3.7		25±2.3		1.98±0.21	

Before and after nutrition rehabilitation.

FIGURE 4-23. A, Lymphocyte counts in Colombian children with protein–energy malnutrition (PEM). The total lymphocyte count did not change significantly as a result of protein energy malnutrition. **B,** Lymphocyte subpopulations in PEM. Circulating T-lymphocyte counts are reduced in individuals with PEM. The CD3+T (T3+), CD4+T (T4+), and CD8+ (T8) subset frequencies are significantly decreased in malnourished children compared with controls. However, after nutrition rehabilitation, the frequencies return to normal levels. This decrease is thought to account for the reduction in cell-mediated immunity observed with malnutrition. T-cell function is modulated by nutrition status [10]. (*Adapted from* Keusch [10].)

Role of Vitamins and Minerals

RESULTS OF EIGHT VITAMIN A INTERVENTION TRIALS ON MORTALITY IN YOUNG CHILDREN IN DEVELOPING COUNTRIES*

Location	Effect, %
Aceh, Indonesia	-27
Sudan	4
Hyderabad, India	-6
Jumla, Nepal	-26
Sarlahi, Nepal	-29
Ghana (VAST study)	-20
Bogor, Indonesia	-30
Tamil Nadu, India	-50

*Mean relative risk, 0.77; 95% confidence interval, 0.68, 0.84

FIGURE 4-24. Results of vitamin A intervention trials on mortality in young children. Vitamin A deficiency causes a four- to 12-fold increase in the mortality rate of young children in developing countries as summerized in this table [13]. This increased mortality is linked to a two- to threefold higher incidence of respiratory disease and diarrhea in children with preexisting vitamin A deficiency.

The mechanisms of vitamin A in immunity were examined in mice, and the findings demonstrate that vitamin A mediates at least three activities: It balances T-helper 1 (Th1) and T-helper 2 (Th2) functions, downregulates Th1 secretion of interferon-γ (IFN-γ) and decreases activated antigen-presenting cell factors, and promotes Th2 cell growth and/or differentiation for antibody production [13].

Vitamin A and related retinoids play an important role in the regulation of immune function. Vitamin A deficiency compromises immunity, resulting in major morbidity and mortality. The link between clinical vitamin A deficiency (xerophthalmia) and infectious disease morbidity and mortality has been known for hundreds of years. The underlying basis for the use of vitamin A is that it acts via all *trans*- or 9-*cis* retinoic acid and nuclear retinoic acid receptors (PAR, PXR) to regulate gene transcription or may use a pathway involving 14-hydroxy-4, 14-retro retinol. Retinoids influence many aspects of immunity, including mucin and keratin expression; hematopoiesis; apoptosis; growth and differentiation and function of neutrophils, natural killer cells, monocytes/macrophages, Langherhans' cells, and T and B lymphocytes; balance between Th1 and Th2 immune responses; immunoglobulin production; and expression of cytokines (transforming growth factor–β, tumor necrosis factor–α, IFN-γ, interleukin-1, -2, -3, -4, -6, -10) and adhesion molecules such as intracellular adhesion molecule–1. The findings with retinoids depend on cell type and culture, and extrapolation to *in vivo* conditions must be made with caution. The impact of vitamin A deficiency on immunity is well established in some immune compartments, including components of mucosal immunity by alterations of keratins and mucin, compromised function of accessory cells, alteration of cytokine networks (which influence immune responses) and altered antibody response. High-dose supplementation reduces morbidity and mortality in acute measles [14] and has become recommended therapy for measles in both developed countries and the United States. (*Adapted from* Scrimshaw and San Giovanni [13].)

DECREASES IN IMMUNE FUNCTION CAUSED BY VITAMIN E DEFICIENCY STUDY

Decreased Immune Function	Study Animals	Humans
Humoral response, B-cell function	Mice, rats	—
Immunoglobulins	Mice	—
T-lymphocyte response	Mice, rats, pigs, sheep, dogs	Severe vitamin E deficiency, premature infants respond to vitamin E supplementation
Delayed cutaneous hypersensitivity	—	Severe vitamin E deficiency, vitamin E–deficient patients with tropical sprue
Phagocytic function	Mice, rats, pigs	Severe vitamin E deficiency, glutathione-deficient neonates
Hemagglutination titers	Mice	—
Cytokine of lymphokine function or production	Rats	Severe vitamin deficiency

FIGURE 4-25. Decreases in immune function caused by vitamin E deficiency [13]. Vitamin E is the most effective chain-breaking, lipid-soluble antioxidant in the biologic membranes of all cells. Free radical damage to immune cell membrane lipids may ultimately damage the ability of immune cells to respond normally to antigenic challenges. Several animal and human studies have shown that vitamin E deficiency is associated with an inadequate immune response [13]. Vitamin E deficiency impairs B- and T-cell–mediated immunity as well as phagocytic cell function. Supplementation with higher than recommended levels of vitamin E has been shown to enhance immune response in older adults and animals [13]. (*Adapted from* Scrimshaw and San Giovanni [13].)

EFFECT OF VITAMIN E SUPPLEMENTATION ON ANTIBODY TITER TO HEPATITIS B IN THE ELDERLY*

Group (subjects, n)	Geometric Mean, U/ml				P value†	Subjects with Detectable Hepatitis B Titer, %‡
	Baseline	Post 1	Post 2	Post 3		
Placebo (16)	4.0	4.0	4.6	7.3	.20	19
Vitamin E, mg						
60 (18)	4.0	4.0	6.2	10.4	.12	28
200 (18)	4.0	7.2	12.1	23.9	.05	41
800 (18)	4.0	4.0	4.4	9.2	.03	42

*A standard dose of hepatitis B vaccine was administered on day 156 of the study. Two additional hepatitis B booster dose were administered on days 186 and 216. Blood for serum antibody level measurement was collected before vaccination, 1 month after vaccination (post 1), and 1 month following second (post 2) and third (post 3) hepatitis B booster administrations. Serum samples with undetectable levels were assigned 4 IU/mL for the purpose for calculating geometric means.
†Post 3 compared with baseline using Wilcoxen's signed rank test followed by Bonferroni correction for multiple comparisons.
‡Detectable level set at 8 IU/mL or higher as detected by radioimmunoassay after the third hepatitis B vaccine booster.

FIGURE 4-26. Effect of vitamin E supplementation on antibody titer to hepatitis B in the elderly [15]. Vitamin E supplementation has been shown to enhance immunity in elderly populations. Using a double-blind, randomized assay, Meydani et al. [15] supplemented elderly individuals (older than 65 years of age) with placebo or 60, 200, or 800 mg/d of α-tocopherol for 235 days. All three vitamin E doses significantly enhanced delayed-type hypersensitivity. In addition, a significant increase in antibody response to hepatitis B was observed in subjects consuming 200 or 800 mg/d of α-tocopherol. Those consuming 200 mg/d also had a significant increase in antibody response to tetanus toxoid vaccine. The mechanisms behind the immunostimulatory effect of vitamin E are not known.

Vitamin E has long been recognized as an essential element for humans and animals. It is the most effective chain-breaking, ligand-soluble antioxidant in the biologic membranes of all cells. It is found in the membranes of immune cells because their high polyunsaturated fatty acid content puts them at high risk for oxidative damage. Free radical damage to immune cell membrane lipids may ultimately damage the ability of immune cells to respond normally to challenge. In some instances, higher than recommended vitamin E levels may improve immunity. (Adapted from Meydani et al [15].)

DECREASES IN IMMUNE FUNCTION CAUSED BY VITAMIN C DEFICIENCY*

Decreased Immune Function	Study	
	Animals	Humans
T-lymphocyte response	Guinea pig	Elderly subjects
Delayed cutaneous hypersensitivity	Guinea pig	Experimentally induced deficiency, elderly subjects
Phagocytic function	Guinea pig	—
Killing power	Guinea pig	—
Complement formation or function	Guinea pig	Gupta in Cunningham-Rundles, states: "Vitamin C deficiency in humans is associated with...an impairment of complement activity."
Epithelial integrity	Guinea pig	Spongy gums, subcutaneous hemorrhages

*Vitamin C may also act by increasing iron absorption.

FIGURE 4-27. Decreases in immune function caused by vitamin C deficiency [13]. Associated neutrophil functions, impaired delayed cutaneous hypersensitivity, and abnormal serum complement concentrations have been documented in studies with vitamin C deficiency in both experimental and human subjects. Reduced phagocytic responses and killing power as well as reduced antibody response have been described in clinical studies [13]. (Adapted from Scrimshaw and San Giovanni [13].)

DECREASES IN IMMUNE FUNCTION CAUSE BY IRON DEFICIENCY

Decreased Immune Function	Study	
	Animals	Humans
Humoral response, B-cell function	+	+
Immunoglobulins	+	—
Thymic structure or function	+	—
T-lymphocyte response	+	+
Delayed cutaneous hypersensitivity	—	+
Phagocytic function	+	—
Killing power	+	+
Cytokine or lymphokine function or production	+	—

FIGURE 4-28. Decreases in immune function caused by iron deficiency. Iron deficiency is the most widespread nutrient deficiency in the world and is associated with increased morbidity from infectious diseases. Iron supplementation of cross-deficient populations results in decreased frequency of infectious episodes. The mechanisms identified in association with iron deficiency are impaired phagocytic killing power, less response to lymphocyte stimulation, fewer natural killer cells associated with reduced interferon production, and depressed delayed cutaneous hypersensitivity [13]. *Adapted from* Scrimshaw and San Giovanni [13]; with permission.

DECREASES IN IMMUNE FUNCTION CAUSED BY ZINC DEFICIENCY

Decreased Immune Function	Study	
	Animals	Humans
Humoral response, B-cell function	+	—
T-cell–dependent antigens (SRBC)*	+	—
T-cell–independent antigens (dextran)	+	—
Immunoglobulins	+	+
Thymic structure or function	+	+
Cell-mediated immunity functions	+	+
T-lymphocyte response	+	+
Delayed cutaneous hypersensitivity	+	+
Phagocytic function	+	+
Killing power	+	—
Cytokine or lymphokine function or production	+	+

SRBC—sheep red blood cells.

FIGURE 4-29. Decreases in immune function caused by zinc deficiency. Zinc, a ubiquitous trace metal essential to the development and maintenance of the immune system, influences both lymphocyte and phagocytic cell functions [13]. (*Adapted from* Scrimshaw and San Giovanni [13].)

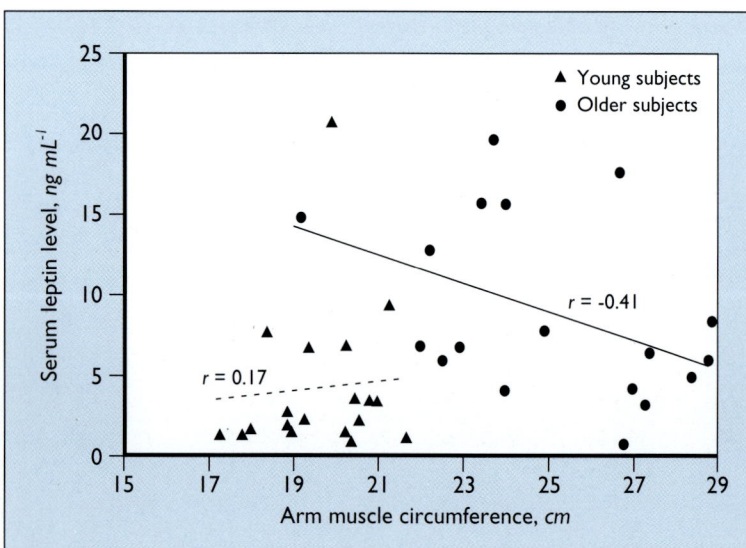

FIGURE 4-30. Serum leptin level and arm muscle circumference in humans [16]. Leptin is a 16-kD protein that is produced by adipocytes. In humans, serum leptin levels are highly correlated with measures of body fat content. Leptin is thought to be important in the control of appetite and metabolic rate. The injection of leptin into mice could shrink mice that were bloated with fat because they lacked the gene for the hormones [16]. These researchers suggest that fat cells normally produce leptin to tell the brain how fat the body is and, therefore, whether an organism should continue to eat. (*Adapted from* Cederholm et al. [16].)

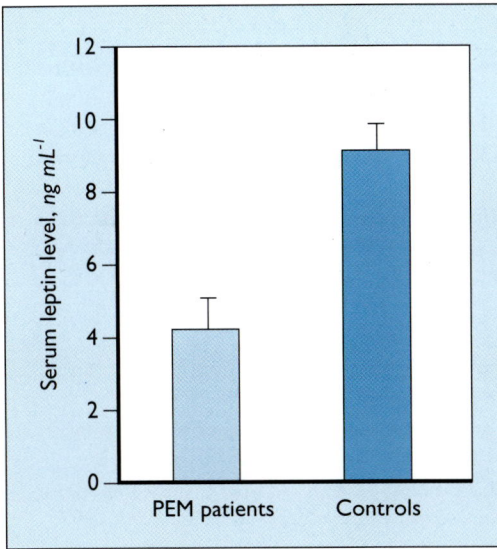

FIGURE 4-31. Circulating leptin concentrations in protein–energy malnourished (PEM) chronically ill elderly and age-matched controls. Clearly, leptin levels are significantly decreased in PEM patients compared with controls. (*Adapted from* Cederholm *et al.* [16].)

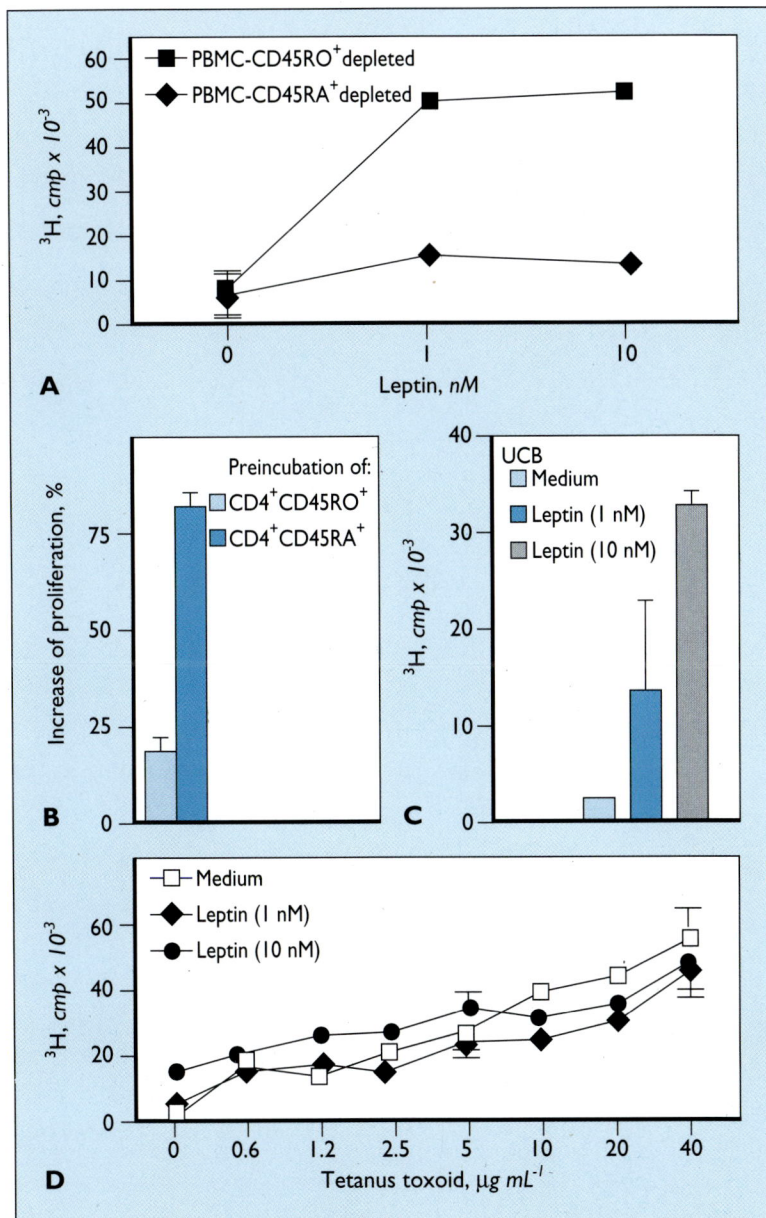

FIGURE 4-32. Regulation of the immune response by leptin. Leptin has also been shown to regulate the immune response. Researchers at the Imperial College, School of Medicine in London [17] have found that mice that have been starved for 48 hours had an impaired immune response. However, when the starved mice were given leptin, they reacted as strongly as did the fed mice. This finding may explain why underweight, malnourished humans have an increased susceptibility to infectious diseases. Most researchers also find that T lymphocytes express leptin receptors on the cell surface and also respond to leptin in culture by secreting cytokines. These findings might also explain why vaccines are ineffective in people experiencing famine.

Experiments were done and determined the modulating effect of leptin on naive T lymphocytes, but there was no effect on memory T lymphocytes. **A,** Mixed lymphocyte reaction (MLR) with either human CD45RO+ (memory)- or CD45RA+(naive)-depleted peripheral blood mononuclear cells (PBMCs) as responders. **B,** Preincubation with leptin (10 nM) of either CD4+CD45RA+ T cells or CD4+CD45RO+ T cells before an MLR in the absence of leptin. **C,** MLR using human umbilical cord blood (UCB) responder cells. **D,** An adult T-cell recall antigen response to tetanus toxoid. (*Adapted from* Lord *et al.* [17].)

References

1. Heber D: *Endocrinology, vol 3, part XI,* edn 3. Edited by DeGroot, Cahill, Martini *et al.* Philadelphia: WB Saunders; 1995:2663–2678.

2. Chandra RK: *Contemporary Issues in Clinical Nutrition, vol 11, Nutrition and Immunology.* Edited by Chandra R. New York: Alan R. Liss, Inc; 1988:1–8.

3. Janeway CA, Travers P, eds: *Immunobiology: The Immune System in Health and Disease,* edn 3. New York: Current Biology Ltd/Garland Publishing; 1998.

4. Rodewald HR: The thymus in the age of retirement. *Nature* 1998, 396:630–631.

5. Brandtzaeg P, Farstad IN, Helgeland L: Phenotypes of T Cells in the Gut. In *Chemical Immunology, vol 71, Mucosal T Cells.* Edited by MacDonald TT. Basel: Karger; 1998:1–26.

6. Lesourd BM, Mazari L, Ferry M: The role of nutrition in immunity in the aged. *Nutr Rev* 1998, 56(suppl):S113–S125.

7. Curtiss LK: Cholesterol, apolipoprotein E, and immune cell function. In *Nutrient Modulation of the Immune Response.* Edited by Cunningham-Rundles S. New York: Marcel Dekker; 1993.

8. Calder PC: Dietary fatty acids and the immune system. *Nutr Rev* 1998, 56(suppl):S70–S83.

9. Fernandes G, Jolly CA: Nutrition and autoimmune disease. *Nutr Rev* 1998, 56(suppl):S161–S169.

10. Keusch GT: Malnutrition and the thymus gland. In *Nutrient Modulation of the Immune Response.* Edited by Cunningham-Rundles S. New York: Marcel Dekker; 1993.

11. Lesourd BM: Nutrition and immunity in the elderly: modification of immune responses with nutritional treatments. *Am J Clin Nutr* 1997, 66:478S–484S.

12. Chandra RK: Nutrition and the immune system: an introduction. *Am J Clin Nutr* 1997, 66:460S–463S.

13. Scrimshaw NS, SanGiovanni JP: Synergism of nutrition, infection, and immunity: an overview. *Am J Clin Nutr* 1997, 66:464S–477S.

14. Hussey GD, Klein M: A randomized controlled trial of vitamin A in children with severe measles. *N Engl J Med* 1990, 323:160–164.

15. Meydani SN, Meydani M, Blumberg JB, *et al.*: Vitamin E supplementation and in vivo immune response in healthy elderly subjects. *JAMA* 1997, 277:1380–1386.

16. Cederholm T, Arner P, Palmblad J: Low circulating leptin levels in protein–energy malnourished chronically ill elderly patients. *J Intern Med* 1997, 242:377–382.

17. Lord GM, Matarese G, Howard JK *et al.*: Leptin modulates the T-cell immune response and reverses starvation-induced immunosuppression. *Nature* 1998, 394:897–901.

5

CAUSES AND METABOLIC CONSEQUENCES OF OBESITY

David Heber and Morton Maxwell

*O*besity is defined as excess body fat and results from an interaction between genes and the environment. It is normal for fat deposition to occur when the intake of energy exceeds the expenditure. Humans are well-adapted to starvation as the result of thousands of years of exposure to irregular food supplies. However, we are poorly adapted to overnutrition. In fact, it would be surprising if adaptation to overnutrition had occurred because it is only in the past one hundred years that humans have had a surplus of food. The modern high-fat diet combined with physical inactivity has resulted in an epidemic of obesity and overweight that affects one of every two Americans. Clearly, individual differences in metabolism and energy efficiency exist that are partly inherited. Therefore, although genetics determines the potential for obesity, the factors that determine whether and to what extent obesity develops are diet, exercise, and lifestyle.

The metabolic consequences of obesity are highly dependent on fat distribution. Increased abdominal fat accumulation is associated with insulin resistance. Although this type of fat distribution is called android obesity, it can occur in both men and women. Lower-body obesity, called gynoid obesity, however, occurs only in women and castrated men. Abdominal adipocytes release free fatty acids more readily under the influence of catecholamines. These fatty acids in the portal circulation may engender insulin resistance. Women with abdominal obesity have higher levels of male hormones than do women with gynoid obesity. In fact, visceral obesity is associated with hyperinsulinemia, hypertriglyceridemia, glucose intolerance, hypertension, and common forms of cancer. In addition, polycystic ovarian syndrome—characterized by insulin resistance, dysmenorrhea, hirsutism, and obesity—is more common in women with upper-body obesity. Infertility also is more common in overweight women.

The health consequences of obesity include some of the most common chronic diseases in our society. Obesity is an independent risk factor for heart disease, the most common fatal disease in the United States. Non–insulin-dependent diabetes mellitus, hypertension and stroke, hyperlipidemia, osteoarthritis, and sleep apnea all are more common in persons with obesity. A weight loss of only 20 pounds can be associated with a marked reduction in the risks of these chronic diseases. Conversely, adult weight gain is associated with increased risk of breast cancer in postmenopausal women. Psychiatric disorders are no more common in persons with obesity. The incidence of mild depression and anxiety, however, is increased in persons who are obese compared with those who are not. It has not been determined how much of the increased risk is secondary to the negative reaction of our society to persons who are obese versus endogenous differences associated with obesity.

Obesity is the most common nutritional disorder in the United States. A 30% increase in its incidence has been observed over the past 10 years. The exact cause of this epidemic has not been determined. A more hectic lifestyle, with accompanying reduced time for exercise and increased caloric intake, has been identified as a potential factor. Our fat intake has increased over the past 80 years and an increased incidence of obesity has been observed, despite the recent availability of over one thousand so-called fat-free foods. Consumption of these foods does not reduce caloric intake when sugar is used as a substitute for flavor. Often, there is no difference in the caloric content of fat-free foods compared with the full-fat version.

Obesity is a complex disorder for which no simple single solution will suffice.

Etiology of Obesity

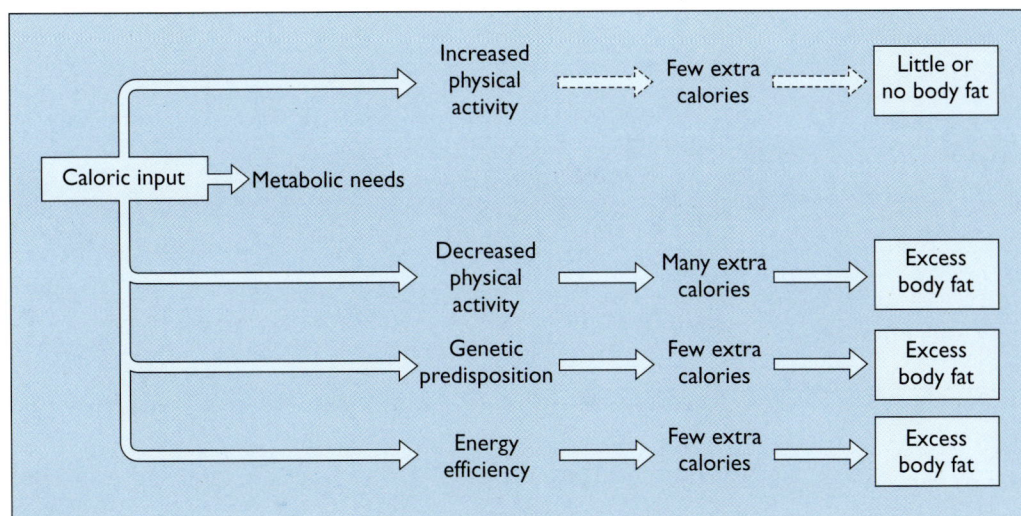

FIGURE 5-1. Causes of obesity. *Obesity* is defined as excess body fat. It can result from a combination of genetic and environmental factors. In most persons, it is clear that overnutrition and underactivity cause accumulation of excess body fat. However, individual differences exist in energy efficiency and in the tendency to store excess calories as fat.

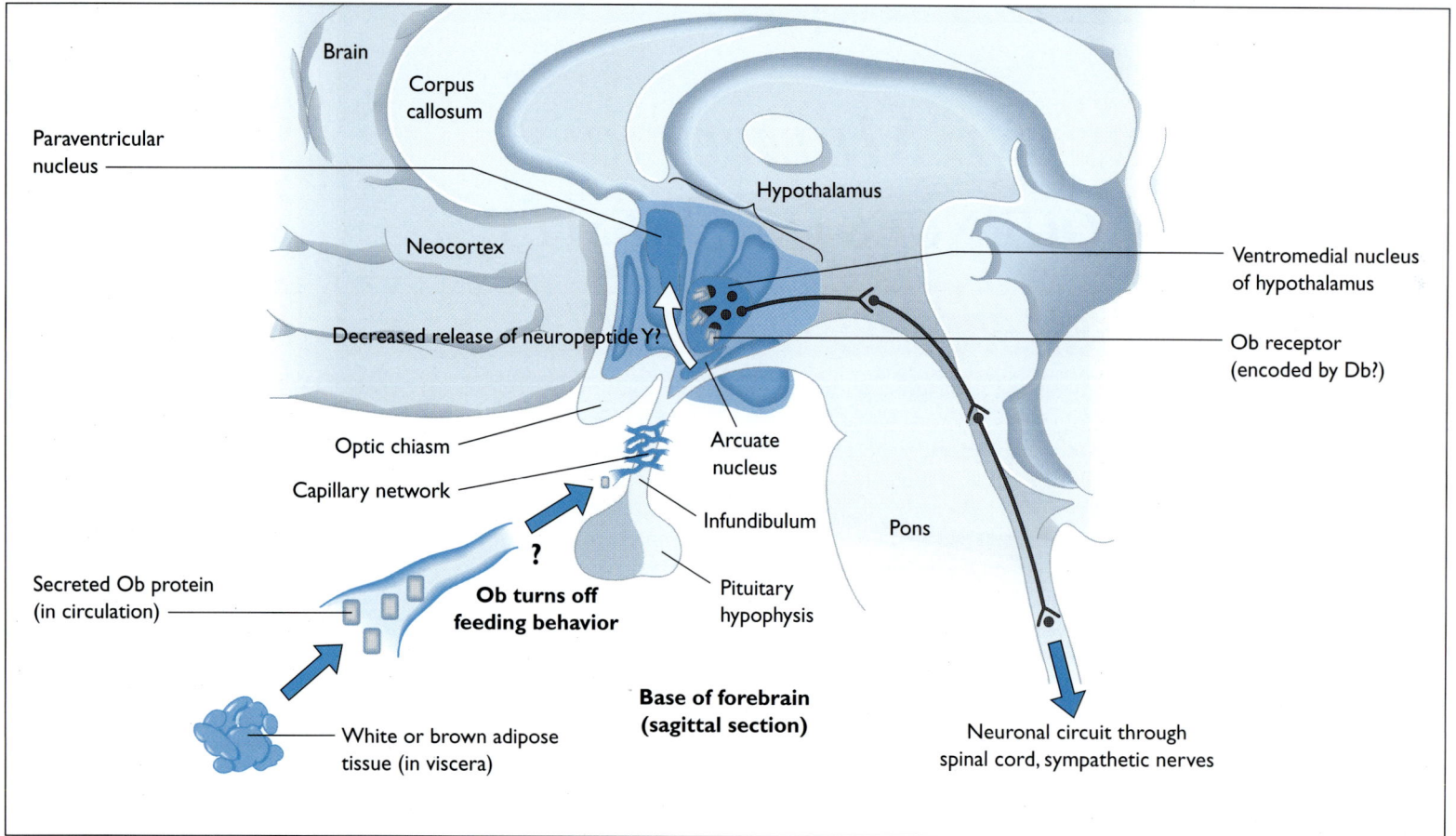

FIGURE 5-2. Role of the hypothalamus in controlling food intake, satiety, and thermogenesis. The arcuate nucleus involved in reproductive hormone home-ostasis has receptors for leptin as does the ventromedial nucleus, which controls satiety. Destruction of the ventromedial hypothalamus leads to obesity because leptin is unable to suppress food intake at a hypothalamic level when its receptor is missing. (*From* Ezzell [1].)

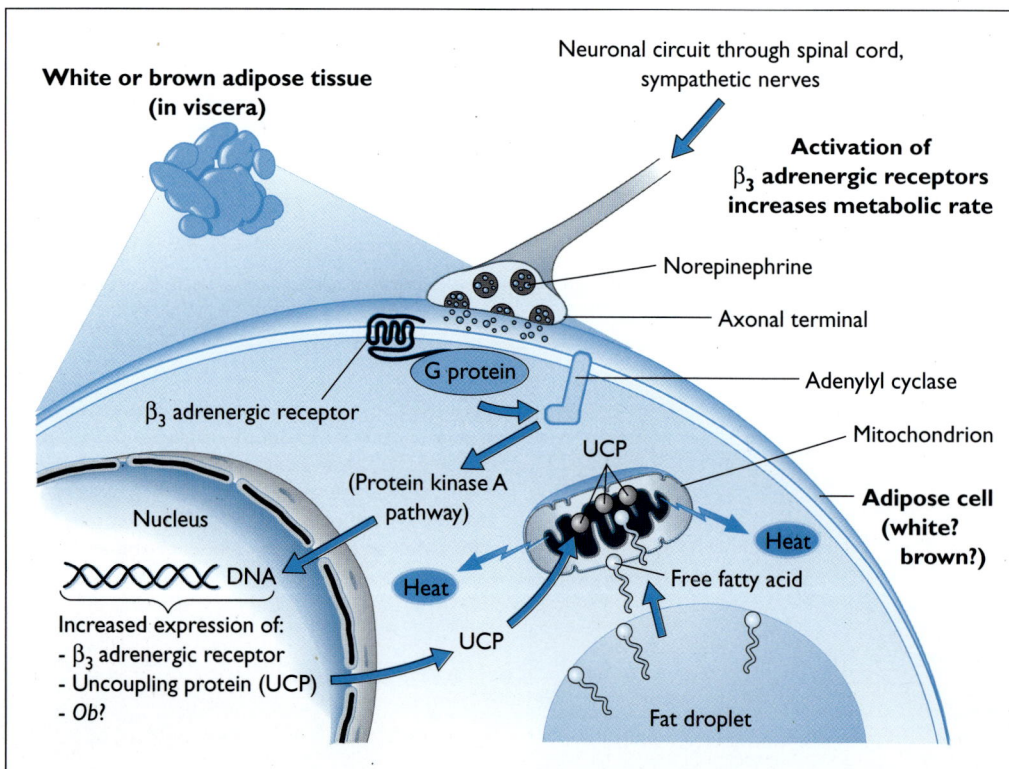

FIGURE 5-3. The fat cell. The fat cell is an endocrine organ. It has receptors for insulin and other adipogenic hormones as well as adrenoreceptors for neurotransmitters released under the influence of leptin at a central level. The fat cell and the hypo-thalamus form a classic endocrine feedback loop such that adipogenesis and lipolysis are highly regulated processes. (*From* Ezzell [1].)

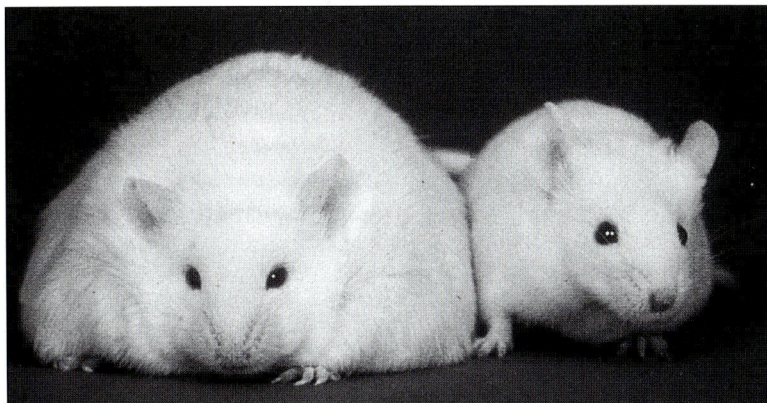

FIGURE 5-4. The ob/ob mouse and its normal counterpart. The ob/ob mouse has a genetic mutation inherited in an autosomal recessive fashion, resulting in nonfunctional leptin. As a result, this mouse is underactive and stores fat more efficiently than does its normal (congenic) counterpart. Its counterpart is identical in every way except for the ob protein (leptin) mutation. The ob/ob mouse also is infertile as a result of hypogonadotropic hypogonadism. Administration of leptin to this animal will correct obesity and restore fertility. (*From* Ezzell [1]; with permission.)

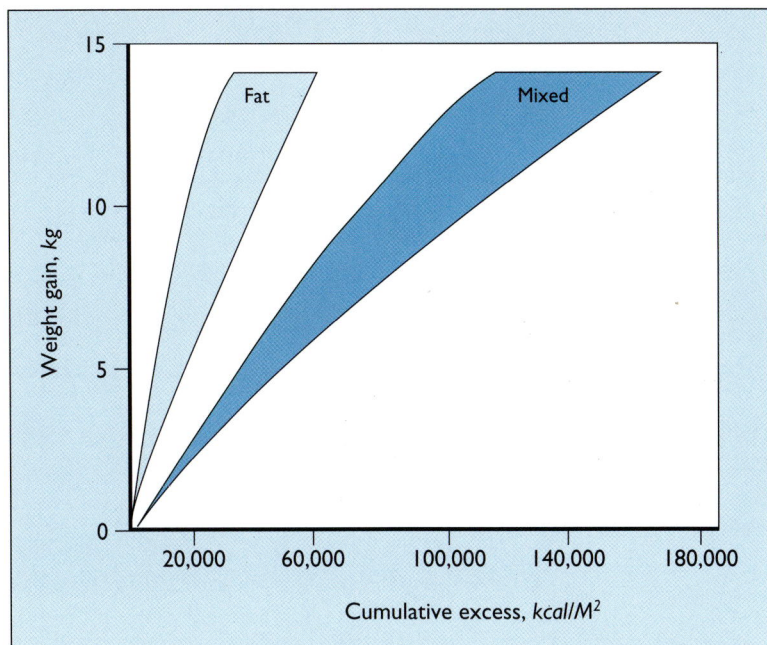

FIGURE 5-5. Weight gain experienced by animals fed either a high-fat or mixed diet. Fat is a primary determinant of caloric density and weight gain in animals and humans. As shown, there is much greater weight gain on the high-fat diet. In humans, dietary fat usually is correlated with fat intake, except for the greater than one thousand so-called fat-free foods. If the fat is replaced with sugar in these foods, with no decrease in caloric content, they are an exception to the above general principle. (*From* Bray [2].)

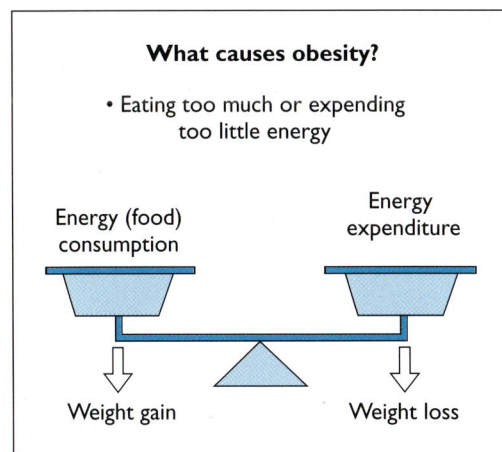

FIGURE 5-6. What causes obesity? Obesity results from an imbalance of energy input and energy expenditure. Genetics sets the stage for obesity; however, it is diet, exercise, and lifestyle factors that determine whether and to what extent obesity occurs.

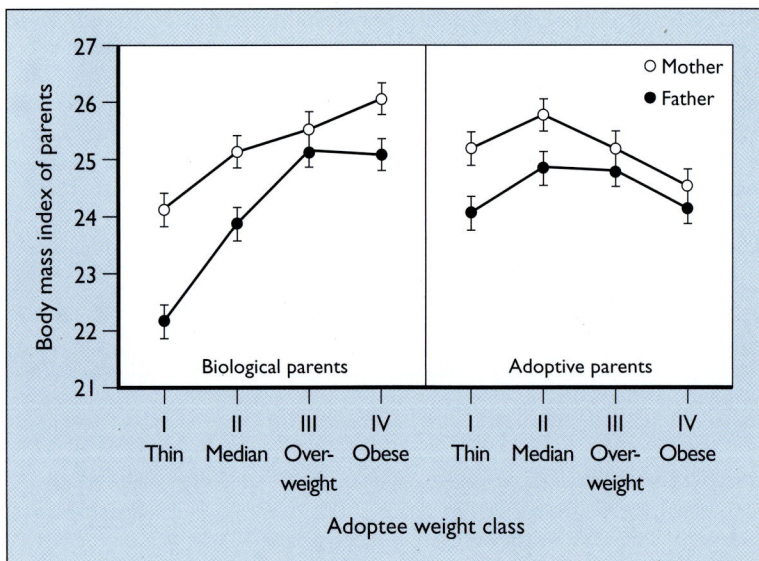

FIGURE 5-7. The role of genetics in obesity. Based on studies in identical twins, the impact of genetics on the causation of obesity is estimated to be 35%, whereas the impact of the environment is 67%. In these studies, the incidence of obesity is examined in identical twins reared apart and obesity is compared in biologic and adoptive families. A child reared by two parents with obesity has a tenfold increased risk of obesity based on both genetics and diet. Obese families tend to have obese pets. Therefore, environment is important, especially for many persons with obesity in our society without a genetic predisposition. (*From Stunkard et al.* [3].)

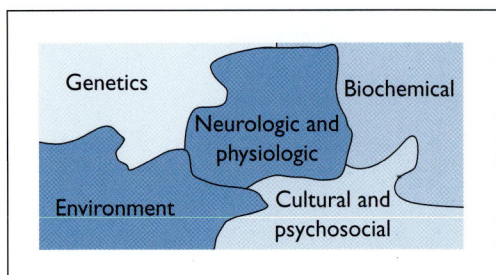

FIGURE 5-8. Causes of obesity. Obesity is caused by numerous complex and interrelated factors. The causes may even represent a collection of syndromes based on different causes. Some classifications use the categories shown here and classify obesity in an orderly fashion. Unfortunately, a combination of factors pertain to many persons with obesity. (*Adapted from* Clinical Guidelines [4]; with permission.)

Health Consequences of Obesity

HEALTH CONSEQUENCES OF OBESITY

Cardiovascular disease
Cancer, some common types
Degenerative joint disease
Dyslipidemia
Gallstones
Gynecologic irregularities
Hypertension
Sleep apnea syndrome
Type II diabetes mellitus

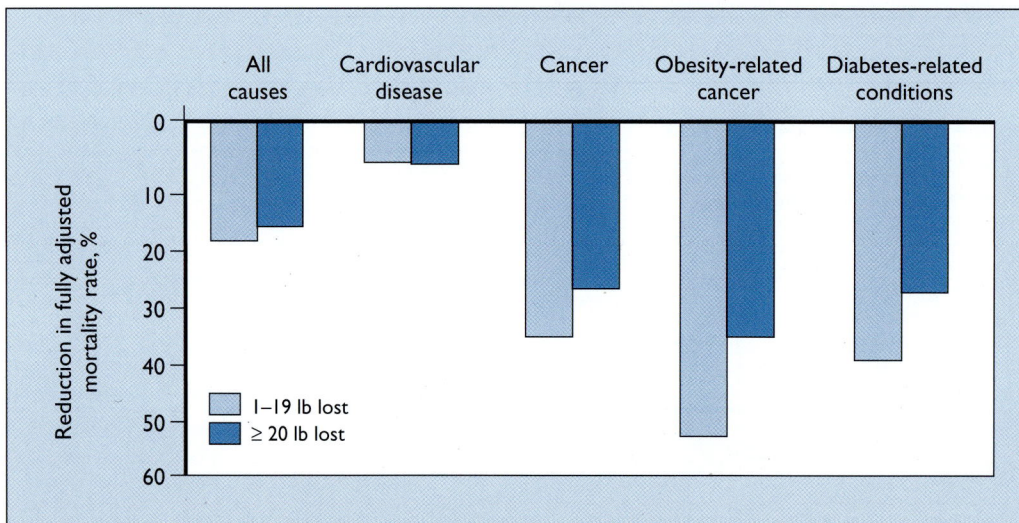

FIGURE 5-9. The health consequences of obesity include some of the most common diseases in our society: heart disease, diabetes, hypertension, and many common forms of cancer. The psychosocial morbidity of obesity also is a major factor often ignored in considering the economic and personal impact of obesity.

FIGURE 5-10. A prospective study of intentional weight loss and mortality in women. A study in a large population of women who have intentionally lost weight has demonstrated that overall mortality is reduced significantly by weight loss, either less than 20 lb (*light blue*) or greater than 20 lb (*dark blue*). The largest effects shown were on diabetes and cancer, especially obesity-related cancer. (*From* Williamson et al. [5]; with permission.)

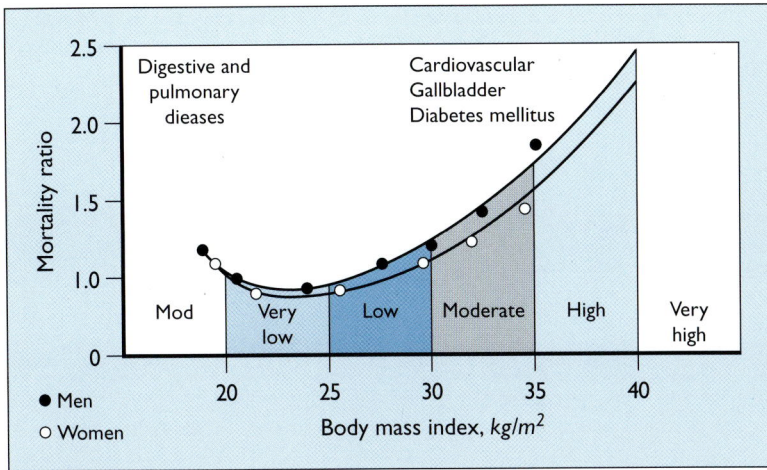

FIGURE 5-11. Obesity and the risk of mortality. Obesity clearly increases the overall mortality risk when the body mass index (weight divided by height, squared [wt/h^2]) is used as an indicator of excess body fat. These results from an epidemiologic study of over 750,000 persons by the American Cancer Society also demonstrate the increased risk of common forms of cancer associated with obesity. BMI—body mass index. (*From Gray [6].*)

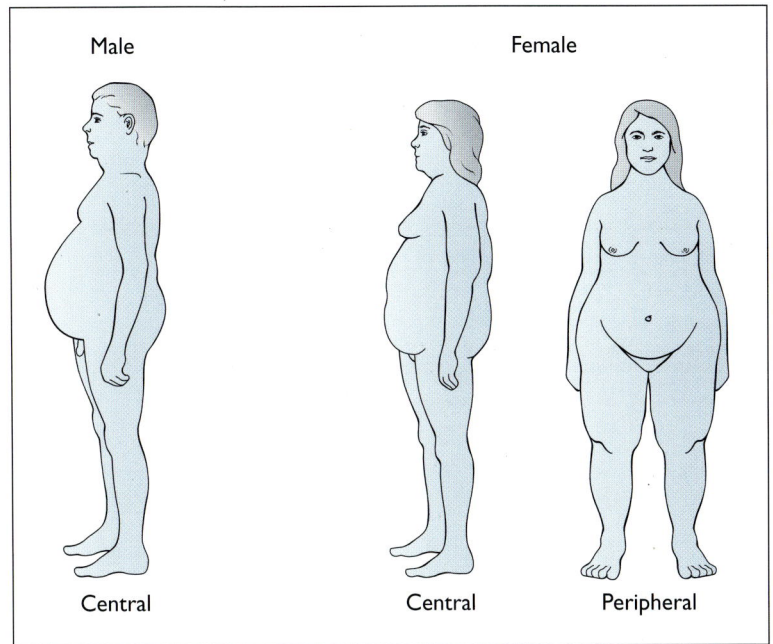

FIGURE 5-12. Differing body fat distributions in men and women. Women tend to have lower-body fat, called gynoid fat; whereas men tend to have upper-body fat. Women can have upper-body as well as lower-body fat patterns; however, men do not have lower-body fat unless castrated. As a rule, women with upper-body fat have higher male hormone levels and responsiveness than do women with lower-body fat. Upper-body obesity is associated with polycystic ovarian disease. (*From Greenwood and Pittman-Waller [7].*)

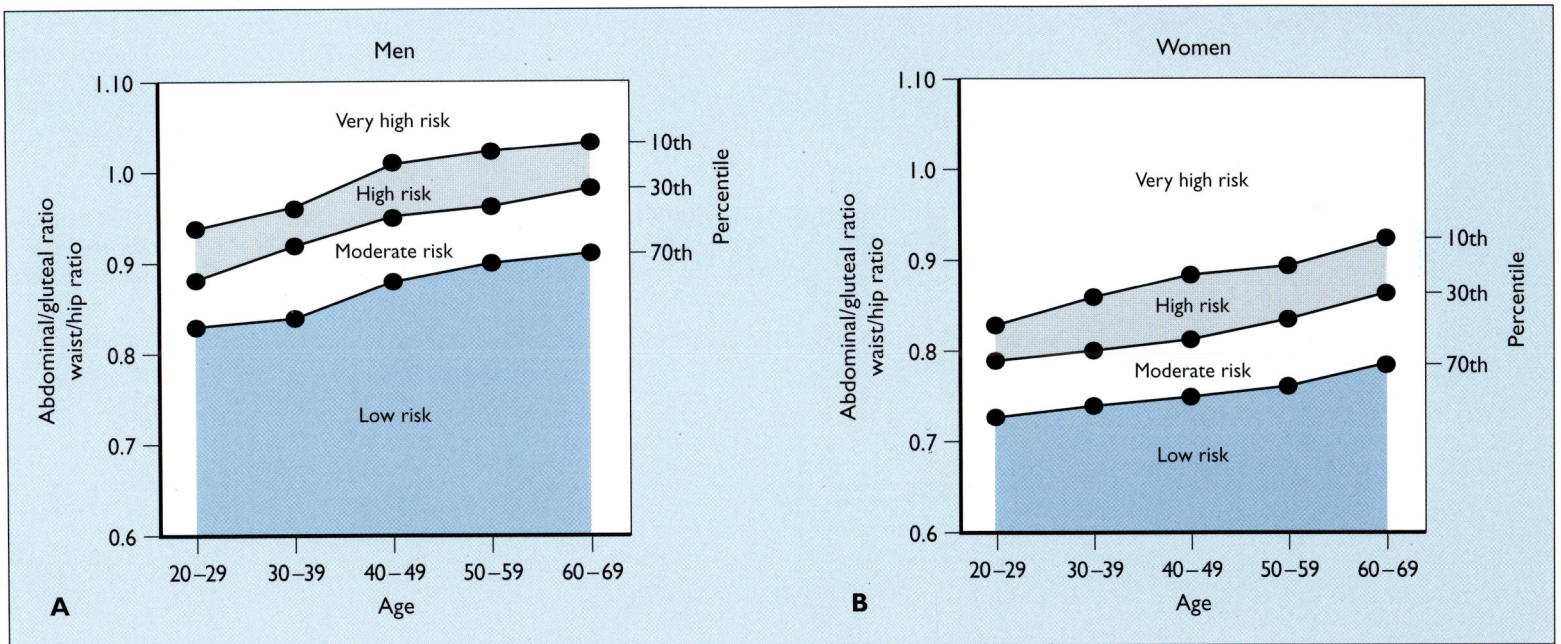

FIGURE 5-13. Upper-body fat measured by waist circumference or waist-to-hip ratio in men (**A**) and women (**B**). These measurements correlate with an increased risk of chronic diseases such as hypertension, gallbladder disease, and diabetes. At any given degree of body fat, the waist-to-hip ratio (a surrogate for visceral fat) has an independent effect on increasing the risk. (*From Kissebah et al. [8].*)

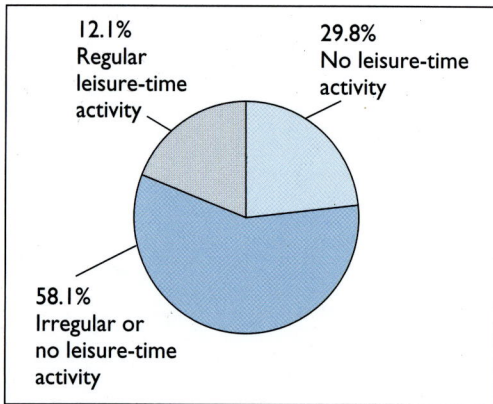

FIGURE 5-14. Lifestyle and obesity. Americans are too inactive, with 29.8% reporting no leisure activity and 58.1% reporting irregular or no leisure time activity. This inactivity magnifies the effects of overeating as a result of reduced caloric expenditure. (*From* Morbidity and Mortality Weekly Reports [9].)

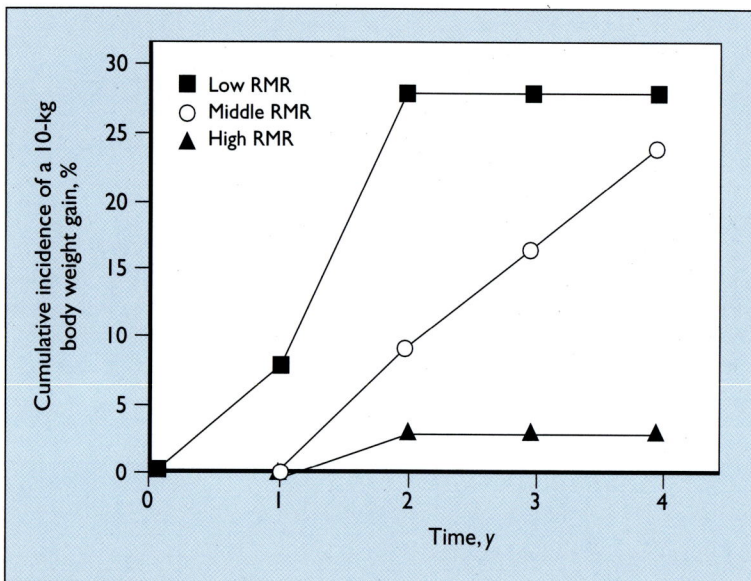

FIGURE 5-15. Data from Pima Indian families studied by Ravussin *et al.* [10]. Within the population, families were characterized as having high, low, or midrange metabolic rates. Those with the lowest metabolic rates were at greatest risk for gaining 10 kg over 4 years. This weight gain presumably is mediated by genetics, because other factors do not explain the differences in metabolic rates among families. RMR—resting metabolic rate. (*From* Ravussin *et al.* [10].)

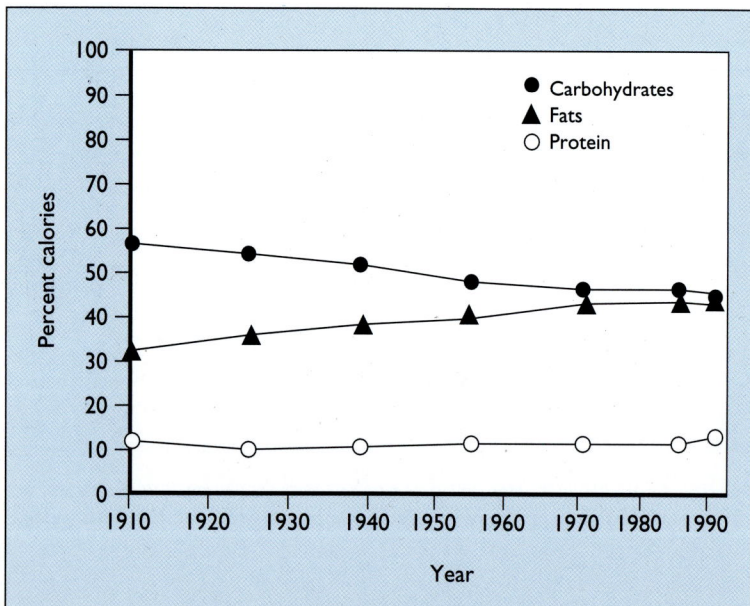

FIGURE 5-16. Macronutrient intake in the United States has changed markedly in the twentieth century and has contributed to obesity. Our intake of fat and sugar has increased, whereas our intake of complex carbohydrates has decreased. (*From* USDA National Food Consumption Surveys [11].)

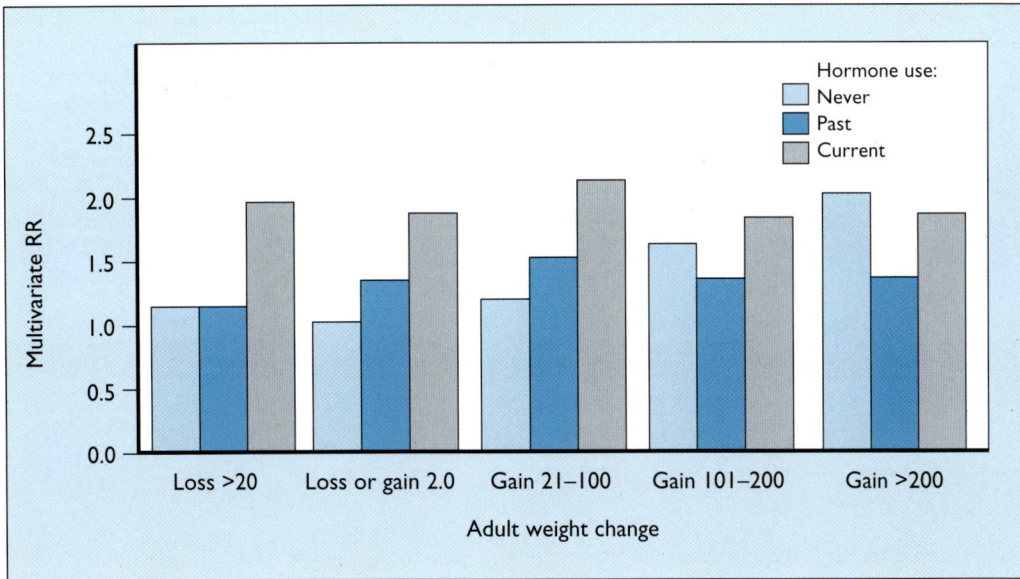

FIGURE 5-17. Relative risk (RR) among post-menopausal women: adult weight change and hormone use. The relative risk of breast cancer increases with adult weight gain in women. There is a twofold higher risk in women who gain more than 20 pounds compared with those whose weigh varies by less than 2 pounds. (*From* Huang *et al.* [12].)

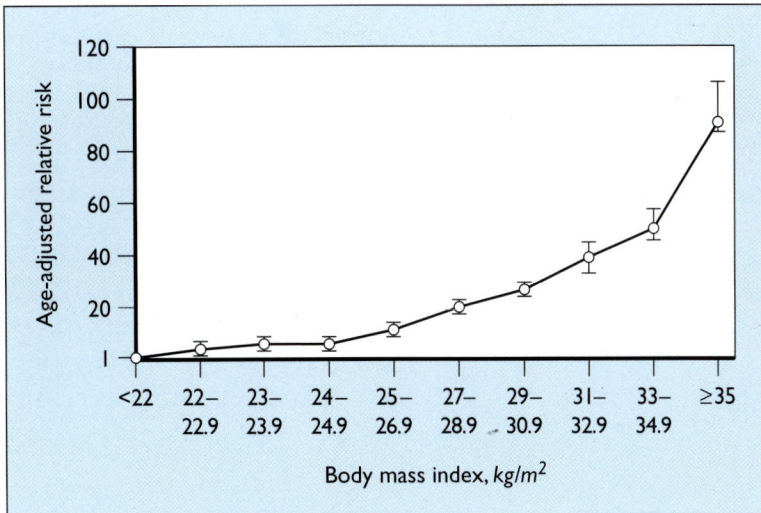

FIGURE 5-18. Body mass index and the risk of non–insulin-dependent diabetes (NIDDM). The relative risk of NIDDM is increased even at low levels of obesity in women. The accumulation of visceral fat is more important than overall weight in the pathogenesis of diabetes in obesity. (*From* Colditz *et al.* [13].)

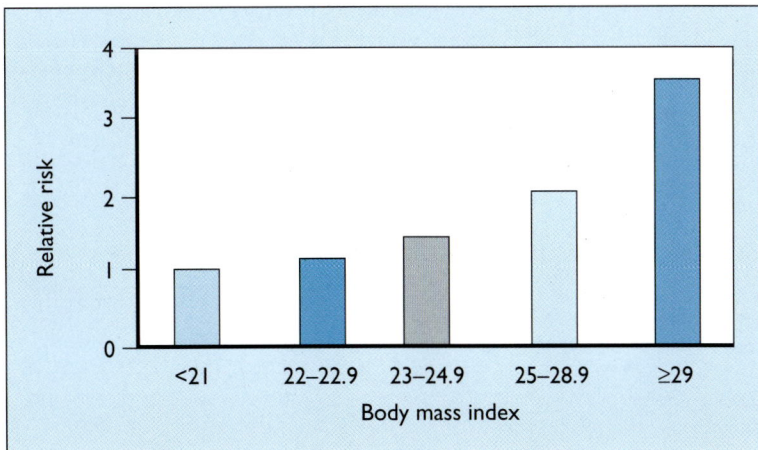

FIGURE 5-19. Obesity and cardiovascular disease. The relative risk of heart disease in women increases markedly with increased body weight. (*Adapted from* Willett *et al.* [14].)

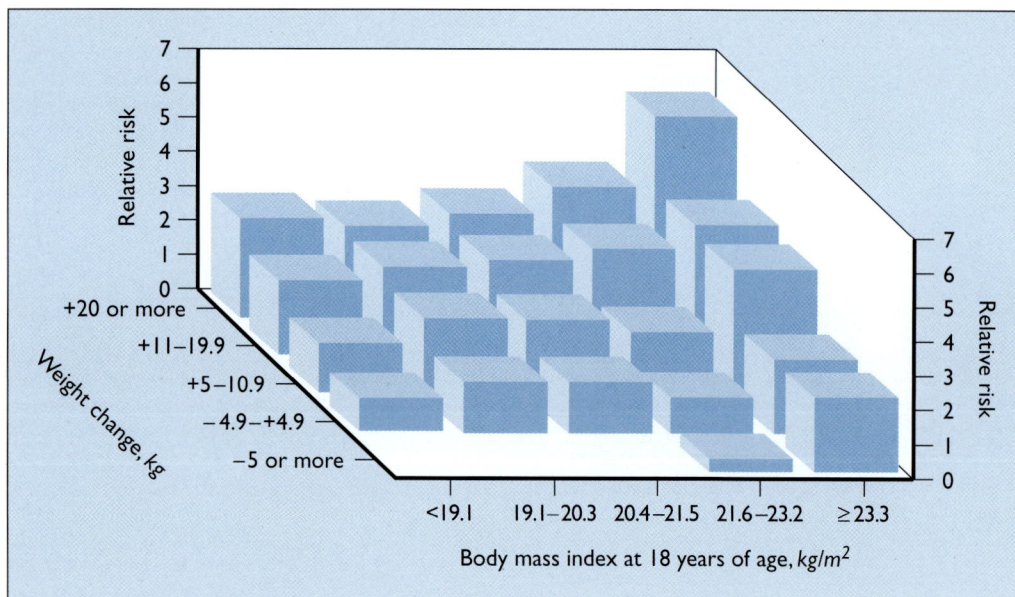

FIGURE 5-20. Body mass index and the risk of coronary heart disease. This risk is related both to the body weight at 18 years of age and amount of weight gain during adulthood in this prospective study from a large cohort. In fact, obesity is now accepted as an independent risk factor for cardiovascular disease. (*From* Willett *et al.* [14].)

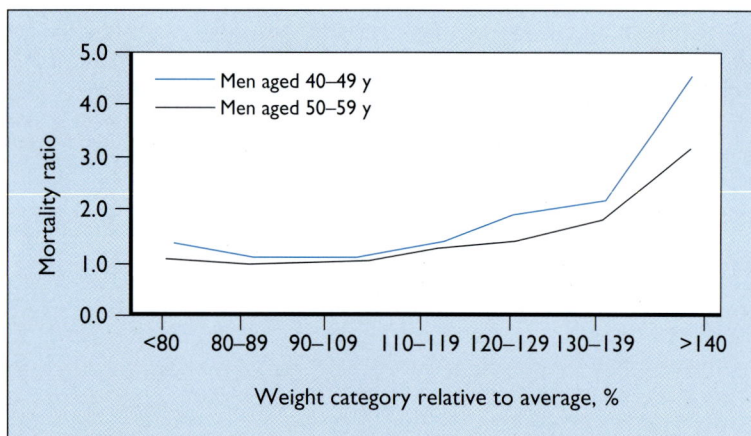

FIGURE 5-21. Mortality ratios from cerebrovascular lesions in middle-aged men. (Relative to death rates in middle-aged men at 90% to 100% of average weight.) The relative risks of stroke and cerebrovascular disease increase with increasing relative weight above 130%, which is roughly equivalent to a body mass index of 30. (*Adapted from* Lew and Garfinkel [15].)

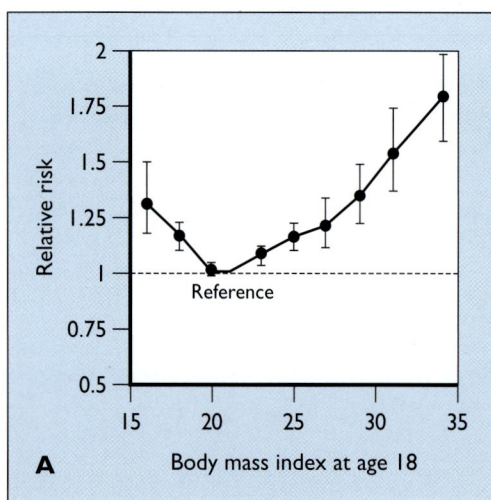

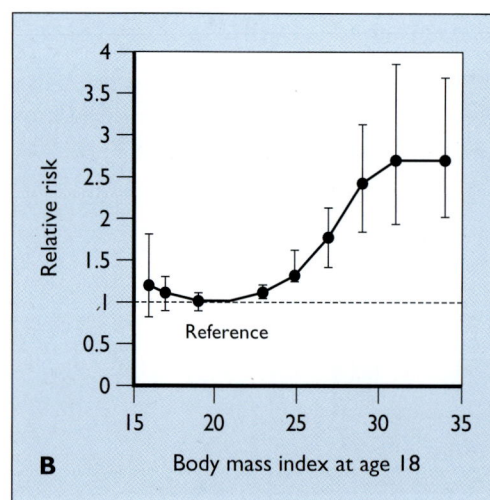

FIGURE 5-22. Obesity and infertility in women. The relative risks of menstrual cycle irregualrity (**A**) and ovulatory infertility (**B**) are increased in women with obesity. Abnormal menses and infertility are common complaints among women with obesity, often in association with polycystic ovarian syndrome and hirsutism. (*From* Rich-Edwards [16].)

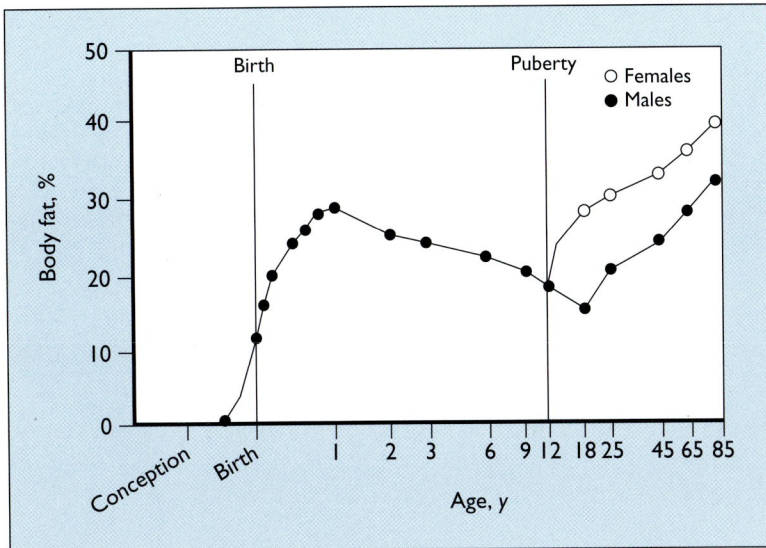

FIGURE 5-23. Changing body composition from gestation to adulthood. The percentage of body fat is higher in women than in men at all ages after puberty. Because metabolism is related to lean body mass and not fat mass, women also have lower metabolic rates than do men at any given height and weight. (*From* Friss-Hansen [17].)

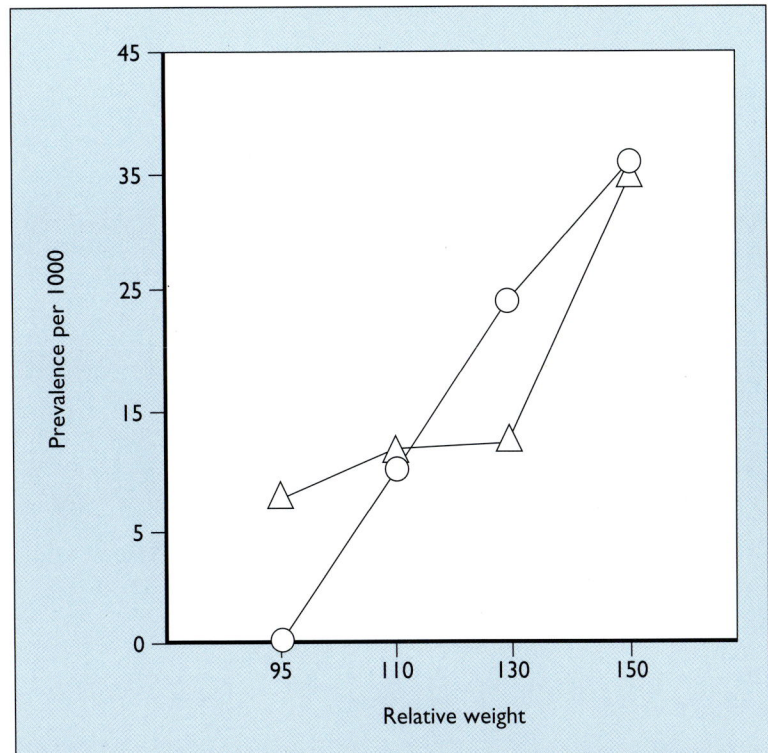

FIGURE 5-24. Increased prevalence of gout in obesity. The genetics of hyperuricemia are well understood and are associated with genes for hypertriglyceridemia. Increased dietary intake of purines from red meat and other protein sources also are likely to play a role in the pathogenesis of gout in patients with obesity. (*From* Rimm et al. [18].)

FIGURE 5-25. Actual and expected rates of osteoarthritis by weight in men and women. An increased incidence of osteoarthritis in the hands and feet is observed as body weight increases. (*From* Engel [19].)

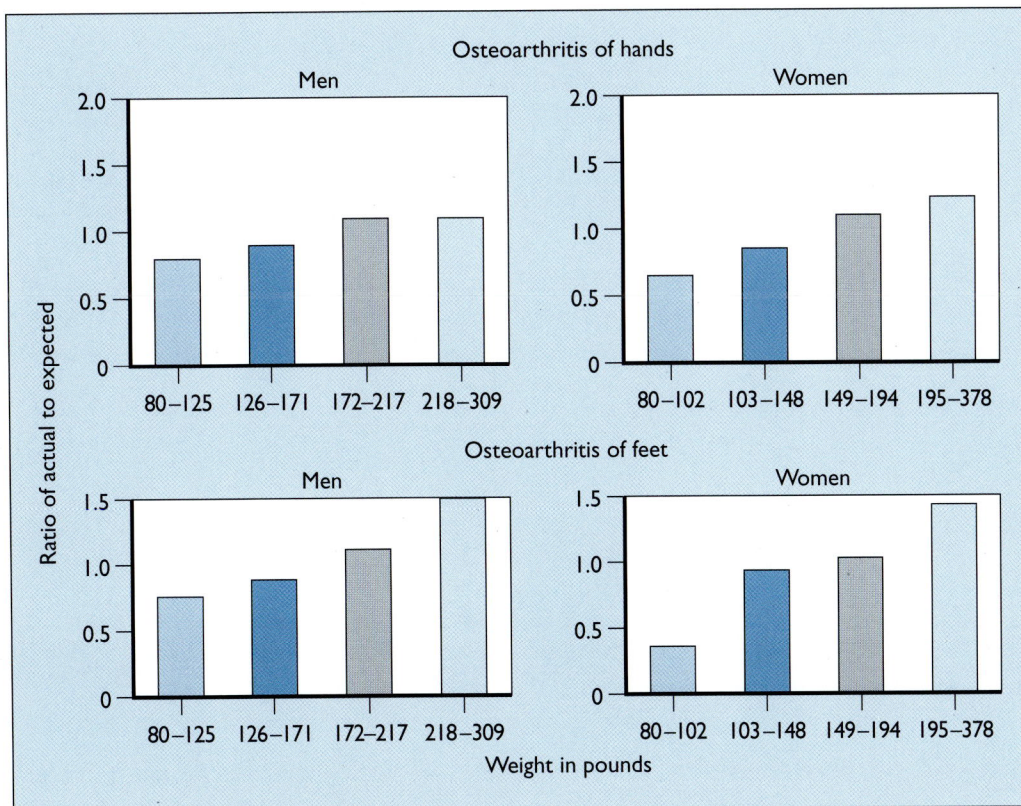

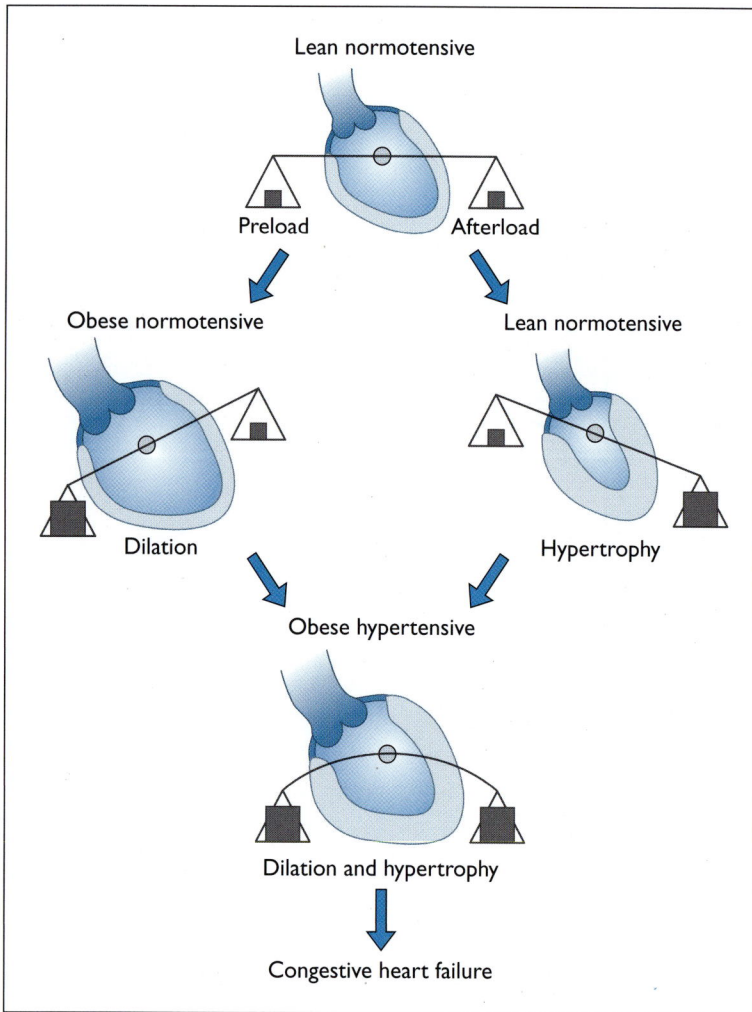

FIGURE 5-26. Adaptation of the heart to obesity and hypertension. Adaptation involves both hypertrophy and dilation of the heart. These abnormalities originate with left ventricular hypertrophy and dilation. The former is caused by hypertension and the latter by increased extracellular fluid volume. In some patients with obesity, these changes combined with protein and trace mineral depletion as a result of dieting can contribute to increased ventricular premature contractions and other arrhythmias. (*From* Blumberg and Alexander [20].)

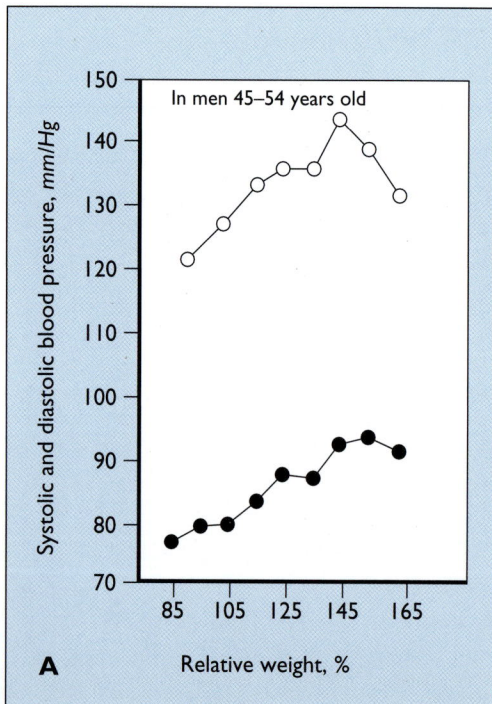

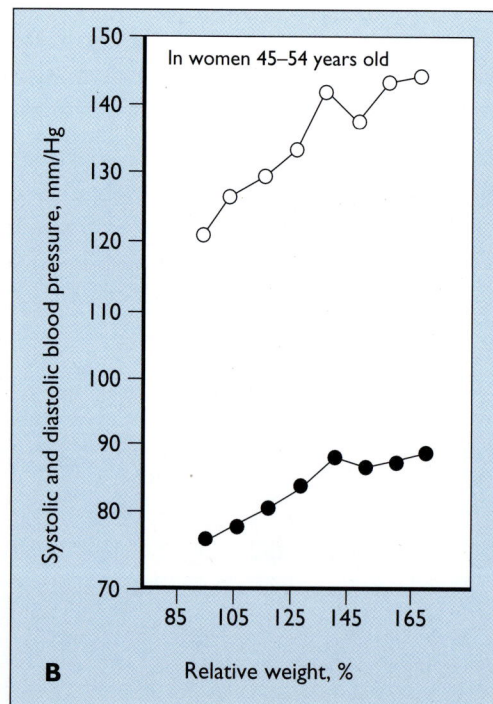

FIGURE 5-27. Increases in systolic and diastolic blood pressures with increasing relative weight in men (**A**) and women (**B**). Obesity is a common cause of hypertension by a number of metabolic and hormonal mechanisms, including insulin resistance, sodium retention, and increased extracellular fluid volume. (*From* Rimm *et al.* [18].)

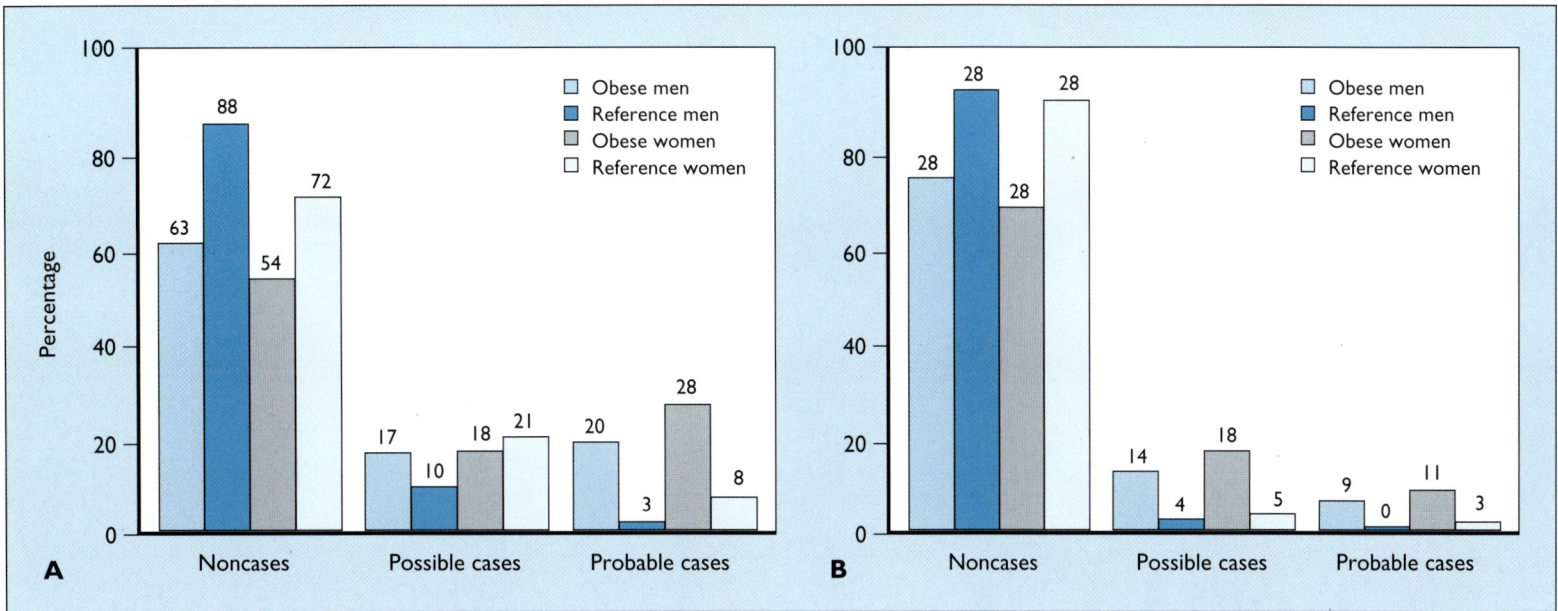

FIGURE 5-28. Increased anxiety (**A**) and depression (**B**) among patients with obesity. Most frequently these patients have no evidence of significant mental disorders but, rather, score in a range in which dysthymia or atypical depression is diagnosed. (*From* Sullivan *et al.* [21].)

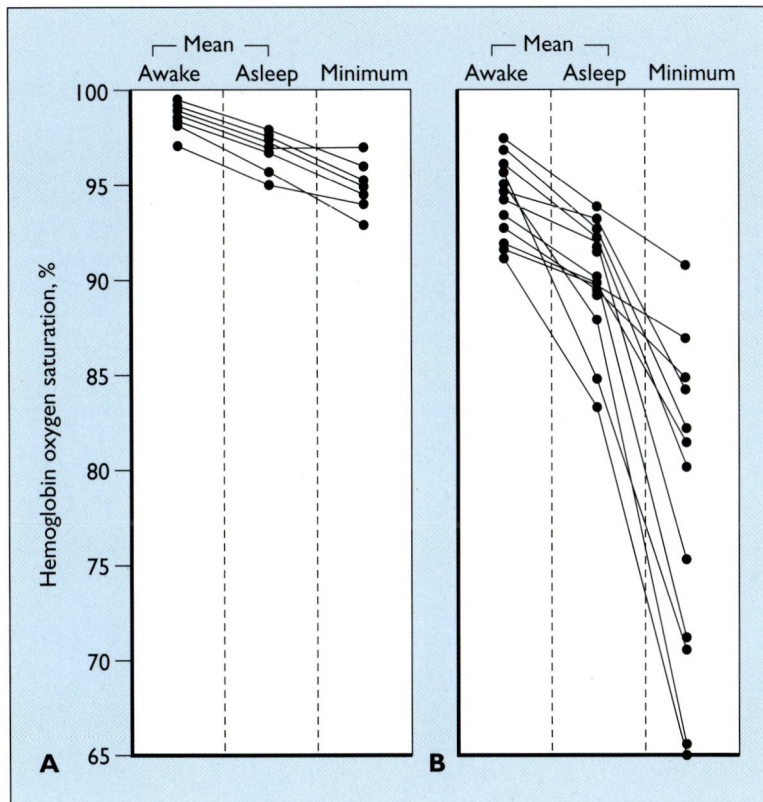

FIGURE 5-29. Measured decreased oxygen saturation during sleep in lean (**A**) versus obese (**B**) men. At least two mechanisms exist for the observed increase in symptoms of sleep apnea with increased body fat. First, fat accumulation occurs in the tissues of the pharynx that, combined with the anatomy of many patients with severe obesity, can lead to obstruction. Second, the restriction on breathing imposed by severe obesity can lead to resetting of respiratory control center sensitivity to stimulation by arterial carbon dioxide. In this situation a higher threshold of arterial carbon dioxide is necessary to stimulate ventilation, leading to carbon dioxide retention. This metabolic abnormality leads to cor pulmonale (right heart failure) with pulmonary hypertension. (*From* Kopleman [22].)

New Approaches to Understanding Obesity

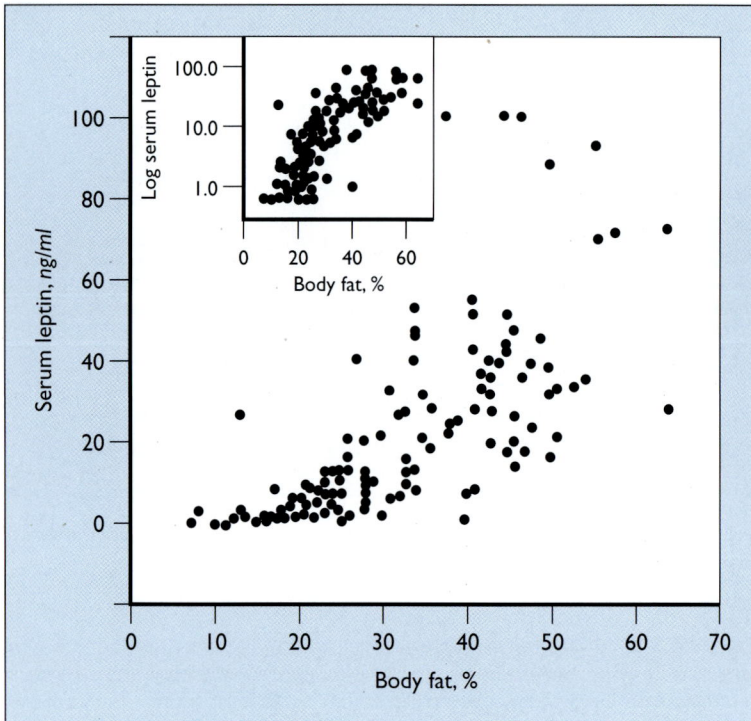

FIGURE 5-30. Serum leptin and its relationship to percentage of body fat as measured by bioelectric impedance. This relationship is shown by a typical sigmoid curve, with most patients who are obsese having elevated levels of leptin and body fat. This observation has led to the conclusion that patients with obesity may have resistance to the effects of leptin by analogy to insulin resistance. (*From* Rosenbaum, *et al.* [23].)

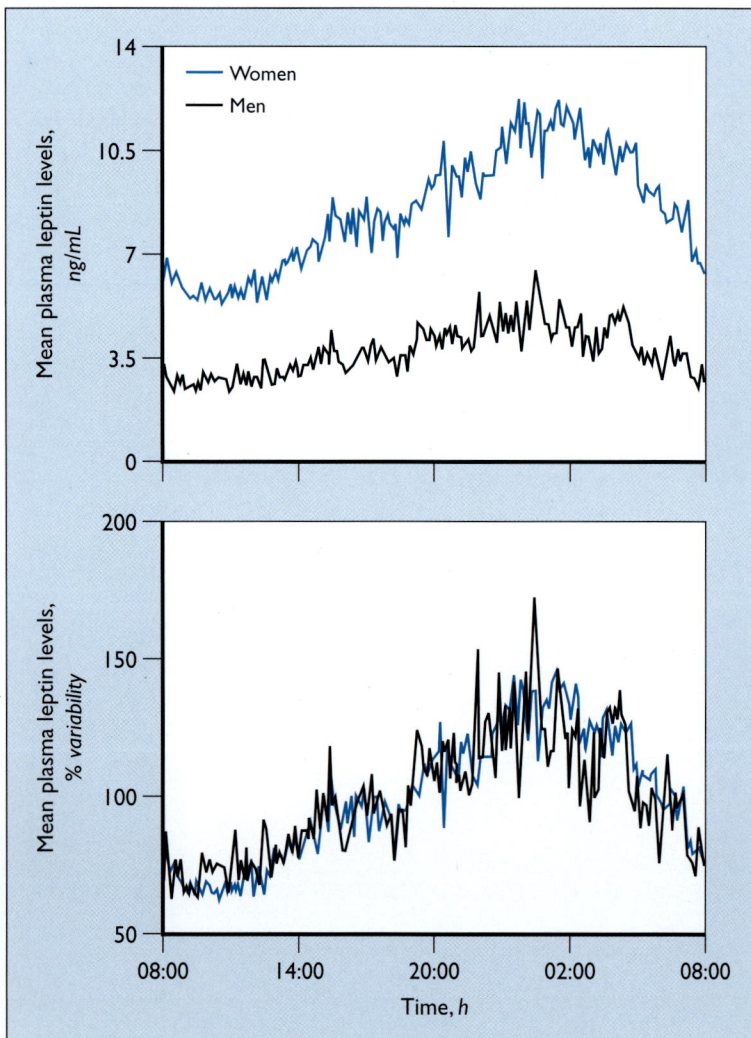

FIGURE 5-31. Plasma leptin concentrations over a 24-hour period for men and women. Fat cells secrete leptin with a periodicity of 7 minutes, and a diurnal variation in men and women exists. These facts suggest that significant interaction occurs between the hypothalamus and the periphery and that this interaction is influenced by nutritional and endocrine signaling. The diurnal variation of leptin is the inverse of the daily cortisol rhythm, suggesting a feedback inter-relationship between leptin and the hypothalamic-pituitary-adrenal axis. (*From* Licinio *et al.* [24].)

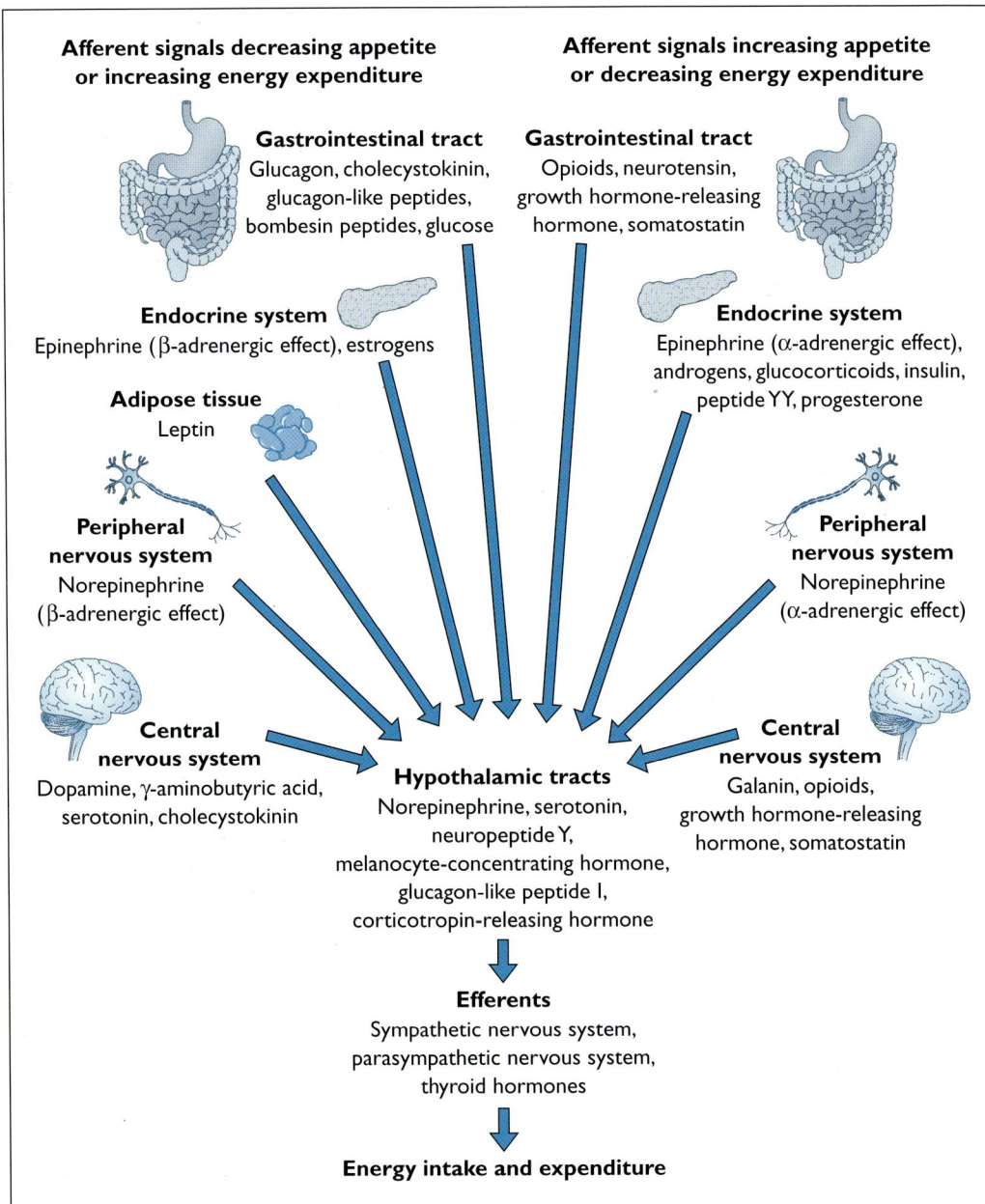

FIGURE 5-32. The many afferent signals affecting energy intake and expenditure. The input from the fat cell through leptin is complemented by a significant amount of information from the gastrointestinal tract, peripheral nervous system, and endocrine system. The integrated system is geared toward retention of energy because man is well-adapted to starvation but poorly adapted to overnutrition. (*From* Rosenbaum *et al.* [25].)

Afferent signals decreasing appetite or increasing energy expenditure

Gastrointestinal tract
Glucagon, cholecystokinin, glucagon-like peptides, bombesin peptides, glucose

Endocrine system
Epinephrine (β-adrenergic effect), estrogens

Adipose tissue
Leptin

Peripheral nervous system
Norepinephrine (β-adrenergic effect)

Central nervous system
Dopamine, γ-aminobutyric acid, serotonin, cholecystokinin

Afferent signals increasing appetite or decreasing energy expenditure

Gastrointestinal tract
Opioids, neurotensin, growth hormone-releasing hormone, somatostatin

Endocrine system
Epinephrine (α-adrenergic effect), androgens, glucocorticoids, insulin, peptide YY, progesterone

Peripheral nervous system
Norepinephrine (α-adrenergic effect)

Central nervous system
Galanin, opioids, growth hormone-releasing hormone, somatostatin

Hypothalamic tracts
Norepinephrine, serotonin, neuropeptide Y, melanocyte-concentrating hormone, glucagon-like peptide I, corticotropin-releasing hormone

Efferents
Sympathetic nervous system, parasympathetic nervous system, thyroid hormones

Energy intake and expenditure

References

1. Ezzell C: Fat times for obesity research: tons of new information, but how does it all fit together? *J NIH Res* 1995, 7:39–41.

2. Bray GA: *The Obese Patient.* Philadelphia: WB Saunders; 1976.

3. Stunkard AJ, Sorensen TI, Hanis C, *et al.*: An adoption study of human obesity. *N Engl J Med* 1986, 314:193–198.

4. Clinical Guidelines: Weighing the options: National Heart, Lung, and Blood Institute; 1995:52.

5. Williamson DF, Pamuk E, Thun M, *et al.*: Prospective study of intentional weight loss and mortality in overweight white men aged 40–64 years. *Am J Epidemiol* 1999, 149:491–503.

6. Gray DS: Disgnosis and prevalence of obesity. *Med Clin North Am* 1989, 73:1–13.

7. Greenwood MRC, Pittman-Waller VA: Weight control: a complex, various and controversial problem. In *Obesity and Weight Control: The Health Professional's Guide to Understanding and Treatment.* Edited by Frankle, Yang. Rockville, MD: Aspen Publishers; 1988:3–15.

8. Kissebah AH, Freedman DS, Peiris AN: Health risks of obesity. *Med Clin North Am* 1989:111–138.

9. Prevalence of sedentary lifestyle: behavioral risk factors surveillance system, United States, 1991. *MMWR* 1993; 42:576–579.

10. Ravussin E, Lillioja S, Knowlder W, *et al.*: Reduced rate of energy expenditure as a risk factor for body-weight gain. *N Engl J Med* 1988, 318:467–472.

11. USDA National Food Consumption Surveys.

12. Huang Z, Hankinson SE, *et al.*: Dual effects of weight and weight gain on breast cancer risk. *JAMA* 1997, 278:1407–1411.

13. Colditz GA, Willett WC, Rotnitzky A, Manson JE: *Ann Intern Med* 1995, 122:481–486.

14. Willett WC, Manson JE, Stampfer MJ, Colditz GA: Weight, weight change and coronary disease in woman. Risk within normal weight range. *JAMA* 1995, 273:461–465.

15. Lew EA, Garfinkel L: Variations in mortality by weight among 750,000 men and women. *J Chronic Dis* 1979, 32:563–576.

16. Rich-Edwards JW, Goldman MB, Willett WC, *et al.*: Adolescent body mass index and infertility caused by ovulatory disorder. *Am J Obstet Gynecol* 1994, 171:171–177.

17. Friss-Hansen: In *Human Body Composition.* Edited by Brozek J. Oxford: Pergamon Press; 1965:191–209.

18. Rimm AA, Werner LH, Yserloo BV, Bernstein RA: Relationship of obesity and disease in 73,532 weight-conscious women. Framingham data. *Public Health Rep* 1975, 90:44–54.

19. Engel: Vital Health and Statistics.

20. Blumberg VS, Alexander J: Obesity and the heart. In *Obesity.* Edited by Bjorntorp, Brodoff. Philadelphia: JB Lippincott; 1992: 517–531.

21. Sullivan M, Karlsson J, Siostrom L, *et al.*: Swedish obese subjects–an intervention study of obesity. Baseline evaluation of health and psychosocial functioning in the first 1743 subjects examined. *Int J Obes Rel Metab Disord* 1993, 17:503–512.

22. Kopleman PG: Altered respiratory function in obesity: sleep-disordered breathing and the Pickwickian syndrome. In *Obesity.* Edited by Bjorntorp, Brodoff. Philadelphia: JB Lippincott; 1992: 568–578.

23. Rosenbaum M, Nicolson M, Hersch J, *et al.*: Effects of gender, body composition, and menopause on plasma concentrations of leptin. *J Clin Endocrinol Metab* 1996; 81:3424–3427.

24. Licinio J, *et al.*: Sex differences in circulating human leptin pulse amplitude: clinical implications. *J Clin Endocrinol Metab* 1998, 83:4140–4147.

25. Rosenbaum M, Liebel RL, Hirsch J: Obesity. *N Engl J Med* 1997, 337:396–407.

BOTANICAL DIETARY SUPPLEMENTS

David Heber

6

Sales of botanical dietary supplements now exceed $1.5 billion a year and are increasing annually by about 25%. Although herbal products have been used for many years in other countries (notably Germany, where approximately $3 billion a year is spent on botanicals), their popularity in the United States has grown dramatically within the past 6 years. Studies have shown that about one third of the U.S. population now uses some form of alternative therapy. Consumers here are seeking alternative therapies to supplement modern conventional medicine. There are approximately 150,000 to 200,000 edible plant species in the world, and of these some 1200 to 1800 are available as botanical dietary supplements in this country.

The growing popularity of botanical dietary supplements can be ascribed to increased appreciation of products termed "organic" and "all natural," disenchantment with traditional medicine, fewer side effects perceived or observed with many gentle herbal remedies, and the relatively low cost of herbal products. German physicians have far greater experience with botanical dietary supplements than do their US counterparts. It is part of their formal medical school curriculum, and competence in this field is required for licensure. Seventy percent of German physicians prescribe botanicals, and so-called phytomedicines make up 30% of all drugs sold in German pharmacies. From 1978 to 1994, the German Federal Health Authority (equivalent to the US Food and Drug Administration) evaluated more than 80% of the herbs available on their market and compiled their findings in the *Commission E Monographs*, which provide taxonomic, pharmacologic, and clinical information of 410 herbal products. The monographs were recently translated into English and are now available in the United States from the American Botanical Council. Not all recommendations contained in the report are based on scientific data; no data are given after 1994, no references are cited, and "approval" did not require proof of "absolute" safety.

In the United States, the Dietary Supplement Health and Education Act of 1994 established a federal framework for the regulation of product labeling and information about dietary supplements. Dietary supplements are, for the first time, specifically defined to include vitamins, minerals, herbs and other botanicals, amino acids, and other dietary substances used to supplement the diet. The Act also allows product labeling to contain a statement describing how the product's consumption affects "structure or function" or general well-being in humans. However, it does not permit a manufacturer to make a specific health claim for a product. For example, product promotional material and packaging cannot claim to treat or prevent benign prostatic hypertrophy, but they can assert promotion of urinary tract health. The product label must carry the disclaimer: "This statement has not been evaluated by the Food and Drug Administration. This product is not intended to diagnose, treat, cure, or prevent any disease." The total quantity of all ingredients and the phrase "dietary supplement" must also be included on all labels [1]. Interdisciplinary research interactions among natural product chemists, agriculture and botany experts, and physician scientists are needed to integrate all of the relevant information into appropriately designed mechanistic and clinical studies in the future. Until this occurs, it will be important for physicians to have some familiarity with botanical dietary supplements to be able to advise their patients appropriately.

Overview

US HERBAL SUPPLEMENT SALES IN FOOD, DRUG, AND MASS MARKET RETAIL OUTLETS—1997			
Supplement	**Sales, $**	**Supplement**	**Sales, $**
Total herbal supplements	441,502,560	Grapeseed extract	9,965,772
Ginkgo	90,197,288	Evening primrose oil	7,299,353
Ginseng	86,048,080	Cranberry	6,182,210
Garlic	71,474,288	Valerian	6,104,450
Echinacea/Goldenseal	49,189,576	Bilberry	4,555,723
St. John's wort	47,774,792	Milk thistle	3,037,672
Saw palmetto	18,381,592	Kava kava	2,950,132

FIGURE 6-1. Herbal supplement sales in the United States in 1997. The legal definition of a dietary supplement according to the Dietary Supplement Health Education Act is a product (other than tobacco) that is intended to supplement the diet and bears or contains one or more of the following ingredients: a vitamin, a mineral, an herb or other botanical, an amino acid, a dietary substance for use by humans to supplement the total dietary intake; or a concentrate, metabolite, constituent, extract or any combination of any of the above ingredients. Consumer use of herbs and medicinal plants is one of the fastest-growing segments in retail pharmacies and mass market outlets. In the United States, herb supplement sales through mass market outlets in 1997 exceeded $441 million, which represents a dramatic 79.5% increase over the total 1996 sales of $246 million [2].

FIGURE 6-2. Therapeutic uses of herbal supplements. Herbs often contain several active substances that work synergistically to modify the effects of one another. The therapeutic effect of herbal preparations depends in part on purity, potency, and dosage. Herbs are generally used as tonics or adaptogens (substances that are believed to offer increased resistance to stress and to balance and normalize bodily functions). Other herbals are used more specifically, eg, as antibiotics, anti-inflammatory agents, astringents, digestive aids, emetics, emollients, expectorants, laxatives, sedatives, and stimulants.

THERAPEUTIC USES OF HERBAL SUPPLEMENTS

Adaptogens	Emollients
Expectorants	Antibiotics
Laxatives	Anti-inflammatory agents
Digestive aids	
Sedatives	Astringents
Stimulants	Emetics

Herbal Supplements

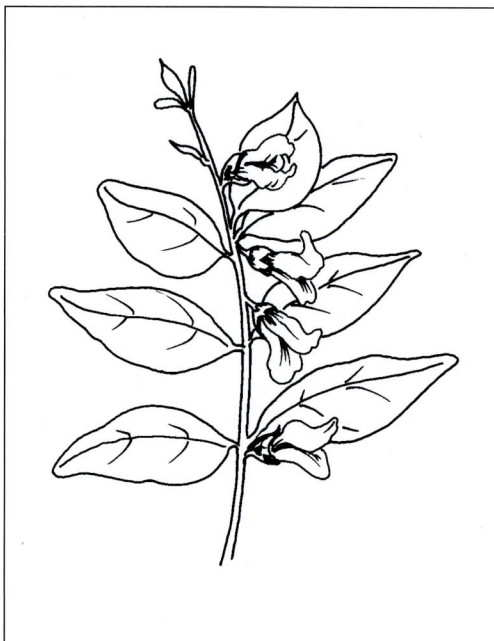

FIGURE 6-3. Astragalus. This member of the legume family is native to Northern China and Mongolia. The customary dosage is 3 to 6 g of dried root/day or the equivalent: 250 mg, twice a day, of a 10:1 root extract standardized to 0.4% 4'-hydroxy-3'-methoxy-isoflavone-7-glycoside, and greater than 10% total polysaccharides [3,4]. In traditional Chinese medicine it is used as a tonic, especially for the spleen and lungs; for treating infections of the mucous membranes of the urinary and respiratory tracts; and in combination with other herbs. Astragalus contains saponins, polysaccharides, and flavonoids, but the bioactivity of these constituents in mediating putative immune system-enhancing effects has not been established. It is also said to possess moderate diuretic activity and to cause vasodilation, but these actions (which are said to improve blood circulation) are also unproven. Astragalus has no known side effects or drug interactions, and the only contraindications (found in traditional Chinese medicine literature) are acute sickness with fever and thirst. No strong body of clinical trial evidence supports the use of astragalus at this time.

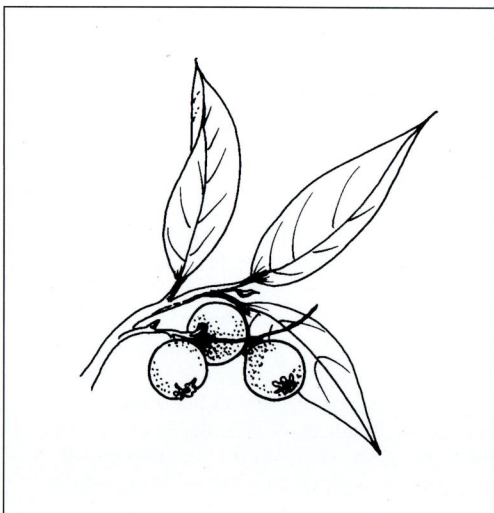

FIGURE 6-4. Bilberry (*Vaccinium myrtillus*). This small perennial shrub is related to the blueberry. Most members of this family grow well in the forests of Europe and also in temperate regions of the United States. Traditionally, bilberry has been used for many disorders, including poor night vision, scurvy, urinary infections and stones, digestive disorders, and gout. Standardized bilberry extract has low acute toxicity. Rare reports have described digestive disturbances, which can be minimized if the extract is taken with food. Patients with hemorrhagic disorders should use bilberry with caution. The recommended dosage is 80 mg, twice a day, of a fruit extract standardized to contain 25% anthocyanidins. The therapeutic dosage is 240 to 640 mg/d [5,6]. The main constituents are flavonoids in the form of anthocyanidins, which impart color and possess in vitro antioxidant activity. Some studies suggest that the fruit extract may be beneficial in the treatment of a variety of diverse conditions, primarily because of its beneficial effect on the microcirculatory system. Some actions of the extract are said to be vasoprotective, antiedemic, arterial vasomotive, and collagen-stabilizing. The anthocyanosides are active in increasing sensitivity of the retina to light. Clinical studies provide some support for the use of bilberry for peripheral vascular disorders, such as varicose veins and hemorrhoids; for microcirculatory disorders, including diabetic retinopathy; and for improved night vision.

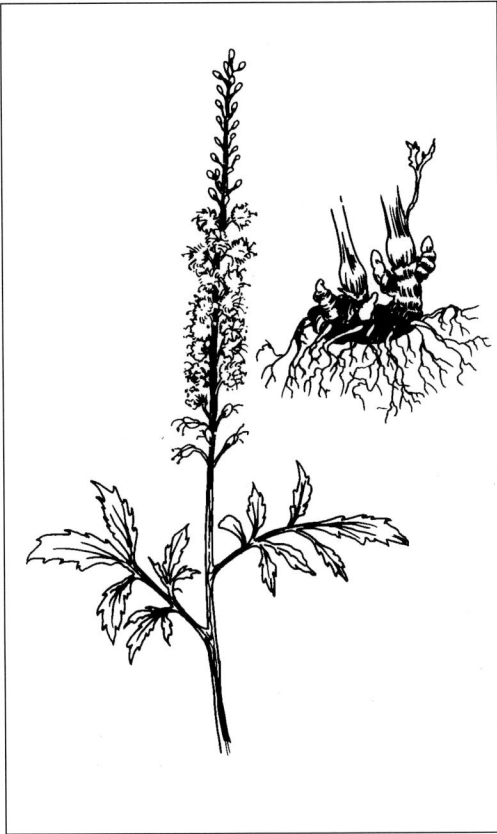

FIGURE 6-5. Black cohosh. This plant is also known as bugbane, a name stemming from a belief that the strong odor of the plant will repel insects. The root of the plant has traditionally been used by Native Americans to treat kidney ailments, malaria, rheumatism, and sore throat; to relieve menstrual cramps; and to ease labor. The chemical makeup of black cohosh is not completely known, but triterpene glycosides are considered the main potentially bioactive constituents. Very low concentrations of salicylates exist in the root, but the small amounts in black cohosh are unlikely to cause an allergic reaction in persons sensitive to acetylsalicylic acid. The primary therapeutic application of black cohosh is the treatment of menopausal symptoms, including hot flashes, headache, irritability, and depressive moods. The customary dosage is the equivalent of 40 mg of dried root, standardized to contain 2.5% triterpene glycosides [7]. There is not a strong body of clinical study data supporting its use for menopausal symptoms. Standardization of products is needed. Occasional gastric discomfort is the only noted side effect, and the root has been used in conjunction with estrogen replacement therapy without adverse effects.

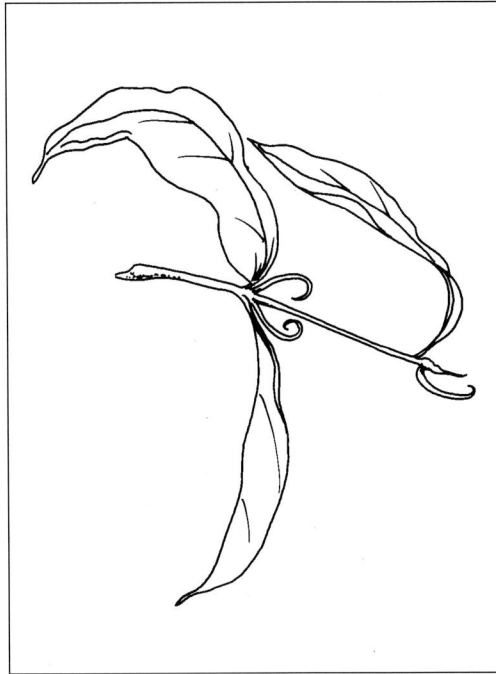

FIGURE 6-6. Cat's claw. The curved, sharp, protruding spines on the branches of the cat's claw vine explain its common name. Nearly all commercially available cat's claw is grown in Peru, where a decoction of the inner bark of the main stem (stem bark) and of the root (root bark) is commonly used to treat gastric ulcers. The bark has also been traditionally used in South America to relieve inflammations, including those associated with rheumatism, arthritis, and urinary tract infections. The customary daily dosage is 20 mg of a standardized root extract containing not less than 1.3% pentacyclic oxindole alkaloids and not more than 0.06% tetracyclic oxindole alkaloids [8–10]. The primary bioactive constituents of the inner barks of the root and stem are thought to be oxindole alkaloids. The root bark also contains proanthocyanidins. The stem bark of cat's claw has been shown to have beneficial effects against nonsteroidal anti-inflammatory drug enteropathy, and one of the primary uses of the bark is as an anti-inflammatory in patients with rheumatoid arthritis. The alkaloids present in cat's claw also have immunopotentiating effects. Possible side effects of cat's claw include increased uric acid excretion, fever, intermittent constipation or diarrhea, and fatigue. No published clinical data support use of this supplement.

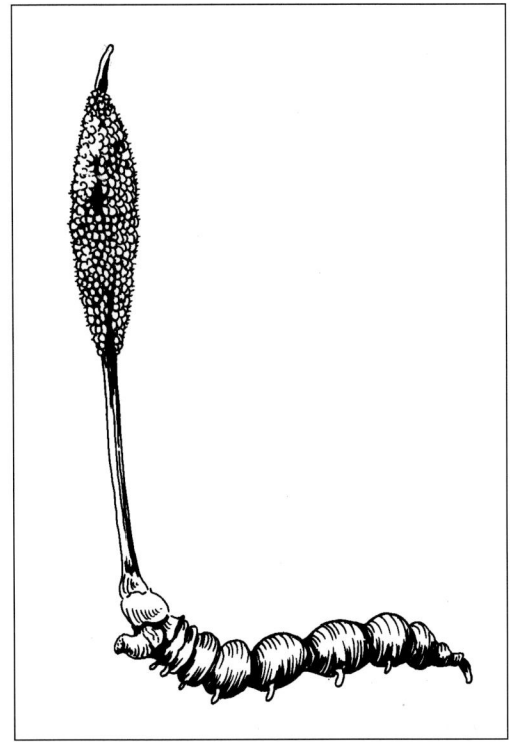

FIGURE 6-7. *Cordyceps sinesis*, also known as caterpillar fungus or vegetable-caterpillar. It is a parasitic fungus on the larvae of bat moths and has been used as a food and a medicine in Asia for thousands of years. Traditionally, it is used to treat fatigue and sexual dysfunction, as well as cough, anemia, tuberculosis, and lower back pain. The polysaccharides present in cordyceps have been shown to be hypolipidemic, and one of the current primary applications is in the treatment of hypercholesterolemia. Cordyceps is said to be useful for treating fatigue and improving tolerance to stress. Some users of the fungus have reported side effects of dry mouth, skin rashes, nausea, diarrhea, and drowsiness. Adenosine present in cordyceps has been shown to inhibit platelet aggregation; therefore, use of the product could potentiate anticoagulant and antithrombotic medications. The customary dosage is 3 to 9 g of fruiting bodies or mycelial fermentation product per day [11,12]. Some research in progress demonstrates a slight increase in anaerobic threshold under controlled exercise conditions.

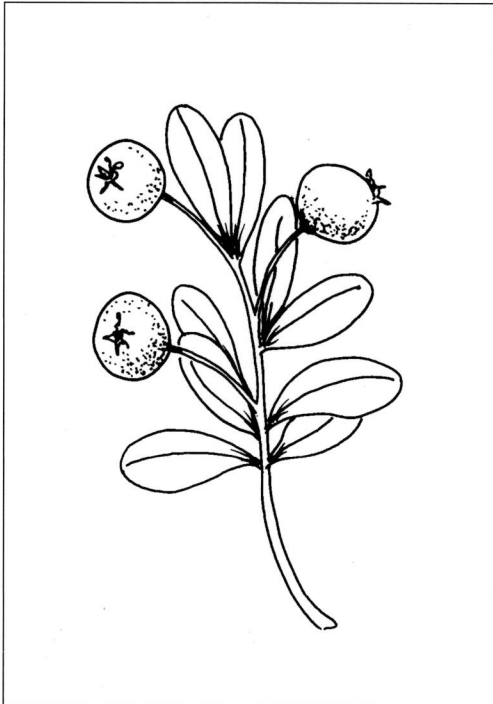

FIGURE 6-8. The American cranberry. This berry grows in damp bogs and mountain forests, with a range that extends as far north as Alaska and as far south as Tennessee. Its use in the United States dates back to 1621, when the pilgrims were said to have eaten them during the first Thanksgiving. New England sailors learned that those who consumed the berries avoided scurvy (because of the presence of vitamin C). More recently, cranberry fruit has been used to inhibit urinary tract infections. Cranberries contain numerous organic acids as active constituents, as well as anthocyanidins and vitamin C. The organic acids and antiadhesion effect of the cranberry (which inhibits adherence of bacteria to the mucosal walls of the urinary bladder) are responsible for its beneficial action. There are no known side effects, but urinary acidification from cranberry juice consumption could render certain antibiotics more effective (tetracycline, cycloserine, novobiocin, methenamine mandelate). The recommended intake is 500 mg of a 15:1 cranberry fruit–dry concentrate, equivalent to 10 ounces of cranberry juice cocktail and 30% total organic acids, or at least 3 to 6 ounces of pure cranberry juice per day [13,14]. Clinical studies have demonstrated the efficacy of cranberry juice and cranberry extracts as a urinary tract disinfectant.

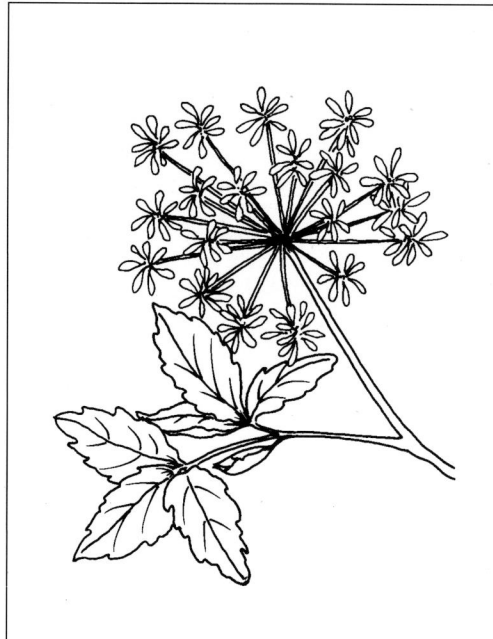

FIGURE 6-9. Dong quai (*Angelica sinesis*). This fragrant perennial herb belongs to the parsley family and grows in mainland China, Korea, and Japan. The dried roots, rich in volatile oils, have been used in China for several centuries as a valuable remedy in the treatment of menstrual disorders, menstrual cramps, and sterility in women. The usual daily dosage is 500 mg of a standardized root extract containing 1% ligustilides, or the equivalent of 3.5 g of powdered root/day [15,16]. Dong quai is generally considered safe, but coumarin derivatives present in the plant may potentiate anticoagulant therapy. All species of dong quai have a high saccharide content; therefore, ingestion may increase blood glucose levels. No published data demonstrate the effectiveness of this supplement for the relief of menstrual symptoms.

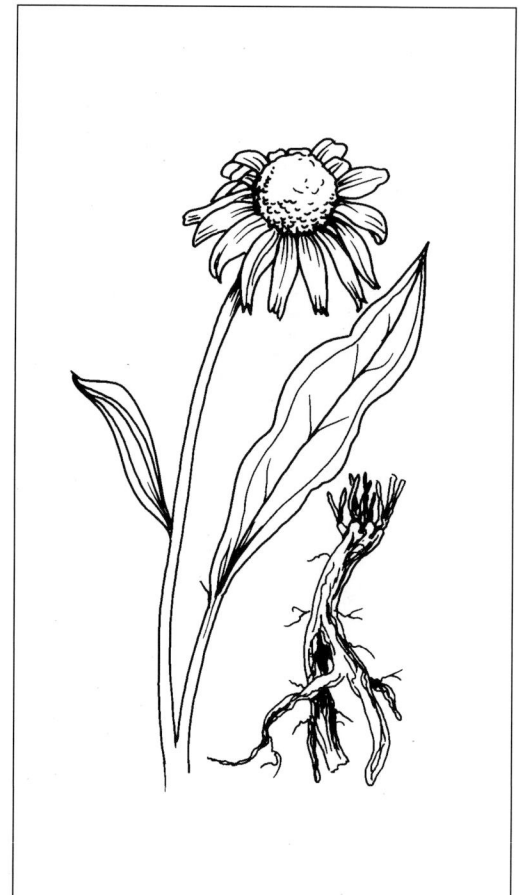

FIGURE 6-10. *Echinacea purpurea, E. angustifolia,* and *E. pallida.* These species are commercially important sources of herbal phytopharmaceuticals. Echinacea is a true native American medicinal plant, used by many American Indian tribes for a variety of ailments, including sore throat, toothache, tonsillitis, stings, and rattlesnake bites. The plant species contain a variety of chemical components that may contribute to their activity, but the identities of the bioactive fractions have not been established. Constituents found in Echinacea species include caffeic acid derivatives, polyacetylenes, flavonoids, and alkylamides, in addition to water-soluble polysaccharides (which have been implicated as one of the primary classes of immunostimulatory compounds). The usual dosage is 225 mg, twice daily, of a 6:1 *E. purpurea* root extract analyzed for content of alkenoic acid amide, cichoric acid, and polysaccharides of molecular weights ranging from 1500 to 50,000 [17–19]. Clinical studies have examined the use of *Echinacea* for acute infections, particularly colds and flu; for acute upper respiratory tract infections (to reduce the length and severity of symptoms); for strengthening and potentiating immune function; and as an anti-inflammatory in the treatment of rheumatoid arthritis. However, the number of supportive studies is small. Reported side effects of nausea, vomiting, and diarrhea occur in less than 0.5% of cases. *Echinacea* is usually used at the onset of acute infections, such as colds and flu. Prophylactic use beyond 6 weeks has traditionally been proscribed because of the potential for down-regulation of the immune-enhancing effects and even immunosuppression. These assertions have not yet been demonstrated in clinical trials.

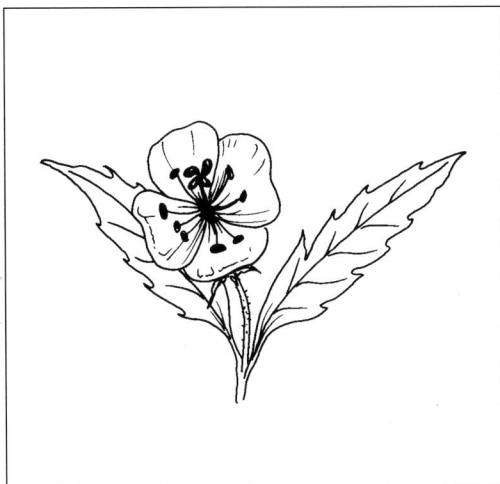

FIGURE 6-11. Evening primrose. This tall biennial, native to North America, is related to the fuschia. All parts of the plant are edible, including the leaves, seeds, and roots. The Shakers were known to prepare a tea from the roots for upset stomach. One of the most common modern uses is as a dietary supplement made from the seed oil, which supplies essential fatty acids (particularly omega-6 gamma-linolenic acid, a prostaglandin precursor). These essential fatty acids are thought to be the primary active ingredients in evening primrose oil. The usual daily dosage is 3 to 6 g of seed oil containing at least 9% gamma-linolenic acid [20,21]. No side effects or drug interactions are known. No strong body of published evidence supports the use of evening primrose oil.

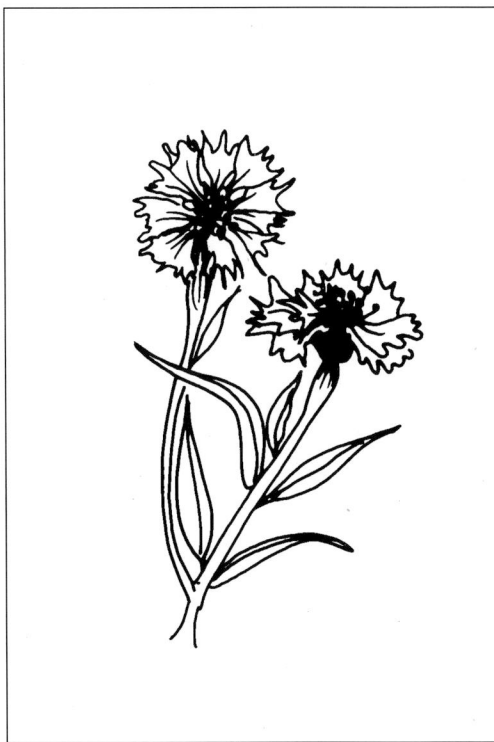

FIGURE 6-12. Feverfew. This bushy, leafy perennial member of the daisy family has been cultivated for centuries throughout Europe and grows throughout the Americas. In traditional medicine, it has been used against inflammation since the first century AD, and it has been used for more than 200 years as a headache remedy. Most of the antimigraine activity of feverfew has been attributed to its content of sesquiterpene lactones, of which parthenolide is the major component. The foliage of feverfew contains both sitosterol and stigmasterol, both of which are widespread plant sterols. Most clinical investigations of feverfew have focused on migraine prophylaxis, the primary application of the herb. No adverse drug interactions have been reported with use of feverfew, but the ingestion of the fresh leaf may cause a dry and sore tongue, swollen lips and mouth, and a loss of taste. Abdominal pain, indigestion, diarrhea, flatulence, nausea and vomiting, and hypersensitivity reactions have also been reported. For prophylaxis against migraine, the recommended daily dosage is 25 to 125 mg of a standardized leaf and flower extract containing a minimum of 0.2% parthenolide. Higher doses of up to 2 g per day may be required for acute treatment of migraine [22,23]. The clinical evidence supporting the use of feverfew for migraine headache prevention is relatively strong.

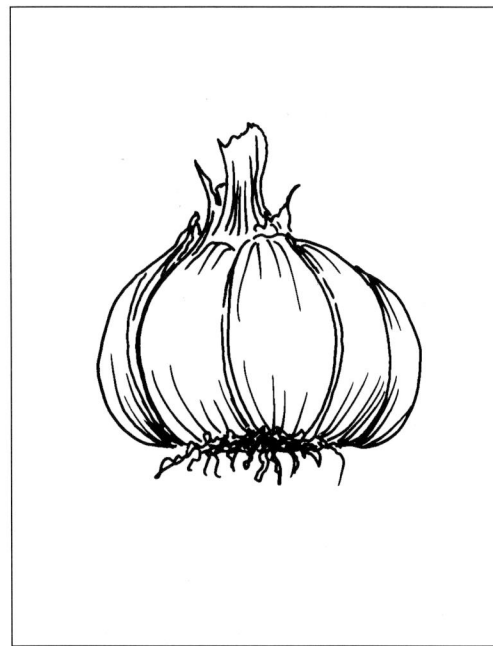

FIGURE 6-13. Garlic. Also called the "stinking rose," garlic is a common food plant used in all parts of the world and is one of the oldest cultivated plants. Hundreds of *Allium* species are known, and the genus includes chives, shallots, and common onion. Garlic has been valued as a flavoring, a food, and a medicine for thousands of years. Traditional and folk medicine uses for garlic have included a wide range of ailments, including colds, coughs, chronic bronchitis, earache, toothache, high blood pressure, arteriosclerosis, dandruff, and hysteria. The sulfur-containing compounds in garlic are the primary active constituents responsible for the therapeutic activity. Many of these compounds are unstable, however, and the chemical composition of garlic and garlic products may vary widely depending on cooking and processing. The usual dosage is 1 clove or 2 g of fresh garlic per day or the equivalent: 650 mg per day of a garlic powder standardized to contain 6 mg of allicin yield plus other garlic constituents [24–26]. Garlic is generally considered nontoxic, although large amounts of raw garlic can irritate the digestive mucosa. The actual occurrence of such side effects has not been well documented. A significant amount of research supports the modest cholesterol-reducing activity of garlic and suggests some potential mechanisms whereby this supplement may reduce blood pressure. A well-publicized study used garlic oil fraction and found no effects on lipids [27], but this study did not exclude an effect by whole garlic or aqueous extracts of garlic.

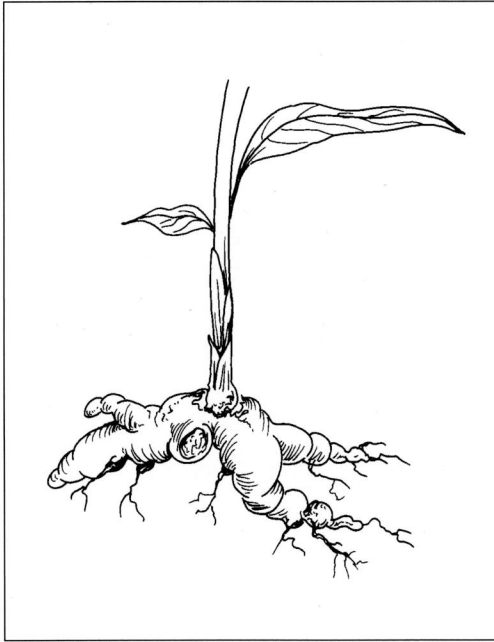

FIGURE 6-14. Ginger. The characteristic odor
and flavor of ginger make this root valued worldwide as a flavoring in foods. The root is often used
fresh but is also the source of the dried spice.
Ginger has been traditionally used in folk medicine
to treat indigestion, flatulence, diarrhea, malaria, and
fever. The primary constituents are the "pungent
principles" (gingerols and shogaols), which give
ginger its characteristic aroma. There are also
numerous volatile oils in the root. The primary uses
of ginger root relate to its antinauseant properties;
it can be effectively used to treat motion sickness,
morning sickness, indigestion, and nausea resulting
from chemotherapy. The usual dosage is one g of
dried, powdered root as needed for nausea, or the
equivalent in extract form standardized to contain
more than 5% gingerols and shogaols [28,29]. There
are no known side effects or drug interactions with
the use of ginger.

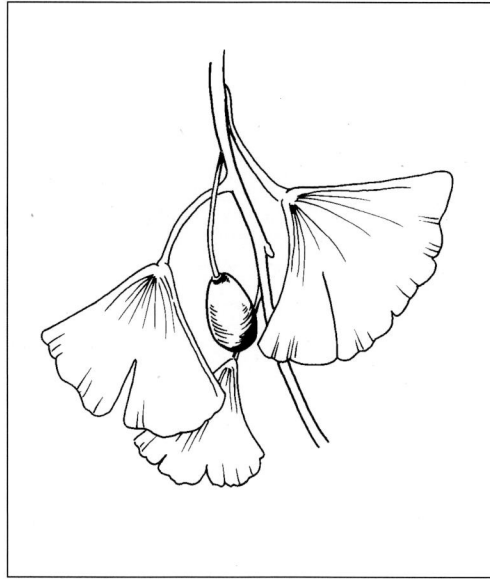

FIGURE 6-15. *Gingko biloba.* The Ginkgo tree has
been called a living fossil because it has existed for
more than 150 million years and is among the
oldest living species on earth. The fruits of nuts of
the tree have been used as medicine for thousands
of years, but Ginkgo extracts currently in use are
derived from the leaves. It is one of the most
widely used herbal preparations, and one of the
most popular botanicals prescribed in Germany.
The two primary active constituents are
ginkgolides and flavonoids. The flavonoids in the
Ginkgo leaf act as antioxidants; the ginkgolides
possess anti-inflammatory and anticoagulant
properties. The usual dosage is 120 to 240 mg/d in
divided doses of 50:1 standardized leaf extract
containing 22% to 27% ginkgo flavone glycosides
and 5% to 7% terpene lactones [30–32]. The efficacy of Ginkgo extract has been examined for
treating cerebral vascular insufficiency and peripheral vascular disorders, including hemorrhoids, varicose veins, phlebitis, and intermittent claudication.
Studies have also supported use of the herb for
mild to moderate dementia, memory deficits,
disturbances in concentration, depression, and
tinnitus associated with impaired cerebrovascular
circulation. No drug interactions or side effects
have been noted with the use of Ginkgo extract.
A recent study of Gingko use in patients with
Alzheimers disease or multi-infarct dementia
showed that cognitive performance and social
functioning stabilized and improved significantly [33].

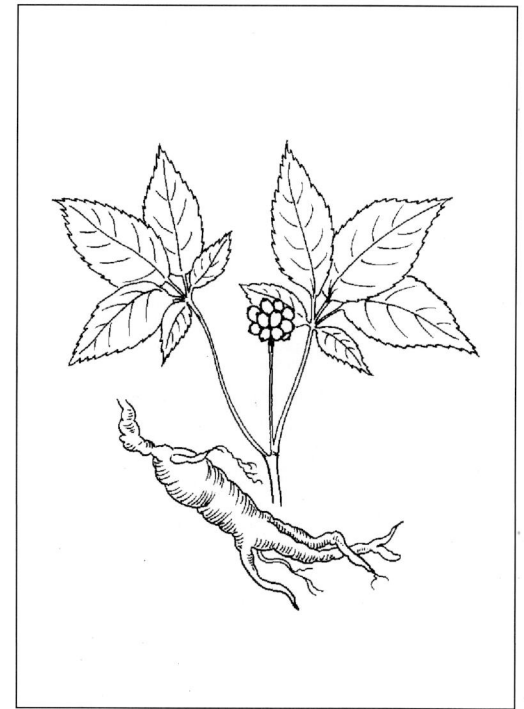

FIGURE 6-16. *Panax ginseng.* Ginseng is
mentioned in the oldest Chinese pharmacopoeia,
and it is estimated that ginseng may have been used
by the Chinese for the past 5000 years. *Panax
ginseng* is also known as Korean, Chinese, Asiatic,
or Oriental ginseng and should not be confused
with Siberian ginseng. The plant is cultivated in
Korea, northeastern China, Russia, and Japan, and
preparations of the root are traditionally used as a
tonic to increase energy and a sense of well-being.
The pharmacologically active components of
ginseng are thought to be the ginsenosides (triterpene saponins). There are 13 ginsenosides, however,
and the relative bioactivity of different preparations
has not been standardized, in part because of the
difficulty in designing studies to demonstrate its
activity in increasing energy. The customary dosage
is 100 mg, twice a day, of a 5:1 standardized root
extract containing more than 5% ginsenosides [34,35].

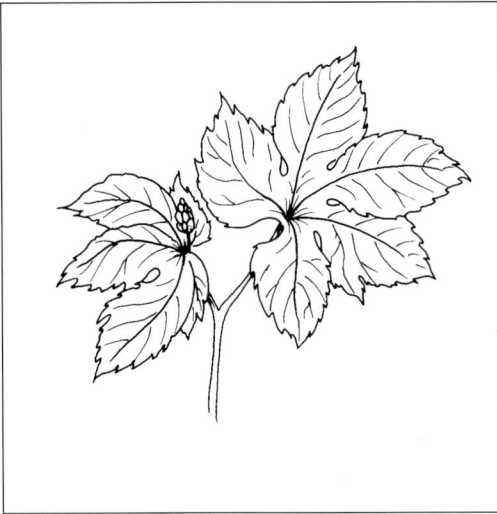

FIGURE 6-17. Goldenseal. This perennial plant is native to eastern North America. Native Americans have used goldenseal root as a source of brilliant yellow dye and have used it medicinally to treat inflammatory conditions brought on by allergy or infection. Its primary uses today are as a broad-spectrum antibiotic and as an antifungal and antiparasitic preparation. The medicinal effects of goldenseal have been attributed to the active constituents isoquinoline alkaloids, specifically berberine and hydrastine. The usual daily dosage is 250 to 500 mg of a 4:1 standardized root extract containing 5% total alkaloids [36–38]. Despite its reputed properties and its claimed benefit as an antibiotic and digestive aid, no strong research data support its use.

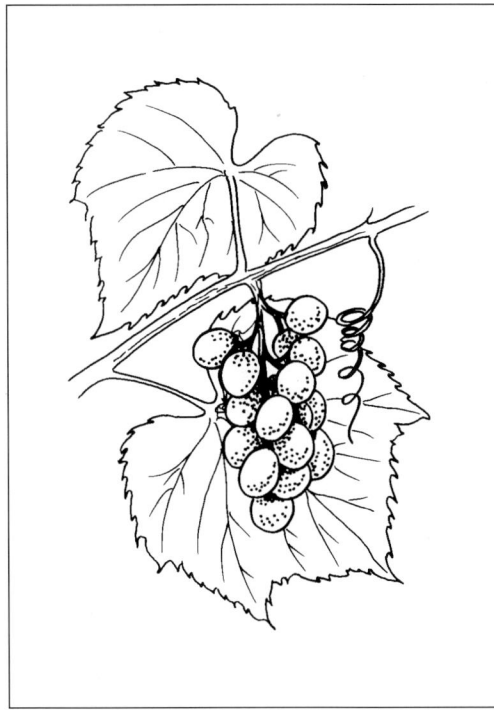

FIGURE 6-18. Grape seed. The medicinal uses of grapes (*Vitis vinifera*) can be traced to ancient times, when the sap, leaves, and juice of unripe fruits were used to treat a variety of conditions. Grape seed oil has also been reported to have beneficial properties, but current interest is focused on the proanthocyanidins (procyanidin oligomers [PCOs]) present in grape seeds. Extracts of grape seed display numerous pharmacologic properties, including cardioprotective, antioxidant, vasorelaxant, anti-mutagenic, and anti-inflammatory properties. The PCOs have been evaluated clinically, and some research supports its use to treat microcirculatory disorders, diabetic retinopathy, and capillary fragility. The PCOs act synergistically with vitamin C and potentiate the activity of the vitamin in wound healing. No side effects or drug interactions are known. The usual daily dosage is 50 to 100 mg of a 100:1 seed extract standardized to contain 80% 85% PCOs [39–42].

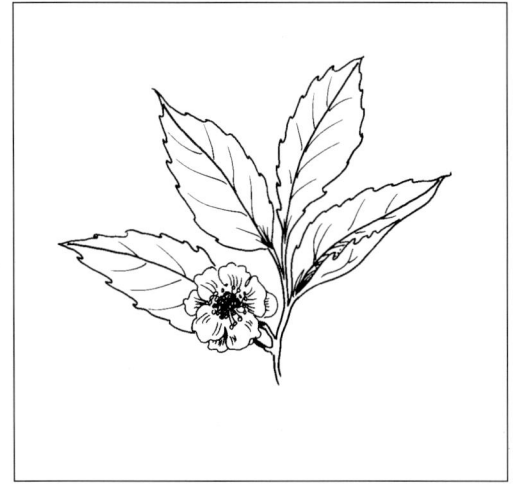

FIGURE 6-19. Green tea. Tea drinking is an ancient practice dating back more than 500,000 years. Green tea is heated or steamed quickly after harvest to arrest the enzymatic oxidation process of the catechins in the leaves. If not arrested, this process results in a reddish or yellow tea (oolong) or black tea depending on the duration of action of the endogenous plant oxidase enzymes in the leaf. The primary active ingredients in green tea are the catechins, or green tea polyphenols, but green tea also contains some caffeine. Preclinical, clinical, and epidemiologic data exist that support the use of green tea for its cancer chemopreventive and anti-carcinogenic properties and as a cellular and tissue antioxidant. Recently, animal studies have demonstrated that green tea inhibits angiogenesis both *in vivo* and *in vitro*, enhancing potential use of the tea in cancer prevention applications. The usual daily dosage of green tea is 250 to 500 mg of a standardized leaf extract containing 60% to 97% polyphenols, standardized on (-)-epigallocatechin-3-gallate (EGCG) content as the primary marker compound, or 4 to 10 cups of brewed tea daily [43–46]. Green tea is rich in potassium and should be avoided by patients who are on potassium-restricted diets.

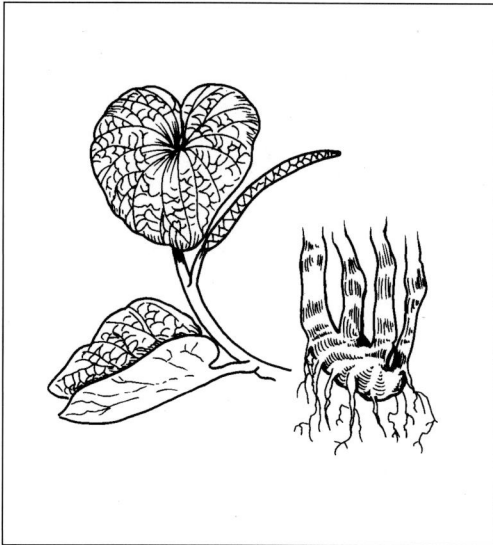

FIGURE 6-20. Kava kava. Kava is a slow-growing perennial and member of the pepper family that is native to Australia and islands of the South Pacific. Prepared kava root has been used for hundreds of years in the South Pacific as a ceremonial drink and has been used medicinally to treat cystitis, relieve headaches, and induce relaxation and sleep. Kava contains several potentially bioactive compounds, referred to collectively as kavalactones, which are centrally acting skeletal muscle relaxants. These constituents appear to have anxiolytic properties and provide relaxation. Thus, the primary uses of kava are to reduce anxiety, relieve stress, and serve as a muscle relaxant and sedative. For anxiety and muscle tension, the usual dosage is a standardized 11:1 root extract equivalent to 709 mg of kava-lactones, 1 to 3 times per day. For sedation, the equivalent of 210 to 500 mg of kavalactones should be taken 1 hour before bedtime [47–49]. Kava may heighten the effects and toxicity of ethanol and may potentiate the effects of barbiturates and benzo-diazepines.

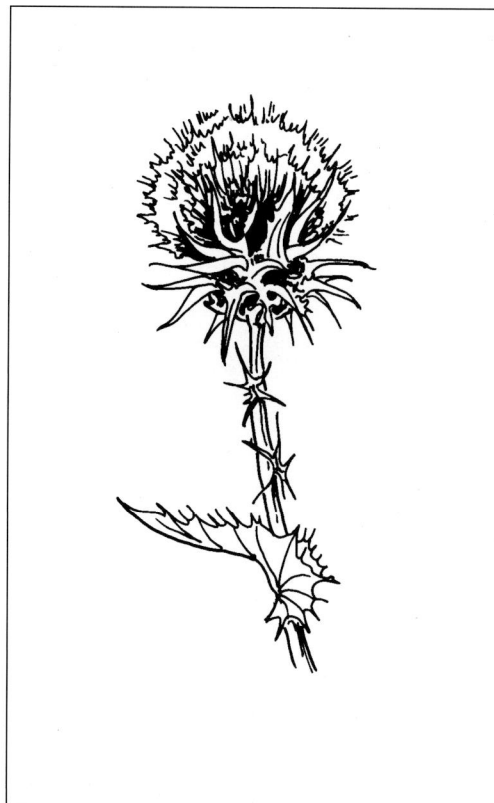

FIGURE 6-21. Milk thistle. Also known as wild artichoke, milk thistle grows wild throughout Europe and North America, often in wastelands and along roadsides. The leaves are edible (much like an artichoke), and roasted seeds of milk thistle can be brewed into a beverage. Its primary use historically was as a therapy for liver ailments. The seeds of milk thistle contain silymarin, the most likely bioactive constituent, and the seed extract is currently in use as a liver protectant. Silymarin has been shown to have hepatoprotective activity against a wide range of toxins that cause liver injury, including carbon tetrachloride and ethanol. Hepatic restoration has been demonstrated by improvements in liver function tests, and decreasing levels of alanine aminotransferase, aspartate amino-transferase, and bilirubin. Milk thistle consumption is considered exceptionally safe. The customary daily dosage, as a liver protectant, is 175 mg of a 30:1 seed extract standardized to contain 80% silymarin [50,51].

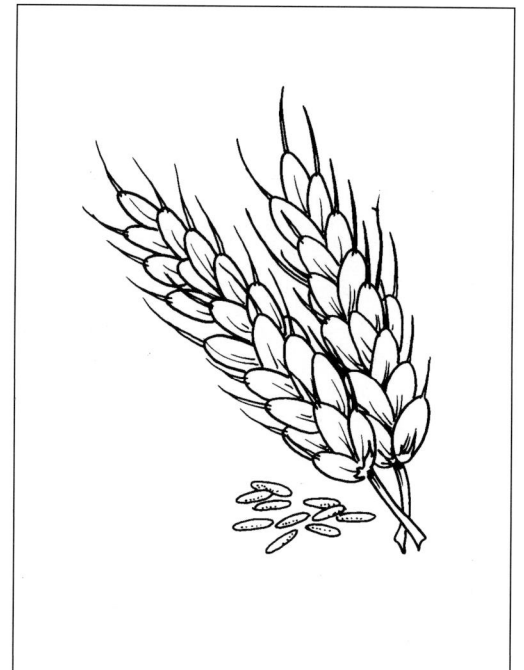

FIGURE 6-22. Red yeast rice. The use of red yeast rice can be traced back as far as 800 AD, during the Tang Dynasty. First recorded use of the product for heart conditions appeared in an ancient Chinese pharmacopoeia written during the Ming Dynasty (1368 to 1644). It was also recom-mended for indigestion and diarrhea and was said to promote the health of the stomach and spleen. Red yeast rice is traditionally prepared by fermenting boiled nonglutinous rice with red wine mash, natural juice of Polygonum grass, and alum water. The red yeast rice is composed of two organisms, *Monascus purpureus*, a mold that breaks down rice starch into simple sugar, and a yeast that allows further conversion into alcohol. The mold is cultivated on rice and develops a rich red pigment that permeates the rice grains, giving it its charac-teristic color. The primary active ingredient in red yeast rice is an hydroxymethylglutaryl coenzyme A (HMG-CoA) reductase inhibitor, monacolin K, which is also known as mevinolin and lovastatin. Other ingredients are a family of eight monacolin-related substances that inhibit HMG-CoA reduc-tase. Red yeast rice also contains sterols (beta-sitosterol, campesterol, stigmasterol, and sapogenin), isoflavones and isoflavone glycosides, and monounsaturated fatty acids. Extensive animal studies and studies in humans have demonstrated the hypercholesterolemic effects of red yeast rice. A recent study in humans found significant reduc-tions in total cholesterol, low-density lipoprotein cholesterol, and triglyceride levels in persons consuming a red yeast rice supplement for 8 weeks compared with those receiving placebo. The frequency of mild side effects (heartburn, flatulence, and dizzi-ness) is extremely low. The recommended dosage of red yeast rice is 1200 mg twice a day [52,53].

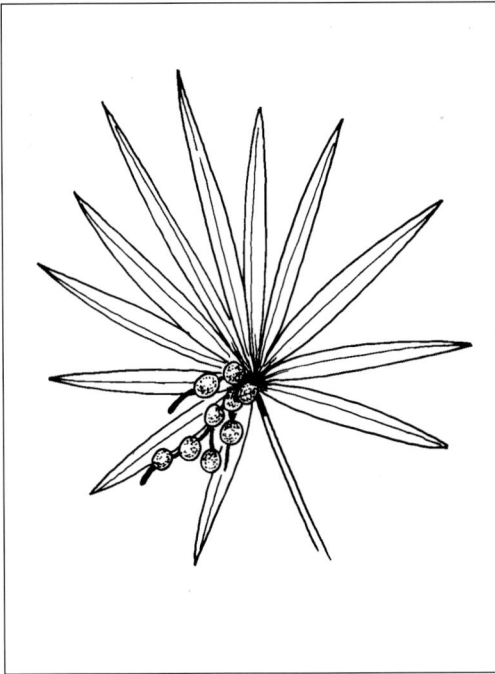

FIGURE 6-23. Saw palmetto (*Serenoa repens*). This evergreen palm is native to the southeastern United States, Central America, and the West Indies. Its stiff, palm-shaped leaves are covered with sharp teeth, which give the plant its common name. The saw palmetto also produces berries that look similar to olives and that turn from green to blue-black when ripe. American Indians and early naturo-pathic physicians prescribed the berries in treating diseases of the genitourinary tract in men. The berries have a long history and list of uses in folk medicine, including tumors, cystitis, epididymitis, diabetes, asthma, chronic bronchitis, kidney diseases, and indigestion. The lipophilic fraction of the oil present in the berries consists of fatty acids and sterols and is considered the active constituent. The primary activity is the inhibition of 5-alpha reductase, an enzyme responsible for the conversion of testosterone to 5-alpha dihydro-testosterone (DHT). An accumulation of DHT in the prostate is believed to contribute to enlarge-ment or hyperplasia of the prostate gland, and the primary use of saw palmetto is to relieve symp-toms of benign prostatic hypertrophy and relieve urination difficulties associated with this condition. The usual dosage is 160 mg, twice a day, of a 10:1 standardized liposterolic berry extract containing 85% to 95% fatty acids and sterols [54,55]. No drug interactions have been reported with saw palmetto.

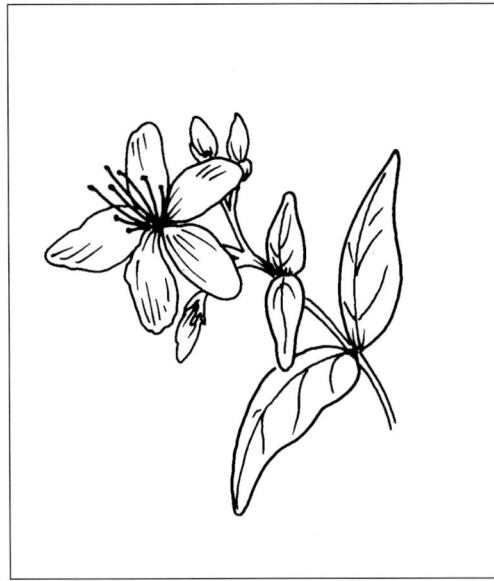

FIGURE 6-24. St. John's wort. Because of its habit of blooming heavily in June, the birth month of St. John the Baptist, *Hypericum perforatum* is commonly known as St. John's wort. There are hundreds of species of *Hypericum* around the world, and the perennial is especially abundant in the northwestern part of the United States. In the middle ages, the herb was used to protect against evil spirits and demonic possession. It was also used throughout history for wound-healing, as a diuretic, and as a treatment for sciatica. Since the late 1700s, herbal-ists have prescribed St. John's wort for treating depression, and current studies support its use to treat mild to moderate depression. The key active constituents are hypericin, a napthodianthrone; flavonoids and proanthocyanidins; and hyperforin. The usual dosage is 300 mg, three times daily, of a 5:1 extract standardized to contain 0.3% hypericin or 3% to 5% hyperforin. The efficacy of St. John's wort in treating depression is reported to be similar to that of standard tricyclic antidepressants, but the herb is associated with a lower incidence and severity of side effects. High doses followed by exposure to ultraviolet or bright sunlight may cause erythema in sensitive persons [56,57].

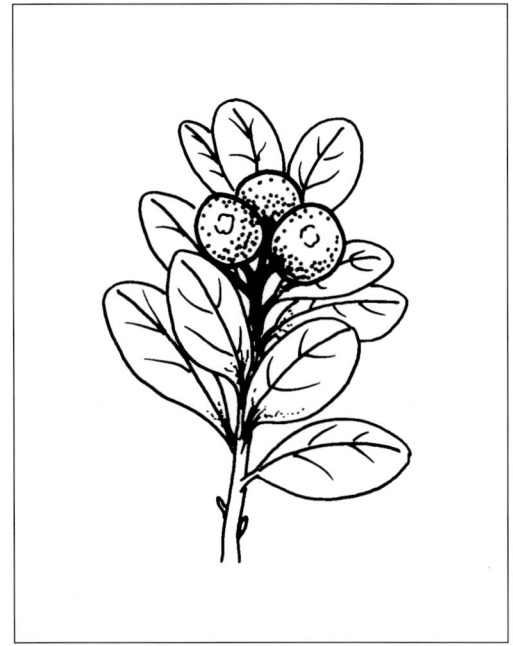

FIGURE 6-25. Uva-ursi. The bearberry, *Arctostaphylos uva-ursi*, is indigenous to the western region of North America. The plants are small and woody, with small leathery leaves and currant-sized berries. The berries are generally not used medici-nally, but the leaves are often employed in botanical medicine. The primary folk medicine uses of the plant have been in the treatment of inflammatory diseases of the urinary tract, including urethritis, chronic cystitis, nephritis, and urinary and renal calculi. Compounds in the leaves that are report-edly responsible for therapeutic activity include arbutin, a hydroquinone derivative; flavonoids; and tannins. The usual daily dosage is 125 to 250 mg of a standardized 5:1 leaf extract containing 20% arbutin [58,59]. Currently, the primary use of uva-ursi is as a urinary tract disinfectant and diuretic, but clinical studies are limited. Because of the high tannin content of uva-ursi, gastric distress can occur in some individuals.

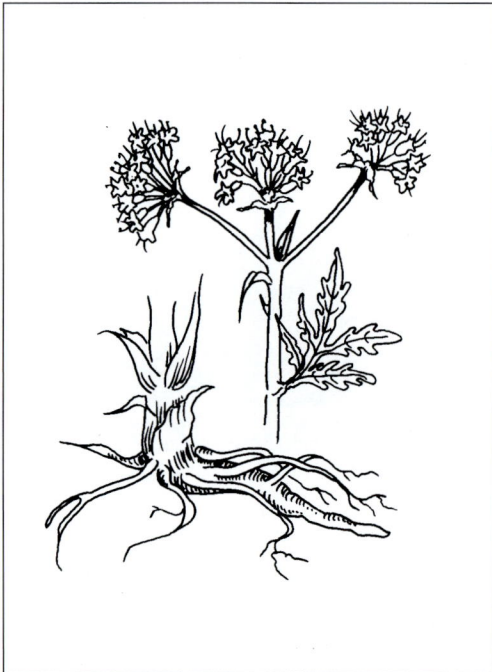

FIGURE 6-26. Valerian. The medieval Latin word, valere, means "to be healthy" or "well-being"; from this derivation comes the common name of *Valeriana officinalis*—allheal. Valerian is native to Europe but is naturalized throughout North America and is cultivated for its root. Traditionally, valerian has been used universally for its sedative properties. It was reportedly used by the ancient Greeks as an aromatic and diuretic and used to treat digestive disorders, flatulence, nausea, and urinary tract disorders. Tincture of the root is the form most often used. Several volatile oils are believed to be the active constituents, with the two major groups being sesquiterpenes and iridoids. Valerian also contains small amounts of flavonoids, triterpenes, and alkaloids. The contribution of the alkaloids to the pharmacologic activity of valerian is unknown. The bulk of clinical studies have investigated the efficacy of valerian as a sleep aid in the treatment of insomnia and for the improvement in the quality of sleep. The customary dosage is 350 to 500 mg of a root extract standardized to 0.8% valerenic acid, taken 40 to 60 minutes before bedtime [60,61]. The herb appears to be an effective sedative; however, it may potentiate other central nervous system depressants and should not be used concurrently with these agents.

Labeling of Herbal Supplements

Dietary Supplement of Amino Acids

Supplement Facts
Serving Size 1 tablet
Servings Per Container 100

Amount Per Tablet

Calories	15
Isoleucine (as L-isoleucine hydrochloride)	450 mg*
Leucine (as L-leucine hydrochloride)	620 mg*
Lysine (as L-lysine hydrochloride)	500 mg*
Methionine (as L-methionine hydrochloride)	350 mg*
Cystine (as L-cystine hydrochloride)	200 mg*
Phenylalanine (as L-phenylalanine hydrochloride)	220 mg*
Tyrosine (as L-tyrosine hydrochloride)	900 mg*
Threonine (as L-threonine hydrochloride)	300 mg*
Valine (as L-valine hydrochloride)	650 mg*

*Daily Value not established.

Other Ingredients: Cellulose, lactose, and magnesium stearate

FIGURE 6-27. Example of "Supplement Facts" box. New dietary supplement labeling regulations, mandated by the Dietary Supplement and Health Education Act of 1994, resulted in the new supplement labels, "Supplement Facts." The format is similar to the "Nutrition Facts" on food products and presents the constituents in the supplement. The products must be identified by the term "dietary supplement" as part of the product name, to distinguish them from conventional food. There are a few key differences between nutrition labels for foods and labels for dietary supplements: 1) serving sizes of foods are based on reference amounts; serving sizes of supplements are determined by the manufacturer; 2) ingredients in food products cannot be included in the "Nutrition Facts" box, but ingredients in supplements may be included in the "Supplement Facts" box; and 3) food product nutrition labeling must follow strict guidelines with regard to type size, spacing, use of bold face, and so forth, whereas supplement labeling has more relaxed formatting requirements [62].

Dietary Supplement Containing Dietary Ingredients with and without RDIs and DRVs

Supplement Facts
Serving Size 1 capsule
Servings Per Container 100

Amount Per Serving	% Daily Value
Calories 20	
Calories from Fat 20	
Total Fat 2 g	3%*
Saturated Fat 0.5 g	3%*
Polyunsaturated Fat 1 g	†
Monounsaturated Fat 0.5 g	†
Vitamin A 4250 IU	85%
Vitamin D 425 IU	106%
Omega-3 fatty acids 0.5 g	†

*Percent Daily Values are based on a 2000-calorie diet.
†Daily Value not established.

Other Ingredients: Cod liver oil, gelatin, water, and glycerin.

FIGURE 6-28. Dietary supplements containing dietary ingredients with and without recommended daily intake and daily recommended value. Some supplements may include ingredients for which a percentage daily value has been established, as well as ingredients that have no established daily value. Both food products and dietary supplements must provide the percentage daily value, based on a 2000-calorie diet, for ingredients that have an established daily value. On food product labels, insignificant amounts of nutrients are listed after the phrase "Not a significant source of...," whereas supplement labels flag nutrients with no daily value by using the statement "+DV [daily value] not established" [62].

PERMISSIBLE AND PROHIBITED CLAIMS

Types of Prohibited Statements	Examples of Prohibited Disease Claims	Examples of Permissible Structure/Function Claims
Effect on a specific disease or class of diseases	Protects against the development of cancer Reduces pain and stiffness associated with arthritis	Helps promote urinary tract health Helps maintain cardiovascular function Promotes relaxation
Drug or substitute for a drug	Antibiotic/antiseptic Laxative Diuretic Antidepressant Herbal Prozac	Energizer Rejuvenative Promotes regularity
Effect on signs or symptoms of a disease	Lowers cholesterol Reduces joint pain	Maintains healthy cholesterol levels Reduces stress and frustration Reduces absentmindedness
Role in body's response to a disease	Supports body's antiviral capabilities Supports body's ability to resist infection	Supports immune system
Treats, prevents, or mitigates adverse effects of a medical therapy or procedure	Helps avoid diarrhea associated with antibiotic use Reduces nausea associated with chemotherapy	Helps maintain healthy intestinal flora

FIGURE 6-29. Permissible and prohibited claims for supplements. The provisions of the Dietary Supplement and Health Education Act of 1994 that relate to claims regulation state that dietary supplements may carry "structure/function" claims, but not claims purporting drug-like effects. An allowable structure/function claim must be truthful and must not contain any misleading statements; it must appear in a context that does not suggest that the product treats, prevents, or mitigates a disease. The claim should contain only statements about the effect of the product on a body system, organ, or function for maintenance of good health and nutrition [62].

References

1. McKenna DJ, ed: *Natural Dietary Supplements: A Desktop Reference.* St. Croix, NM: Institute for Natural Products Research; 1998.

2. *The Complete German Commission E Monographs: Therapeutic Guide to Herbal Medicines.* Edited by Blumenthal M, Busse WR, Goldberg A, *et al.* Austin, TX: American Botanical Council; 1998:11.

3. Kitagawa I, Wang HK, Yoshikawa M, *et al.*: Saponin and sapogenol, XXXIV. Chemical constituents of *Astragali radix,* the root of *Astragalus membranaceus* Bunge. *Chemical and Pharmaceutical Bulletin* 1983, 31:689–697.

4. Morrazzoni PE, Bombardellie E: *Indena Scientific Documentation.* Milan: Indena: March 30, 1994.

5. Murray M: Bilberry (*Vaccinium myrtillus*). *Am J Nat Med* 1997, 4:18–22.

6. Cunio L: *Vaccinium myrtillus. Aust J Med Herb* 1993, 5:81–85.

7. Liske E: Therapeutic efficacy and safety of *Cimicifuga racemosa* for gynecological disorders. *Adv Ther* 1998, 15:45–53.

8. Keplinger K, Laus G, Wurm M, *et al.*: Uncaria tomentosa—ethnomedical use and new pharmacological, toxicological and botanical results. *J Ethnopharmacol* 1999, 64(1): 23–24.

9. Wurm M, Kacani L, Laus G, *et al.*: Pentacyclic oxindole alkaloids from *Uncaria tomentosa* induce human endothelial cells to release a lymphocyte-proliferation-regulating factor. *Planta Medica* 1998, 64(8): 701–704.

10. Sandoval M, Mannick EE, Mahra J, *et al.*: Cat's claw (*Uncaria tomentosa*) protects against oxidative stress and indomethicin-induced intestinal inflammation [Abstract]. *Gastroenterology* 1997, 112:A1091.

11. Zhu JS, Halpern GM, Jones K: *Cordyceps sinensis*: the scientific rediscovery of an ancient Chinese herbal medicine. Part II. *J Altern Complement Med* 1998;4(4): 429–457.

12. Shiao MS, Wang ZN, Lin LJ, *et al.*: Profiles of nucleosides and nitrogen bases in Chinese medicinal fungus *Cordyceps sinensis* and related species. *Botanical Bulletin of Academia Sinica* 1994, 35:161–167.

13. Ahuja S, Kaack B, Roberts J: Loss of fimbrial adhesion with the addition of *Vaccinium macrocarpon* to the growth medium of P-fimbriated *Escherichia coli. J Urol* 1998, 159:559–562.

14. Chernomordik AB, Vasilenko EG: [Increased activity of novobiocin and widening of its antimicrobial spectrum]. *Antibiotiki* 1981, 26:456–460.

15. Belford-Courtney R: Comparison of Chinese and Western uses of *Angelica sinensis. Aust J Med Herb* 1993, 5:87–91.

16. Zhu DP: Dong quai. *Am J Chinese Med* 1987, 15:117–125.

17. Bauer R: Echinacea: biological effects and active principles. In: *Phytomedicines of Europa: Chemistry and Biological Activity.* Edited by Lawson JD, Bauer R. ACS symposium series 691. Washington, DC: American Chemical Society; 1998:140–157.

18. Bauer R, Wagner H. Echinacea species as potential immunostimulatory drugs. In: *Economic and Medicinal Plant Research,* edn 5. Edited by Farnsworth NR, Wagner H. New York: Academic Press; 1991:253–321.

19. Melchart D, Walther E, Linde K, *et al.*: Echinacea root extracts for the prevention of upper respiratory infections: a double-blind placebo-controlled randomized trial. *Arch Fam Med* 1998, 7:541–545.

20. Hudson BJF: Evening primrose (*Oenothera* spp.) oil and seed. *Journal of the American Oil Chemists' Society* 1984, 61:540–543.

21. Horrobin DF: Nutritional and medical importance of gamma-linolenic acid. *Prog Lipid Res* 1992, 31:163–194.

22. Murphy JJ, Heptinstall S, Mitchell JRA: Randomized double-blind placebo-controlled trial of feverfew in migraine prevention. *Lancet* 1988, 2(8604): 189-192.

23. Bohlmann F, Zdero C: Sesquiterpene lactones and other constituents from *Tanacetum parthenium. Phytochemistry* 1982, 21:2543–2549.

24. Warshafsky S, Kramer RS, Sivak SL: Effect of garlic on total serum cholesterol. *Ann Intern Med* 1993, 119:599–605.

25. Abdullah TH, Kandil O, Elkadi A, *et al.*: Garlic revisited: therapeutic for the major diseases of our times. *J Natl MedAssoc* 1988, 80:439–445.

26. Phelps S, Harris WS: Garlic supplementation and lipoprotein oxidation susceptibility. *Lipids* 1993, 28:475–477.

27. Berthold HK, Sudhop T, von Bergmann K: Effect of a garlic oil preparation on serum lipoproteins and cholesterol metabolism: a randomized controlled trial. *JAMA* 1998, 273:1900–1902.

28. Wood CD, Manno J, Wood M, *et al.*: Comparison of ginger with various antimotion sickness drugs. *Clin Res Pract Drug Reg Aff* 1988, 6:129–136.

29. Tanabe M, Chen Y, Saito K, *et al.*: Cholesterol biosynthesis inhibitory component from *Zingiber officinale. Chem Pharm Bull* 1993, 41:710–713.

30. LeBars P, Katz MM, Berman N, *et al.*: A placebo-controlled, double-blind randomized trial of an extract of *Ginkgo biloba* for dementia. *JAMA* 1997, 278:1327–1332.

31. Kleijnen J, Knipischild P: *Ginkgo biloba. Lancet* 1992, 340:1136–1139.

32. Huh H, Staba EJ: The botany and chemistry of *Ginkgo biloba* L. *Journal of Herbs, Spices and Medicinal Plants.* 1992, 1:92–124.

33. LeBars PL, Katz MM, Berman N, *et al.*: A placebo-controlled, double-blind randomized trial of an extract of *Ginkgo biloba* for dementia. North American Egb Study Group. *JAMA* 1997, 278:1327–1332.

34. Shibata S, Tanak O, Shoji J, *et al.*: Chemistry and pharmacology of *Panax.* In: *Economic and Medicinal Plant Research.* Edited by Wagner H, Hikimo H, Farnsworth NR. New York: Academic Press; 1985:217–284.

35. Javetsky K, Morreale AP: Probable interaction between warfarin and ginseng. *Am J Health System Pharm* 1997, 54:692–693.

36. Leung AY, Foster S: *Encyclopedia of Common Natural Ingredients Used in Food, Drugs and Cosmetics.* New York: John Wiley & Sons, Inc.; 1996.

37. Kaneda Y, Torii M, Tanaka T, *et al.*: In vitro effects of berberine sulphate on the growth and structure of *Entamoeba histolytica, Giardia lamblia* and *Trichomonas vaginalis. Ann Trop Med Parasitol* 1991, 85:417–425.

38. Rabbani GH, Butler T, Knight J, *et al.*: Randomized controlled clinical trial for diarrhea due to entertoxigenic *Escherichia coli* and *Vibrio cholerae. J Infect Dis* 1987, 155:979–984.

39. Bombardelli E, Morazzoni P: *Vitis vinifera* L. *Fitoterapia* 1995, 66:291–317.

40. Lanningham-Foster L, Chen C, Chance DS, *et al.*: Grape extract inhibits lipid peroxidation of human low density lipoprotein. *Biol Pharm Bull* 1994, 18:1347–1351.

41. Liviero L, Puglisi PP, Morazzoni P, *et al.*: Antimutagenic activity of procyanidins from *Vitis vinifera. Fitoterapia* 1994, 65:203–209.

42. Schwitters B, Masquelier J: *OPC in Practice. Bioflavonols and Their Application.* Rome: Alfa Omega; 1993.

43. Stoner G, Mukhtar H: Polyphenols as cancer chemopreventive agents. *J Cell Biochem* 1995, 22(Suppl):169–180.

44. Komori A, Yatsunami J, Okabe S, *et al.*: Anticarcinogenic activity of green tea polyphonols. *Jpn J Clin Oncol* 1993, 23:186–190.

45. Mitscher LA, Jung M, Shankel D, *et al.*: Chemoprotection: a review of the potential therapeutic antioxidant properties of green tea (*Camellia sinensis*) and certain of its constituents. *Med Res Rev* 1997, 17:327–365.

46. Cao Y, Cao R: Angiogenesis inhibited by drinking tea. *Nature* 1999, 398:381.

47. Duve RN: Gas-liquid chromatographic determination of major constituents of Piper Methysticum. *Analyst* 1981, 106:160–165.

48. Volz HP, Kieser M: Kava-kava extract WS 1490 versus placebo in anxiety disorders: a randomized placebo-controlled 25-week outpatient trial. *Pharmacopsychiatry* 1997, 30:1–5.

49. *The Complete German Commission E Monographs: Therapeutic Guide to Herbal Medicine.* Edited by Blumenthal M, Busse WR, Goldberg A, *et al.* Austin, TX: American Botanical Council; 1998:156–157.

50. Dehmlow C, Erhard J, deGroot H: Inhibition of Kupffer cell functions as an explanation for the hepatoprotective properties of silibinin. *Hepatology* 1996, 23:749–754.

51. Valenzuela A, Lagos C, Schimdt K, *et al.*: Silymaring protection against hepatic lipid peroxidation induced by acute ethanol intoxication in the rat. *Biochem Pharmacol* 1985, 34:2209–2212.

52. Zhu Y, Li CL, Wang YY, *et al.*: Monascus purpureus (red yeast): a natural product that lowers blood cholesterol in animal models of hypercholesterolemia. *Nutr Res* 1998, 18:71–81.

53. Heber D, Yip I, Ashley JM, *et al.*: Cholesterol-lowering effects of a proprietary Chinese red-yeast-rice dietary supplement. *Am J Clin Nutr* 1999, 69:231–236.

54. Lowe FC, Ku JC: Phytotherapy in treatment of benign prostatic hyperplasia: a critical review. *Urology* 1996, 48:12–20.

55. Rhodes L, Primka RL, Berman C, *et al.*: Comparison of finasteride, a 5 alpha reductase inhibitor, and various commercial plant extracts in vitro and in vivo 5 alpha reductase inhibition. *Prostate* 1993, 22:43–51.

56. St John's wort—*Hypericum perforatum* (Insert). Edited by Upton R. American Herbal Pharmacopeia and Therapeutic Compendium. *Herbal Gram* 1997, 40:32.

57. Linde K, Ramirez G, Mulrow CD, *et al.*: St. John's wort for depression: an overview and meta-analysis of randomized clinical trials. *Br Med J* 1996, 313:253–258.

58. Bradley P, ed: *British Herbal Compensium*, vol I. Bournemouth, England: British Herbal Medicine Association; 1992.

59. Blumenthal MH, Busse WR, Goldberg A et al. (eds). The Complete German Commission E Monograph. Austin, TX: American Botanical Council, 1998: 224–225.

60. Morazzoni P, Bombardelli E: *Valerian officinalis*: traditional use and recent evaluation of activity. *Fitoterapia* 1995, 66:99–112.

61. Dressing H, Reimann D, Low H, *et al.*: Insomnia: are valerian/melissa combinations of equal value to benzodiazepine? *Therapiewoche* 1992, 42:726–736.

62. Storlie J: DSHEA revisited: understanding and using the supplement facts label. *Scan's Pulse* 1996, 15:7–8.

7

DIAGNOSIS AND VERTICALLY INTEGRATED MANAGEMENT OF OBESITY

David Heber

Obesity, defined as excess body fat accumulation, ultimately results from an increase in energy intake over expenditure. However, energy efficiency varies partly on the basis of body composition. Body weight for height or body mass index (BMI, weight in kilograms divided by height in meters squared) is used to diagnose obesity even though these measurements are only indirect measures of body fat. Body fat can be estimated by using bioelectrical impedance analysis; the advantage is that lean overweight persons, such as athletes, can be differentiated from fat overweight persons. In addition, persons of normal weight who have reduced muscle mass because of inadequate protein intake, reduced physical activity, or the effects of drugs that reduce muscle mass can be identified as having excess body fat.

The therapeutic impact of this differentiation is significant. Persons who have increased lean mass will have a higher than average target weight and need to be encouraged to maintain their lean body mass through exercise and adequate protein intake. They must also be encouraged to accept their target weight, which may be higher than what they imagined. Each pound of lean body mass burns about 14 calories per day. Persons with reduced lean body mass can be encouraged to increase lean body mass through heavy resistance exercise in order to increase basal metabolic rate.

Vertically integrated management of obesity is a system in which the method used correlates with the severity of obesity, as measured by body mass index. In overweight and mildly obese persons, diet, exercise, and lifestyle methods are used. The behavioral tools available include confirmation of readiness to change, use of stimulus control to minimize the intake of trigger foods, use of meal replacements and portion-controlled meals to reduce caloric intake, aerobic and heavy resistance exercise, relapse prevention, social support, and stress reduction. Pharmacotherapy is added for persons who have a BMI greater than 30, or greater than 27 with comorbid conditions. Appetite suppressants, satiety agents, and lipase inhibitors are available, and other approaches are still undergoing research. Gastric surgery for obesity can be considered for persons who have a BMI of 35 to 40 and have sleep apnea or other significant morbidity or for persons with a BMI greater than 40. For patients using drugs or undergoing surgery, the same principles of diet, exercise, and lifestyle used for milder forms of obesity are followed. Drugs and surgery are adjuncts to diet and lifestyle change for the treatment of obesity.

Diagnosis of Obesity

WHAT PHYSICIANS SAY ABOUT TREATING OBESITY
"I don't have time during office visits."
"Weight loss is temporary, so why bother?"
"There are no good programs that really work."
"Patients are here to see me for illness."
"I don't get reimbursed for obesity."
"If there were a proven and affordable program available, I would use it!"

FIGURE 7-1. Common reasons given by physicians for failing to recognize and treat obesity as a medical problem in their offices. These include lack of time, lack of knowledge, and economic factors.

PHYSICIAN: AGENT OF CHANGE
Physician is more effective in 10 min than any allied health professional is in 40 min.
Programs prove the success of meal replacements: portion-controlled, affordable, easy, and available.
Doctor can bill for comorbid conditions.
Reduction in costs, increase in patient satisfaction, and retention in practice are associated benefits.

FIGURE 7-2. Arguments for the physician taking a primary role in the management of obesity. These arguments include 1) studies showing that the physician is a more effective agent of behavior change than allied health professionals are; 2) evidence that time-efficient methods, including meal replacements and portion-controlled meals, can be effective in the office setting; and 3) billing for comorbid conditions, cost savings, and increased patient satisfaction result from successful management of obesity in the office setting.

DURING THE OFFICE VISIT

Measure weight, height, and body mass index

Assess comorbid conditions

Communicate to the patient your interest in their undertaking a weight loss program

Outline trigger foods and a simple meal replacement plan for the patient

Provide follow-up and support lifestyle changes

FIGURE 7-3. Components of the office visit for obesity. These include a determination of body mass index, comorbid conditions, communication of physician concern to the patient, counseling on trigger foods, the prescription of meal replacements and portion-controlled meals, and provision for follow-up and lifestyle change.

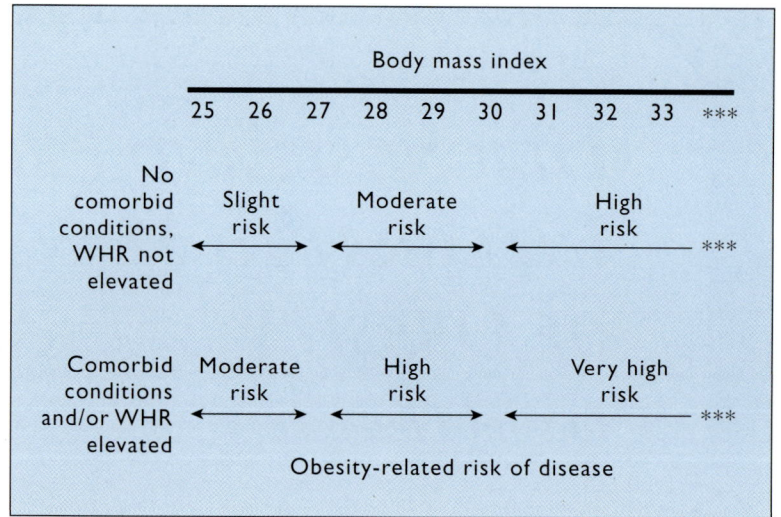

FIGURE 7-4. Influence of comorbid conditions (hypertension, hyperlipidemia, diabetes mellitus, sleep apnea) or elevated waist-to-hip ratio (WHR) (or simply waist circumference) on how body mass index affects disease risk. The diagnosis of obesity must be considered in the context of comorbid diseases, and weight reduction should be used as a part of the therapy for these conditions. Body mass index can be defined by using widely available charts or calculated as the weight in pounds multiplied by the factor 705 and divided by the height in inches squared. (*Adapted from* National Institutes of Health [1].)

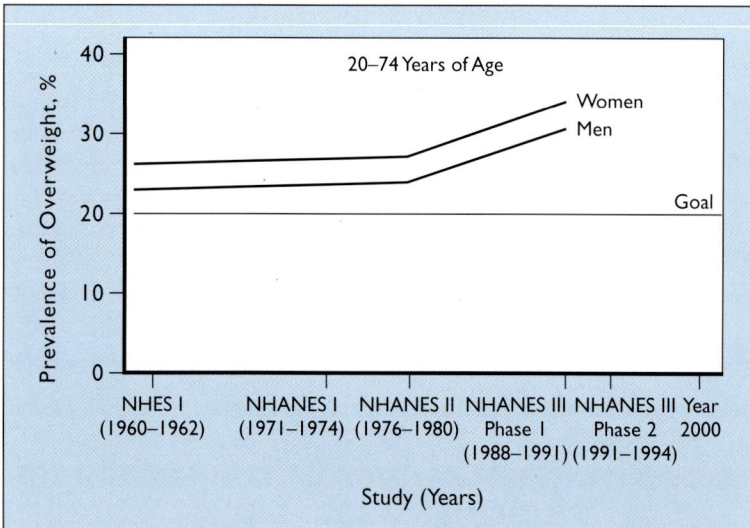

FIGURE 7-5. Age-adjusted prevalence of overweight for US population *vs* year 2000 objective. If body mass index is fixed at an arbitrary level (about 27) to diagnose the presence or absence of obesity in the population, as was done in the National Health and Nutrition Examination Survey (NHANES), there was a 30% increase in the average incidence of obesity (from 24% to 32% of the U.S. population) in the past decade. The reasons for this increased incidence are not fully understood. In some ethnic groups (Hispanic and African-American women), the incidence of obesity approaches 50%. NHES—National Health and Examination Survey. (*From* Kuczmarksi et al. [2].)

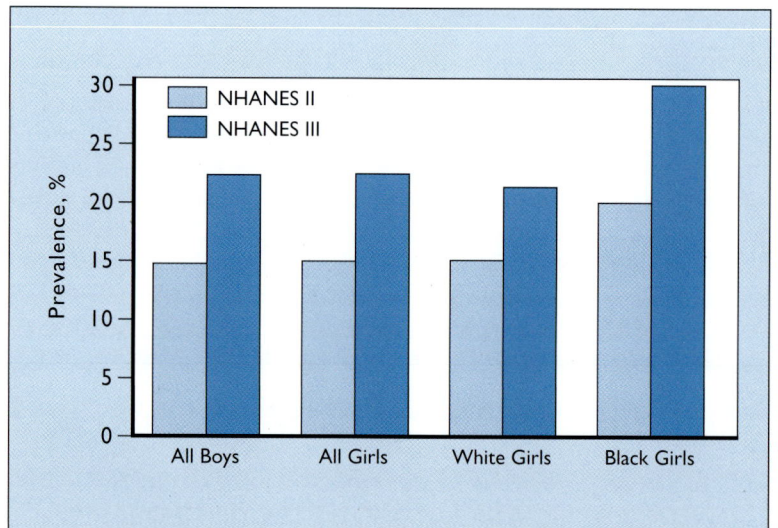

FIGURE 7-6. Age-adjusted prevalence of overweight, ages 12–17 y. An increase in adolescent obesity is seen in the National Health and Nutrition Survey. These changes in body fat during adolescence are being studied to determine their effects on lifetime risks of chronic disease. However, the rate of non–insulin-dependent diabetes mellitus has already increased among adolescents and even preadolescents in certain ethnic groups. The prevention and treatment of adolescent obesity are major public health objectives.

BMI AND THERAPY

BMI, 20–27: Diet, exercise, lifestyle

BMI, 27–30, plus comorbid conditions: Diet, exercise, lifestyle/pharmacotherapy

BMI, 30–40: Diet, exercise, lifestyle/pharmacotherapy

BMI, > 40: Diet, exercise, lifestyle/surgery

FIGURE 7-7. Body mass index and therapy. In the vertically integrated management of obesity, body mass index is used as a guide to therapeutic options while diet, exercise, and lifestyle changes continue to be used with each form of therapy. For patients with comorbid conditions and a body mass index of 27 and for patients without comorbid conditions and a body mass index of 30, pharmacotherapy is an option when diet, exercise, and lifestyle change alone are not adequate. Similarly, surgery is an option for patients with a body mass index of 40 in whom pharmacotherapy has failed; however, diet, exercise, and lifestyle change are used along with the surgical intervention.

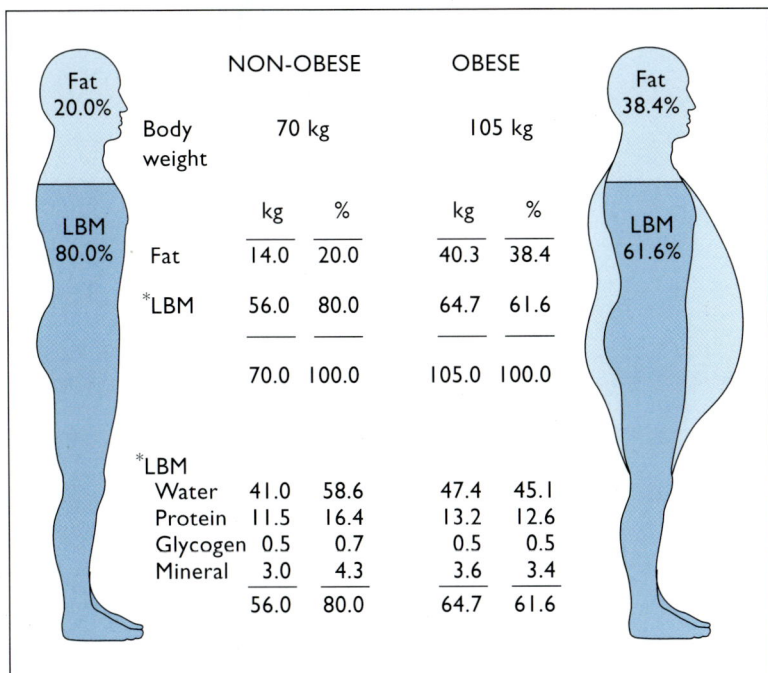

FIGURE 7-8. Body composition of a 70-kg man and a 105-kg man. Both lean body mass and fat mass are increased in obesity, as shown here. The increase in lean body mass (LBM) seen in a large proportion of all obese patients can be masked by factors reducing lean mass, such as previous bouts of crash dieting leading to reductions in lean mass or inadequate protein intake combined with extreme inactivity. (*From* Garrow, *et al.* [3].)

BODY MASS INDEX AND PERCENTAGE BODY FAT IN 28 WOMEN AT INCREASED RISK FOR BREAST CANCER

Age, y	Weight, lb	Height, in	BMI	Body Fat, %
36.8±6.4	137.8±1.9	65.3±2.7	22.9±3.1 (normal < 27)	34.6±4.8 (normal 22%–28%)

Values are the mean ±SD; n=28.

FIGURE 7-9. Sarcopenic obesity occurs when the body mass index (BMI) is low and the percentage of body fat is increased. The weight for height is normal or low, but the person has reduced lean body mass and increased body fat. Bioelectrical impedance measurements done in young women at increased risk for breast cancer demonstrated sarcopenic obesity in 38 of 40 women. As illustrated, although the BMI is normal, the percentage of body fat is increased. This is the operative definition of sarcopenic obesity. Body fat is best reduced in these women by encouraging heavy resistance exercise rather than simply calorie restriction. These patients characteristically have low metabolic rates secondary to their low lean body mass. (*From* Heber *et al.* [4].)

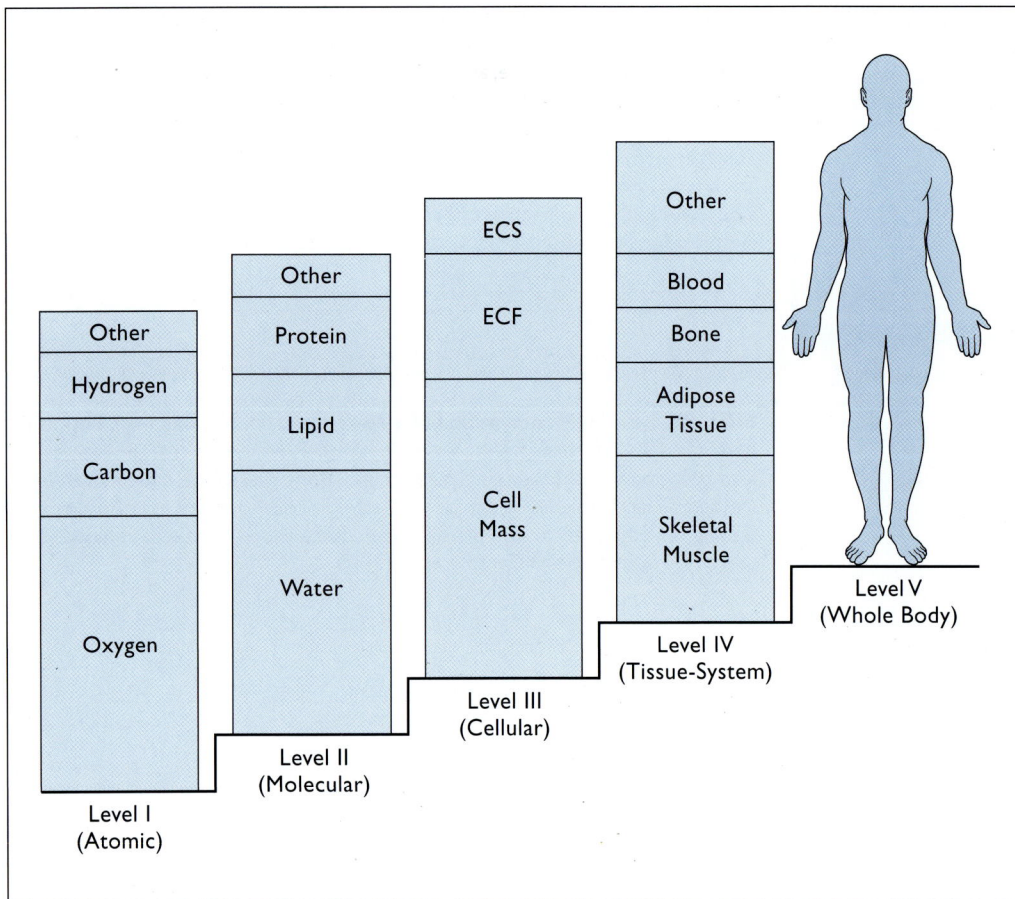

FIGURE 7-10. Human body composition can be described at five levels ranging from elements to the whole body: I, atomic; II, molecular (chemical); III, cellular; IV, tissue-system (including adipose tissue and muscle tissue); and V, whole body. Adipose tissue is distributed as subcutaneous, visceral, interstitial, and yellow marrow. With obesity, adipose tissue distribution in these compartments varies according to sex and age. ECF—extracellular fluid; ECS—extracellular space. (*From* Wang *et al.* [5].)

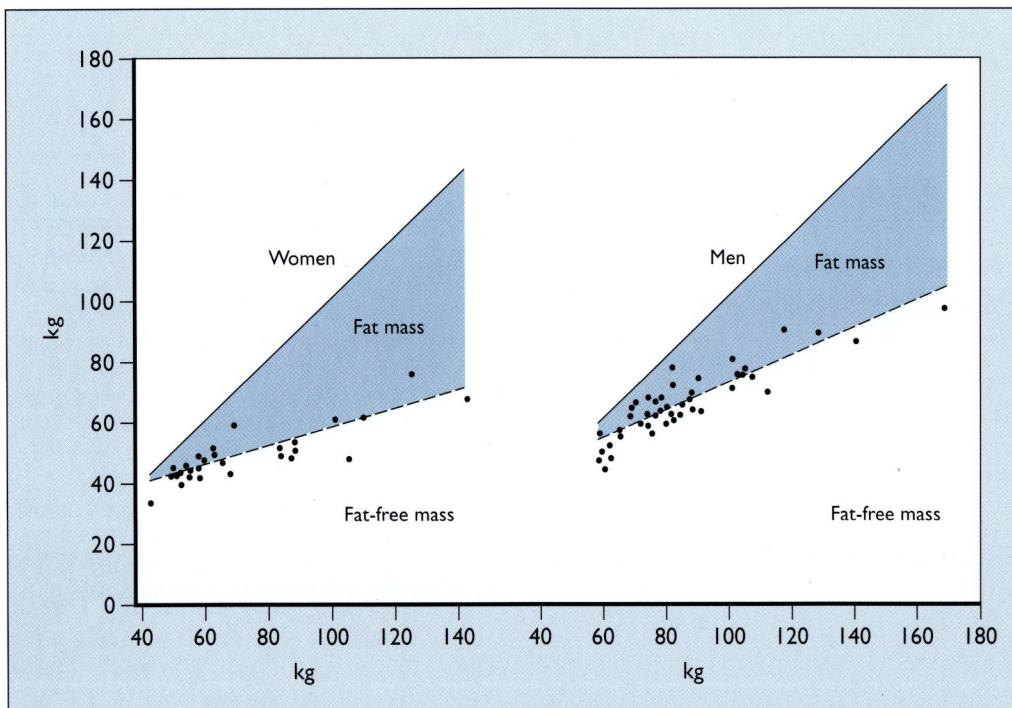

FIGURE 7-11. Relation among fat-free mass, fat mass, and body weight. Fat-free mass increases gradually with increased body weight, but excess fat mass accounts for approximately 75% of the weight increment as body weight increases. With gradual weight loss, fat and protein are lost in these same proportions (75%:25%). However, rapid weight loss due to starvation or semistarvation will be accompanied by protein depletion, with up to 50% of the weight lost from skeletal muscle and visceral protein. (*From* Owen [6].)

Treatment of Obesity

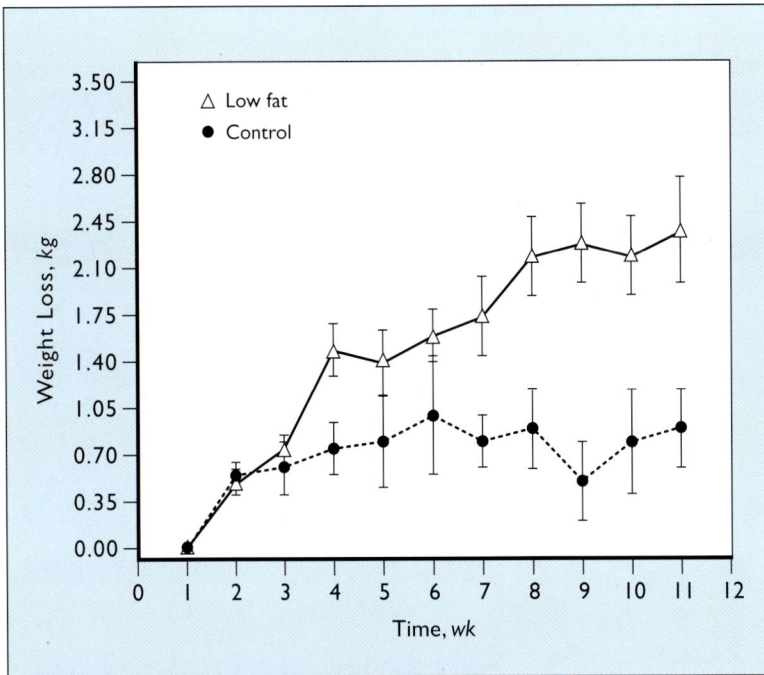

FIGURE 7-12. Mean weight loss as a function of high-fat and low-fat diets during 11 weeks of observation. When eaten ad libitum, high-fat diets in both men and women are associated with weight gain. These observations led to the development of low-fat and so-called nonfat foods. Unfortunately, when the calories saved through fat reduction are replaced with sugar, there is no net reduction in caloric intake or any lasting effect on obesity. To reduce caloric intake, high-fat foods must be eliminated, and meal replacement and portion-control strategies must be instituted. More than 1000 fat-free foods are available, and many of these replace the fat calories with carbohydrates, including refined sugar, to maintain taste. If these foods do not result in the intake of fewer calories, they have no role in a weight-reducing diet. (*From* Kendall-Casella [7].)

REDUCTION OF TRIGGERS

Nuts

Cheese and pizza

Salad dressing

Mayonnaise, margarine, butter

Red meat and fatty fish

Nonfat yogurt, ice cream

FIGURE 7-13. Types of trigger foods. Trigger foods are commonly eaten foods that provide added calories in the diet. They are frequently eaten as snacks in response to stress or boredom. Their identity as a trigger food is not defined by the biochemistry of the food but rather by the behavioral response to its ingestion. Minimizing and controlling intake of the trigger foods that a patient identifies can help control total fat and calorie intake. These are not junk foods to be eliminated but rather represent individual eating behaviors to be modified.

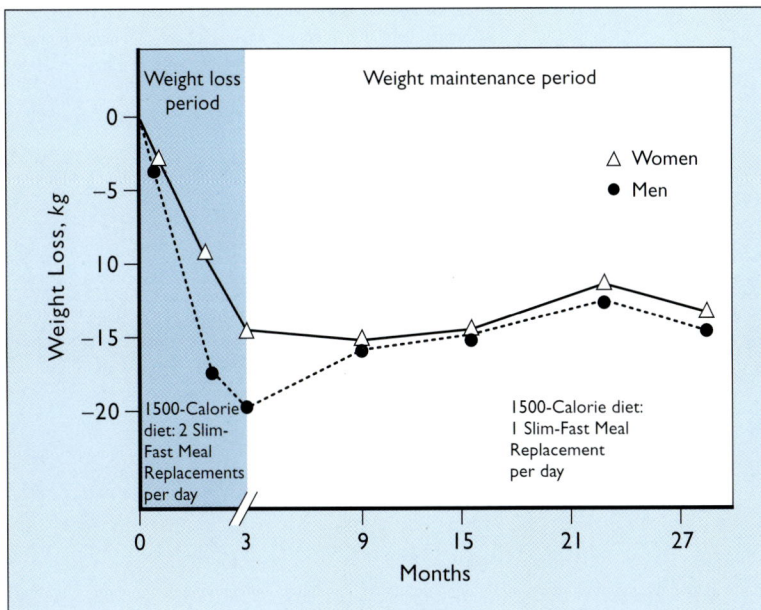

FIGURE 7-14. Weight control with meal replacements (Slim-Fast foods, Co, West Palm Beach, FL). The vertically integrated system of care uses widely available meal replacements and portion-controlled meals to reduce caloric intake effectively. These special foods increase patient confidence in the number of calories they are eating, and the use of meal replacements has been shown to produce results superior to those achieved with calorie-counting. Shown here are findings from an intervention in 300 men and women at six sites throughout the United States. Participants ingested two meal replacement shakes per day as part of a 1200-calorie/d diet for 12 weeks; for the next 24 months, they ingested one shake per day. Weight loss was about 7% of starting weight but about 50% of the excess fat in these mildly overweight patients. Participants continuing to the end of the study (approximately 56% of the initial group) maintained much of their weight loss. (*From* Heber *et al.* [8].)

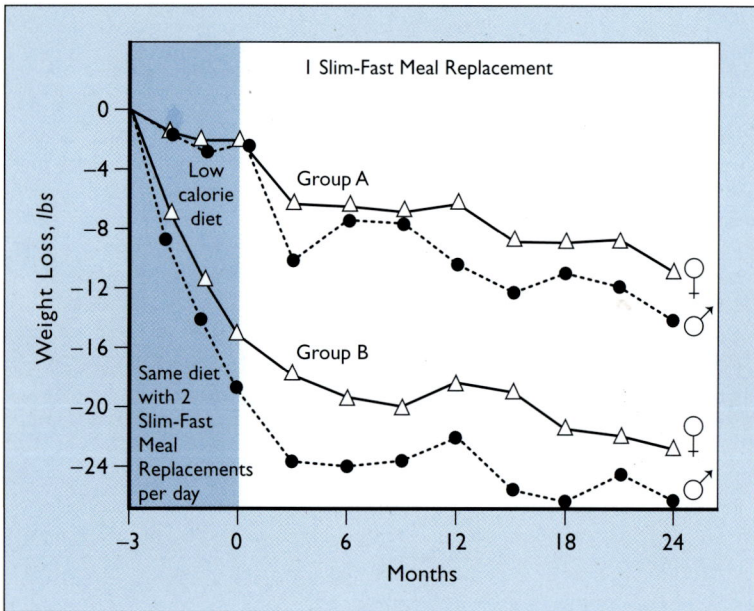

FIGURE 7-15. Weight loss and weight maintenance with daily use of meal replacements (Slim-Fast foods, Co, West Palm Beach, FL). In this study, patients were told to restrict their favorite foods by counting calories between 1200 and 1500 calories per day or to use two meal replacements as part of an overall diet of 1200 to 1500 calories. The markedly increased weight loss in the meal replacement group over the first 12 weeks can be attributed to the enhanced dietary compliance mediated by the use of meal replacements. Both groups then ingested one meal replacement per day over 2 years, and both groups lost additional weight. (*From* Ditschuneit et al [9].)

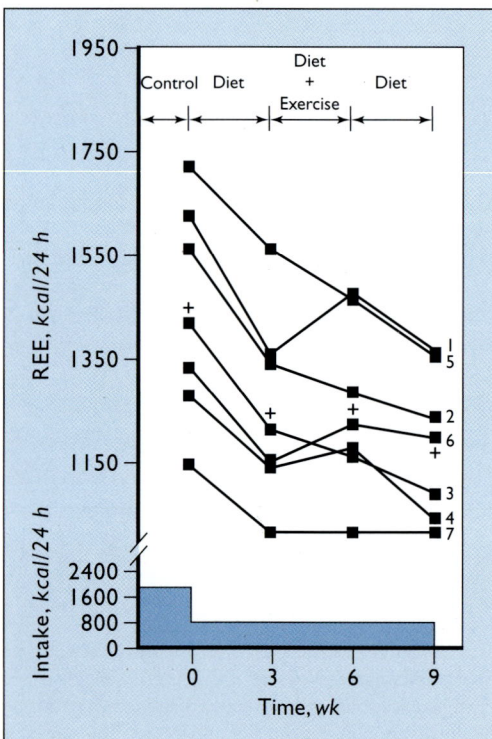

FIGURE 7-16. Caloric restriction accompanied by an adaptive decrease in metabolic rate. The modest effects of exercise on resting energy expenditure (REE) are also shown. However, despite the adaptive decrease in metabolic rate, caloric restriction results in weight loss. Therefore, this adaptation to caloric restriction compensates only partially for the reduction in total calorie intake. Exercise is beneficial from a behavioral standpoint as the single behavior most correlated with continued dietary compliance. However, it leads to modest or no weight loss as an isolated intervention. (*From* Henson et al [10].)

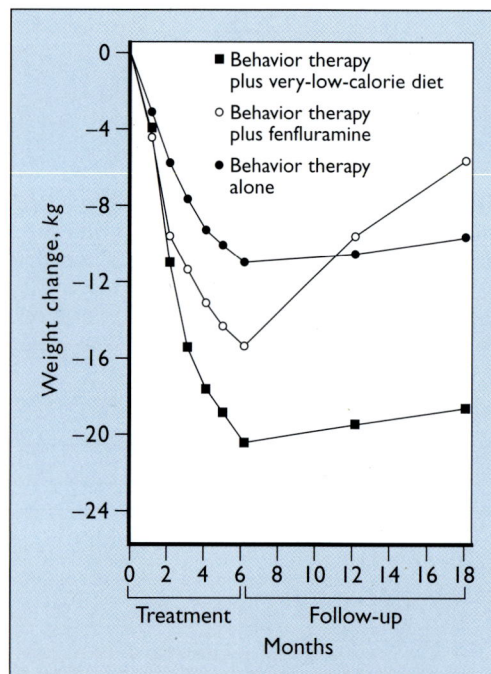

FIGURE 7-17. Reduction in body weight to a minimum at 6 months, with a weight regain over the next 12 months regardless of whether behavior therapy alone, a very-low-calorie diet, or the combination of both was used. All weight loss is due to the reduction of total calorie intake or increased energy expenditure, regardless of whether diet, drugs, or surgery is used. The response shown here is characteristic of most weight loss regimens. (*From* Wadden [11].)

VERTICALLY INTEGRATED SYSTEM

Meal replacements and portion control

Exercise, behavior, lifestyle change

Trigger foods

Drugs and surgery in addition to above for selected patients who do not respond to lifestyle modifications and have a BMI ≥ 27, plus cormorbid conditions (or BMI > 30 without comorbid conditions)

FIGURE 7-18. Components of the vertically integrated system of care for obesity [12–14]. These include diet and lifestyle change plus pharmacotherapy or surgery when indicated. This approach does not define pharmacotherapy or surgery as alternatives to diet and lifestyle change but rather as adjuncts to the basic approaches of recognizing trigger foods, meal replacement, and portion-controlled meals.

PHARMACOLOGY OF ANTIOBESITY AGENTS

Agents	Releasing Agent			Reuptake Inhibitor			Selective Lipase Inhibitor
	5-HT	NE	DA	5-HT	NE	DA	
Dexamphetamine		XX	XX		X	X	
Phentermine		X					
Fenfluramine	XXX			X			
Dexfenfluramine	XXX			X			
Sibutramine				XXX	XXX		
Orlistat							XXX

FIGURE 7-19. Pharmacologic actions of available antiobesity drugs [15,16]. Dexfenfluramine and fenfluramine are no longer available; they were withdrawn by the Food and Drug Administration because of an association with cardiac valvular disease. Most of these drugs work at a central level to affect the hypothalamic appetite centers; the exception is orlistat, which acts in the gastrointestinal tract to inhibit triglyceride breakdown and absorption by about 30%. 5-HT—serotonin; DA—dopamine; NE—norepinephrine.

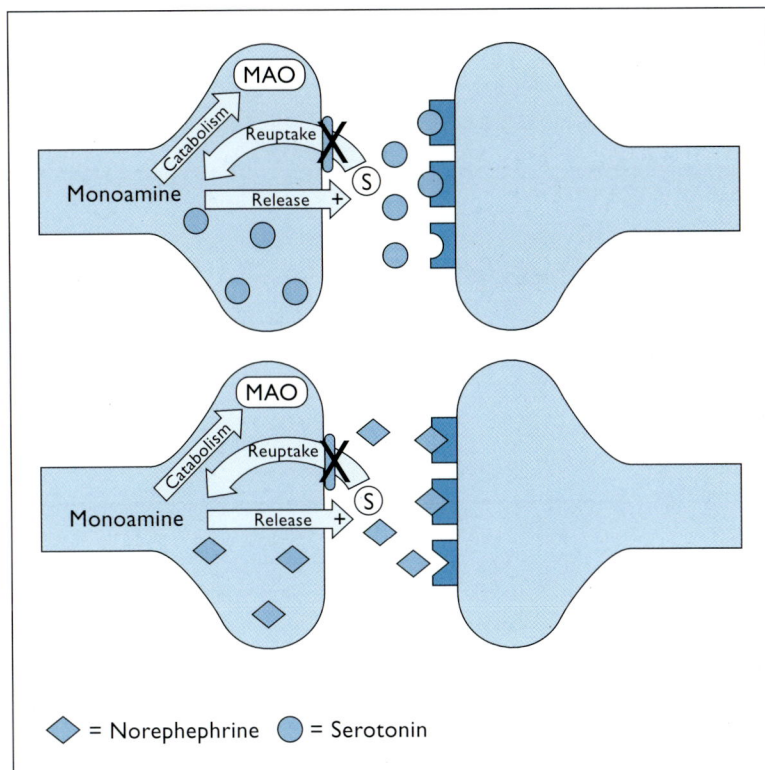

◆ = Norephephrine ● = Serotonin

FIGURE 7-20. Mechanisms of action of sibutramine (S) and active metabolites [15,16]. Sibutramine is a nonselective norepinephrine and serotonin reuptake inhibitor. The normal release and reuptake of neurotransmitters from the synaptic space determine the amount of active neurotransmitter available to bind to the postsynaptic receptor. By inhibiting the reuptake of norepinephrine and serotonin, this drug increases the concentration of both neurotransmitters in the synaptic space. MAO—monoamine oxidase.

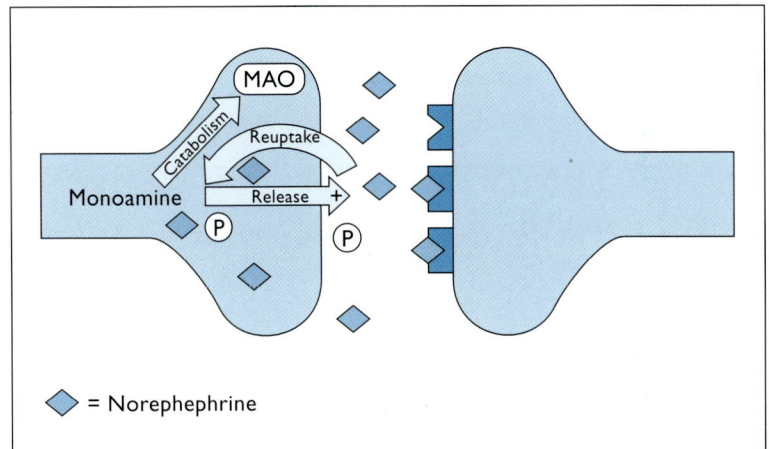

◆ = Norephephrine

FIGURE 7-21. Mechanisms of action of phentermine (P). Phentermine is both a releaser of synaptic stores of norepinephrine and a reuptake inhibitor. It overrides the normal control mechanisms of synthesis-secretion coupling and has a pronounced effect on the levels of norepinephrine in the synapse by comparison to sibutramine. Physicians should be aware that in contrast to sibutramine, this drug is approved only for short-term use in weight management. MAO—monoamine oxidase.

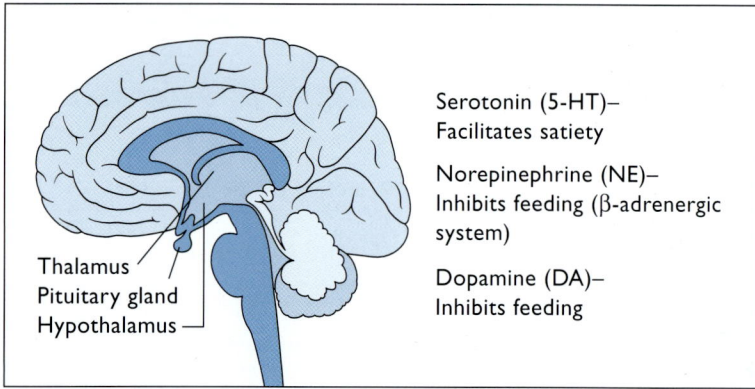

FIGURE 7-22. Monoamine circuits in the hypothalamus governing feeding and satiety. Serotonin facilitates satiety without addictive potential. Norepinephrine inhibits feeding via the beta-adrenergic system, also without addictive potential. Dopamine inhibits feeding but is associated with addictive potential. (*From* Hoebel *et al* [17].)

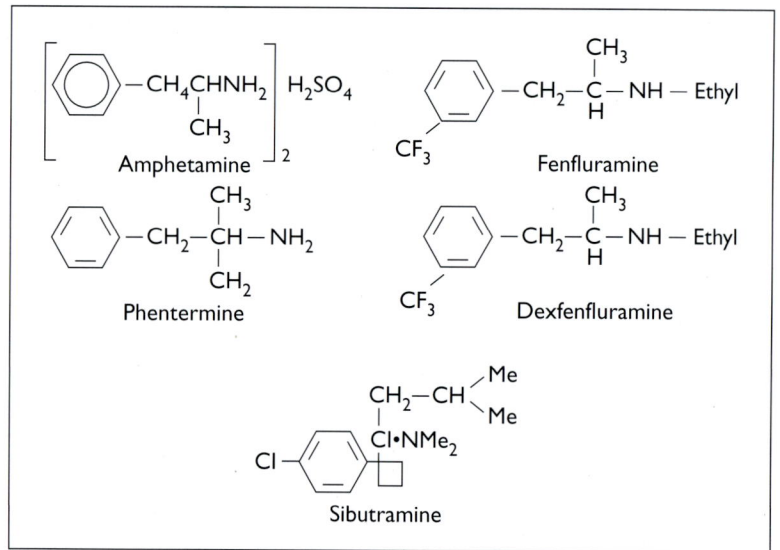

FIGURE 7-23. Chemical structures of centrally acting antiobesity drugs. Phentermine and amphetamines are structurally similar. Sibutramine has structural differences that confer unique properties of nonselective reuptake inhibition for both serotonin and norepinephrine.

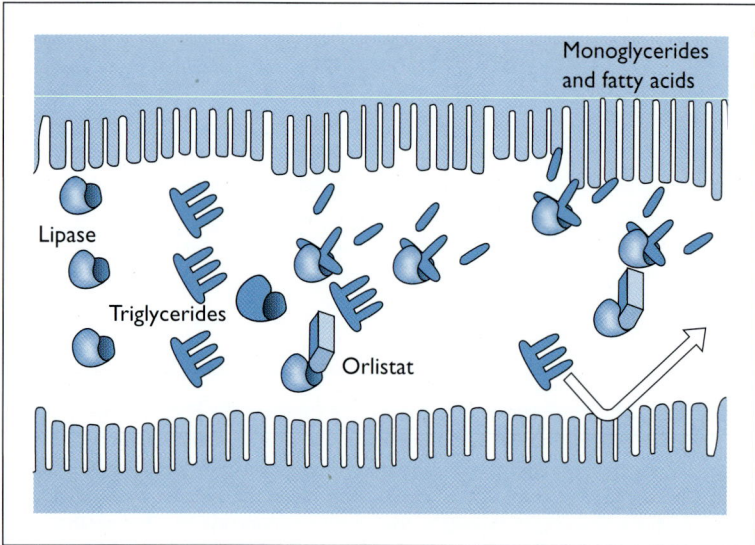

FIGURE 7-24. Effects of orlistat over a 2-year period [18,19]. Inhibition of lipases by orlistat blocks systemic absorption of dietary fat. Up to one third of ingested fat is excreted into the feces. Gastric and pancreatic lipases are the key enzymes that hydrolyze triglycerides into free fatty acids and monoglycerides, which are then absorbed. Orlistat inhibits these lipases.

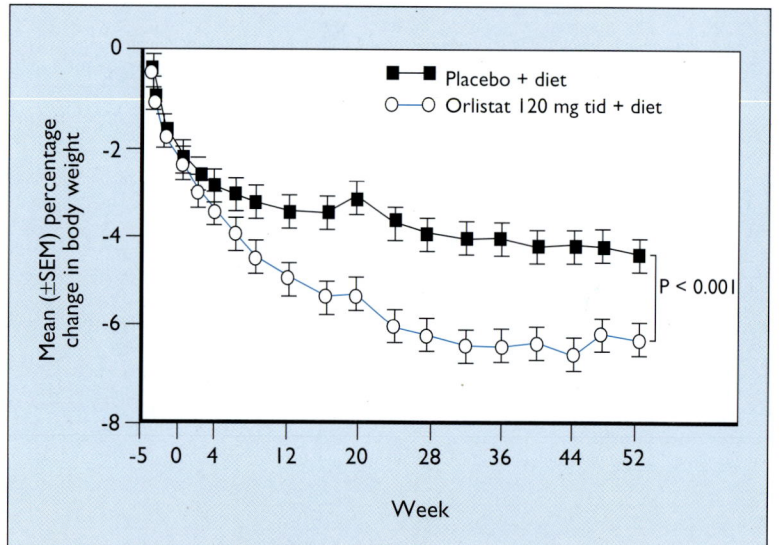

FIGURE 7-25 After 1 year, patients receiving orlistat, 120 mg three times daily, had a mean weight loss of 8.8%, compared with a mean weight loss of 5.8% in the placebo group (*P* < 0.0001). After 2 years, the participants in the orlistat group who had a waist circumference greater than 39 inches had a mean loss of 2.3 inches; similar participants in the placebo group had a mean loss of 1.1 inches. (Data obtained from Roche Laboratories.)

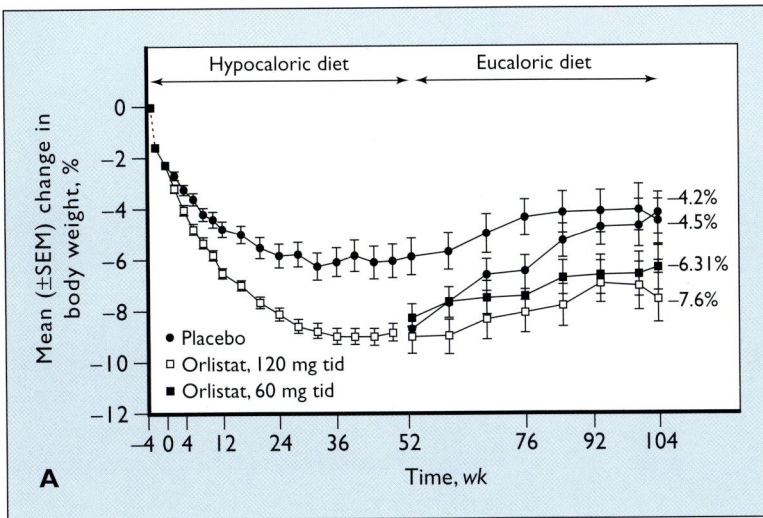

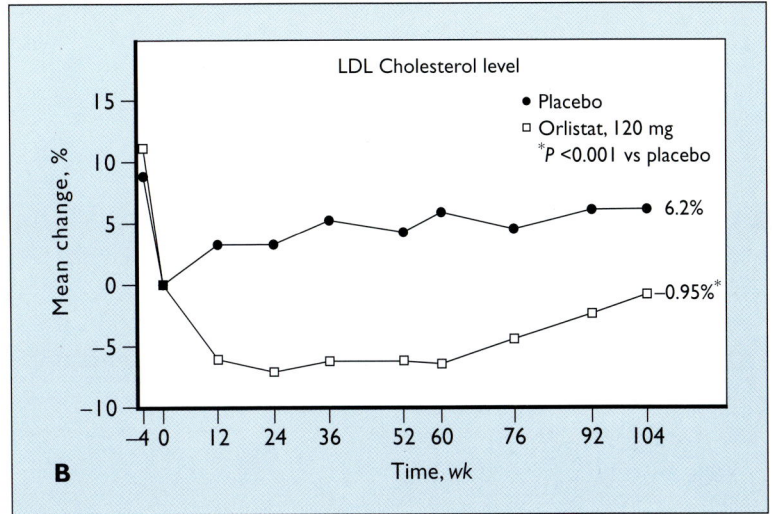

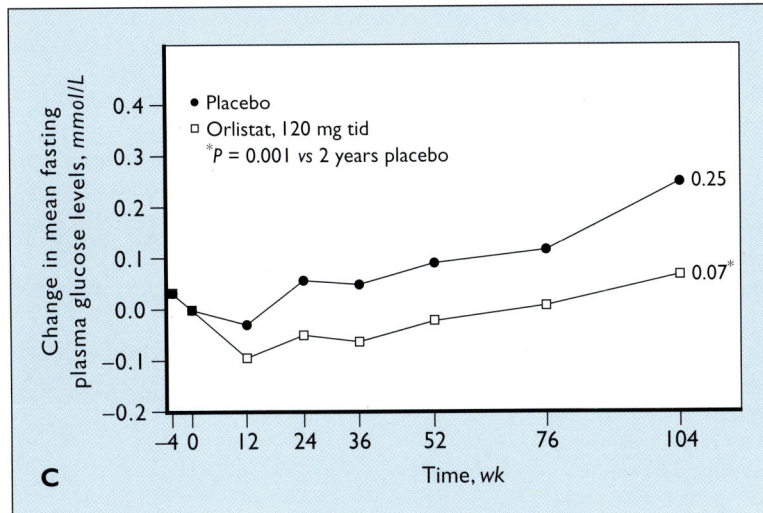

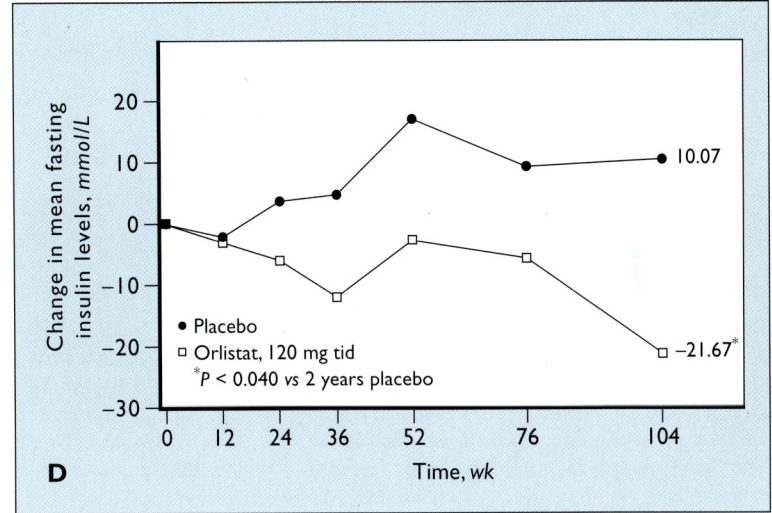

FIGURE 7-26. The weight loss resulting from orlistat positively affected lipids, blood pressure, and glycemic control [20]. After a 2-year clinical trial of obese patients, orlistat was associated with weight loss (**A**), and a hypocaloric diet resulted in decreases in low-density lipoprotein (LDL)

cholesterol levels (**B**), fasting blood glucose levels (**C**), and fasting insulin levels (**D**). The effects of weight loss compared with those of orlistat could not be differentiated: all the effects may be due to the observed weight loss.

SURGICAL TREATMENT

Gastric surgery
  Roux-en-Y bypass
  Vertical-banded gastroplasty

FIGURE 7-27. Surgical treatment. The National Institutes of Health Consensus Conference, reported in 1991, established gastric bypass operations as the only recommended surgical approaches to obesity. Extensive data supported the utility of these approaches. Ileo-jejunal bypass was recommended only under strict control with research protocols. The two most common operations are vertical banded gastroplasty and roux-en-Y gastric bypass.

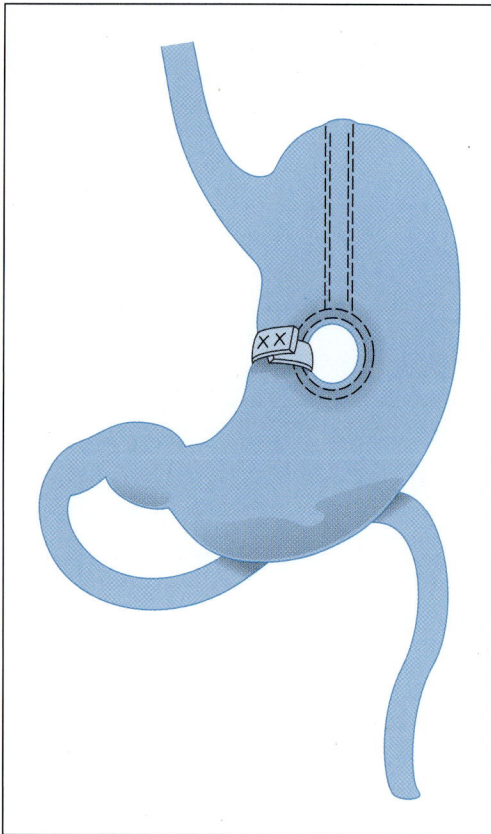

FIGURE 7-28. Vertical banded gastroplasty. This surgery creates a narrow channel for food to pass through in the stomach. The major complications include nausea and vomiting, stretching of the channel with weight regain, and stricture and obstruction. The results of the operation are similar to those achieved with very-low-calorie diets, and the patients require significant diet and lifestyle change to maintain their weight loss. (*From* Mason and Ito [21].)

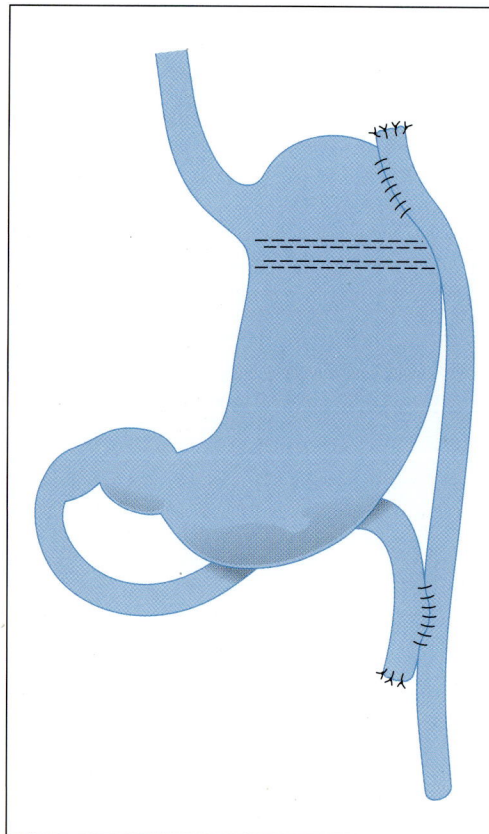

FIGURE 7-29. Roux-en-Y gastric bypass. This surgery creates a small gastric pouch the size of a hard-boiled egg, where food that is well-chewed can enter the intestine. This results in a rapid-onset satiety response. The side effects of the operation include dumping syndrome and hypoglycemia. As with vertical banded gastroplasty, diet and lifestyle changes are needed. The side effects are more pronounced than those with vertical banded gastroplasty, but the results are also more predictable. Vitamin B_{12} must be administered bimonthly by injection because the area of the stomach that produces intrinsic factor is bypassed. This operation is preferred as the primary surgery for obesity at many of the academic medical centers that have comprehensive obesity programs. (*From* Shikora et al. [22].)

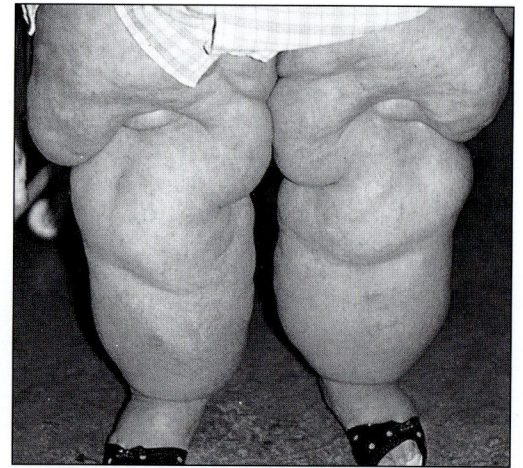

FIGURE 7-30. (*see* Color Plate) Poor result in a patient who regained all of her weight after a liposuction procedure was performed on her thighs. Liposuction and other plastic procedures to remove fat cells are cosmetic procedures. Fat cells in the areas around the sites of fat removal can hypertrophy when weight is regained. This photograph graphically illustrates the principles of vertically integrated management. There are no magical solutions to overeating, and diet and lifestyle must be used with all the approaches discussed in this chapter.

References

1. Clinical Guidelines on the Identification, Evaluation, and Treatment of Overweight and Obesity in Adults. Bethesda, MD: National Institutes of Health; National Heart, Lung, and Blood Institute; 1998:VIII.

2. Kuczmarski RJ, Flegal KM, Cambell SM, et al.: Increasing prevalence of overweight among US adults. The National Health and Nutrition Examination Survey, 1960 to 1991. JAMA 1994, 272:205–211.

3. Garrow JS, Durrant ML, MannS, et al.: Factors determining weight loss in obese patients in a metabolic ward. Int J Obes 1978, 2:441–447.

4. Heber D, Ingles S, Ashley JM, et al.: Clinical detection of sarcopenic obesity by bioelectrical impedance analysis. Am J Clin Nutr 1996, 64:472S–477S.

5. Wang Z, Pierson RN Jr, Heymsfield SB: The five level model: A new approach to organizing body composition research. Am J Clin Nutr 1992, 56:19–28.

6. Owen OE: Obesity. In Nutrition and Metabolism in Patient Care. Edited by Kinney JM, Jeejeebhoy KN, Hill GL, Owen OE. Philadelphia: W.B. Saunders; 1998.

7. Kendall A, Levitsky DA, Strupp BJ, Lissner L: Weight loss on a low-fat diet. Consequences of the imprecision of the control of food intake in humans. Am J Clin Nutr 1991, 53:1124–1129.

8. Heber D, Ashley JM, Wang HJ, et al.: Clinical evaluation of a minimal intervention meal replacement regimen for weight reduction. J Am Coll Nutr 1994, 13:608–614.

9. Ditschuneit HH, Flechtner-Mors M, Johnson TD, et al.: Metabolic and weight-loss effects of a long-term dietary intervention in obese patients. Am J Clin Nutr 1999, 69:198–204.

10. Henson LC, Poole DC, Donahoe CP, et al.: Effects of exercise training on resting energy expenditure during caloric restriction. Am J Clin Nutr 1987, 46:893–899.

11. Wadden TA: Treatment of obesity by behavior therapy and very low calorie diet: a pilot investigation. J Consult Clin Psychol 1984, 52:693.

12. Physician's Desk Reference. Montvale, NJ: Medical Economics; 1996.

13. Garattini S. Biological actions of drugs affecting serotonin and eating. Obes Res 1995, 3(suppl 4):463S–470S.

14. Buckett WR, Thomas PC, Lusscombe GP, et al.: The pharmacology of sibutramine hydrochloride (BTS 54 524), a new antidepressant which induces rapid noradrenergic down-regulation. Prog Neuropsychopharmacol Biol Psychiatry 1988, 12:575–584.

15. Samanin R, Garattini S: Serotonin and the pharmacology of eating disorders. Ann N Y Acad Sci 1989, 575:194–207.

16. Ryan DH, Kaiser P, Bray GA: Sibutramine: a novel new agent for obesity treatment. Obes Res. 1995, 3(suppl 4):553S–559S.

17. Hoebel BG, Leibowitz SF: Brain monoamines in the modulation of self-stimulation, feeding, and body weight. Res Publ Assoc Res Nerv Ment Dis 1981, 59:103–142.

18. Zhi J, Melia AT, Eggers H, et al.: Review of limited systemic absorption of orlistat, a lipase inhibitor in healthy human volunteers. J Clin Pharmacol 1995, 35:1103–1108.

19. Zhi J, Melia AT, Guerciolini R, et al.: Retrospective population-based analysis of the dose-response (fecal fat excretion) relationship of orlistat in normal and obese volunteers. Clin Pharmacol Ther 1994, 56:82–85.

20. Roche Pharmaceutical Data. Nutley, NJ: Roche Laboratories; 1999.

21. Mason EE, Ito C: Gastric bypass in obesity. Surg Clin North Am 1967, 47:1345.

22. Shikora SA, Benotti PN, Forse RA: Surgical treatment of obesity. In: Obesity: Pathophysiology, Psychology and Treatment. Edited by Blackburn and Kanders. New York: Chapman & Hall; 1994:264–282.

8

NON–INSULIN-DEPENDENT DIABETES MELLITUS AND NUTRITION

Ann M. Coulston

Diabetes mellitus affects some 18 million people in the United States and is emerging as a major health problem throughout the world. In the United States, diabetes mellitus is the fourth leading cause of death by disease and a major cause of blindness and kidney disease. The American Diabetes Association (ADA) recognizes two main classifications of diabetes mellitus. Patients with type 1 diabetes have absolute insulin deficiency as a result of beta-cell destruction and rely on exogenous insulin replacement. Patients with type 2 diabetes manifest signs and symptoms of hyperglycemia ranging from predominantly insulin resistance to predominantly an insulin secretory defect with insulin resistance [1]. The latter classification, previously referred to as *non–insulin-dependent diabetes mellitus*, accounts for more than 90% of all patients diagnosed with diabetes [1].

Management of this chronic condition relies on the interplay of three principal therapies: medication, exercise, and nutrition. These therapies interrelate in the management of patients with diabetes in a unique manner such that an alteration in the amount or timing of or compliance with any one therapy has a significant impact on the other therapies and ultimately on the immediate and long-term health outcome.

Because the impact of medication and exercise on the medical management of diabetes is covered elsewhere, this chapter discusses only the nutrition therapy of type 2 diabetes. Whereas medication therapy can be considered the cornerstone of management for patients with type 1 diabetes, nutrition therapy is the cornerstone of management for patients with type 2 disease.

Health professionals and patients recognize nutrition therapy as the most challenging aspect of diabetes management. Adherence to food intake principles and patterns requires an understanding and appreciation of the impact of these specific recommendations. Nutrition therapies often require eating pattern alterations and behavior changes that necessitate individual motivation and a commitment to healthy lifestyle behaviors. The application of nutrition therapy resembles decisions in medication management, in that specific guidelines for nutrition therapy must be individualized for each patient depending on the goals and outcomes of medical management [2].

Rationale for Nutrition Management

MEDICAL NUTRITION THERAPY GOALS

Near-normal blood glucose concentrations

Optimal lipid concentrations

Appropriate caloric intake

Reasonable body weight for adults

Growth and development for children and adolescents

Pregnancy and lactation needs

Meet recommended intakes for vitamins and minerals

FIGURE 8-1. Medical nutrition therapy goals. Control of blood glucose concentration in the near-normal range is related to decreased development and progression of microvascular complications, which are manifest primarily by retinopathy and nephropathy. Postprandial blood glucose concentrations correlate with the amount of carbohydrate consumed in an "eating episode" and can be managed when the amount of carbohydrate consumed is matched with the nutritional needs, medication, and physical activity of the individual. Plasma lipid concentrations reflect overall intake of types and amounts of dietary fats and carbohydrates. Optimal lipid concentration is an important goal because the risk of cardiovascular disease in patients with diabetes is two to three times that in the general population. Body weight and growth and development are directly dependent on daily caloric intake and respond directly (over time) to caloric increases and decreases. Although much of the nutritional management of these patients is devoted to macronutrients, carbohydrate, fat, and protein, age- and lifestyle-specific requirements for vitamins and minerals cannot be overlooked in the medical nutrition therapy plan.

HISTORICAL PERSPECTIVE ON CALORIC DISTRIBUTION

Year	Carbohydrate, %	Protein, %	Fat, %
1921	20	10	70
1950	40	20	40
1971	45	20	35
1986	50–60	12–20	30
1994	*	10–20	*, +

*Based on individual nutrition assessment.

+<10% saturated fatty acids.

FIGURE 8-2. Historical perspective on caloric distribution. Before the discovery of insulin, diabetic patients were treated with "starvation" diets to avoid increased concentrations of glucose in the urine and the accompanying sequelae. As understanding of nutrient metabolism increased, a reliance on the use of fat as a calorie source for this condition was recommended. During these earlier years, nutrition therapy for diabetes was primarily related to patients with type 1 disease. As medication therapies became more sophisticated and exogenous insulin became available for use, the carbohydrate restriction of the diet was gradually relaxed. Before the 1994 ADA nutrition recommendations were made [2], guidelines attempted to apply one nutrient distribution prescription to all patients. With increased understanding of the metabolic abnormalities of insulin resistance and the relationship of both dietary carbohydrate and fat to plasma lipid concentrations, nutrition therapy plans were tailored to specific treatment goals in a manner similar to the selection and adjustment of medication therapies.

METABOLIC ABNORMALITIES ASSOCIATED WITH TYPE 2 DIABETES

Hyperglycemia

Hyerpinsulinemia

Hypertriglyceridemia

Decreased HDL cholesterol

Increased small, dense LDL cholesterol

FIGURE 8-3. Metabolic abnormalities associated with type 2 diabetes. The insulin resistance of type 2 diabetes permits hyperinsulinemia in the face of hyperglycemia. The most frequent lipid abnormalities in patients with type 2 diabetes are hypertriglyceridemia, increased very-low-density lipoprotein (VLDL) cholesterol, and reduced high-density lipoprotein (HDL) cholesterol. Plasma concentrations of total and low-density lipoprotein (LDL) cholesterol are similar to those in the general population. However, about 40% of patients with type 2 diabetes have an elevated LDL cholesterol that cannot be neglected [3]. The hypertriglyceridemia of type 2 diabetes is believed to be due in part to increased hepatic production of triglyceride-rich VLDL particles. The elevation of triglyceride concentrations is also induced by increased dietary carbohydrate intake. The increase in small, dense LDL particles along with the decreased HDL cholesterol and hypertriglyceridemia appear to be sequelae of insulin resistance, although a complete understanding of the mechanism remains to be elucidated [4,5].

RISK FACTORS FOR CARDIOVASCULAR DISEASE

Hyperglycemia

Hyperinsulinemia

Hypertriglyceridemia

Increased low-density lipoprotein cholesterol

Decreased high-density lipoprotein cholesterol

FIGURE 8-4. Risk factors for cardiovascular disease. The risk factors for cardiovascular disease closely parallel the metabolic abnormalities of patients with type 2 diabetes. This is of concern because cardiovascular disease accounts for the majority of deaths in patients with diabetes [6]. In addition, when matched with nondiabetic individuals for plasma lipid concentration, patients with diabetes have a three- to fivefold increase in risk for cardiovascular disease [7]. Fontbonne et al. demonstrated the abnormalities of glucose and lipid metabolism and their impact on increased cardiovascular disease in an 11-year follow-up study [8] and a follow-up examination of the role of hyperinsulinemia associated with abnormal glucose and insulin metabolism and cardiovascular disease [9].

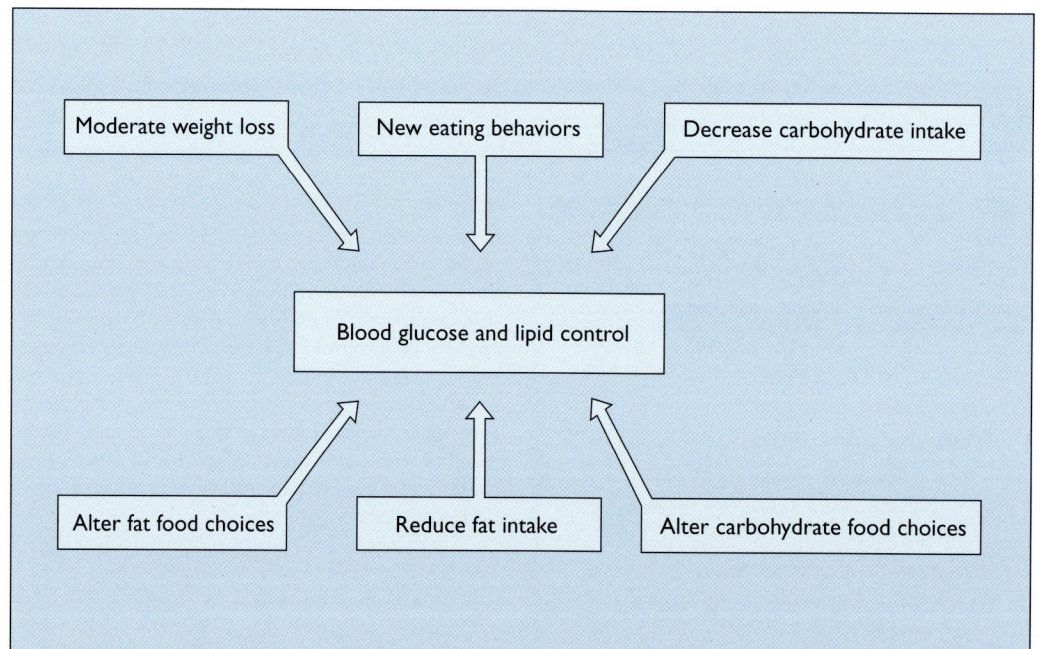

FIGURE 8-5. Strategies for medical nutrition therapy. These are the primary nutrition strategies that can be used to alter blood glucose and lipid concentrations. Everyone agrees that moderate weight reduction leads to improvements in blood glucose and lipid control. Moderate weight loss (in the long-term) and calorie restriction (in the short-term) improve insulin action in insulin-resistant people and improve blood glucose concentration in the face of hyperglycemia. However, for weight maintenance or eucaloric food intake patterns, the impact of the type and amount of dietary carbohydrate and dietary fat on blood glucose and lipid concentration is more meaningful and dietary intervention studies continue to explore this relationship.

Clinical Data to Support Intervention

COMPOSITION OF THE STUDY DIETS*

	Energy Intake Per Day, %	
	High-Carbohydrate Diet	**High–Monounsaturated Fat Diet**
Protein	15	15
Carbohydrate	55	40
Sucrose	10	10
Fat	30	45
Saturated	10	10
Monounsaturated	10	25
Polyunsaturated	10	10

*Nutrient calculations were performed with the General Clinical Research Center (GCRC) Diet Planner Software, Version 2.03, GCRC, University of California–San Francisco, 1990. Supplemental data for fatty acids, fiber, and sucrose were obtained from the Nutrition Coordinating Center, Data Base Version 16.0, School of Public Health, University of Minnesota, Minneapolis, 1989.

FIGURE 8-6. Effects of varying the carbohydrate content: composition of the diet. Because of the strong recommendation to decrease total and saturated dietary fat to protect against heart disease and because patients with type 2 diabetes are at increased risk for cardiovascular disease, diets high in carbohydrates and low in fat have been proposed for patients with type 2 diabetes. Garg et al. [10] studied the metabolic impact of such a diet on 42 patients with type 2 diabetes at four clinical research settings. Because this was a dietary intervention study, the authors wanted to conduct it in an environment in which control over food intake was possible. In these settings, subjects ate one meal each day on the research unit and were provided all other meals for the day. The calorie content for each subject kept them weight-stable during the 12-week study period. Subjects were randomly assigned to the high-carbohydrate or high-monounsaturated diet in a crossover design [10]. (*From Garg, et al.* [10].)

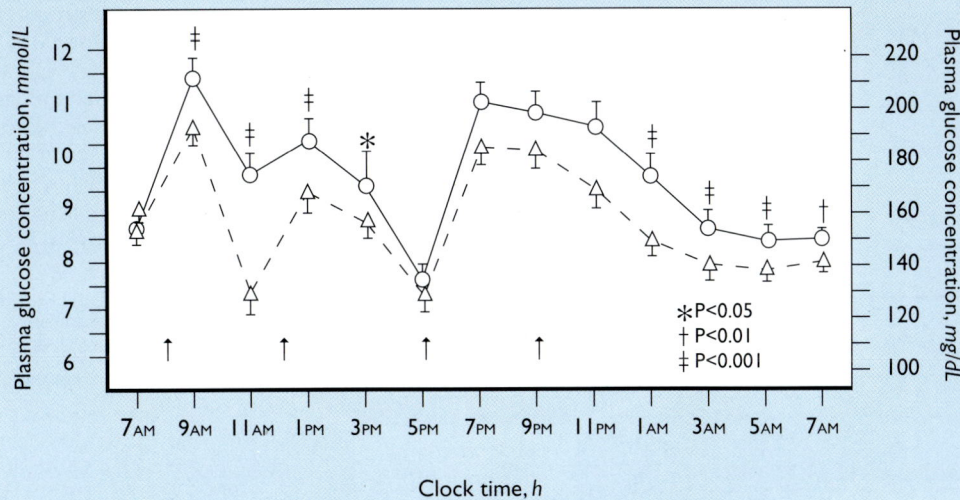

FIGURE 8-7. Plasma glucose concentrations following the two study periods described by Garg et al. [10] (see Fig. 8-6). The *circles* represent the high-carbohydrate diet period and the *triangles* the high–monounsaturated fat diet period. This graph depicts the day-long plasma glucose concentration as determined on the last day of each diet period in response to the diet of that phase. Blood was sampled every 2 hours for 24 hours. *Arrows* represent meal times. With the exception of the fasting blood glucose and the 5:00 PM time point, blood glucose was higher during the high-carbohydrate diet phase. Contrary to accepted dietary management beliefs, the high-carbohydrate diet resulted in postprandial hyperglycemia [10]. (*Adapted from Garg et al.* [10].)

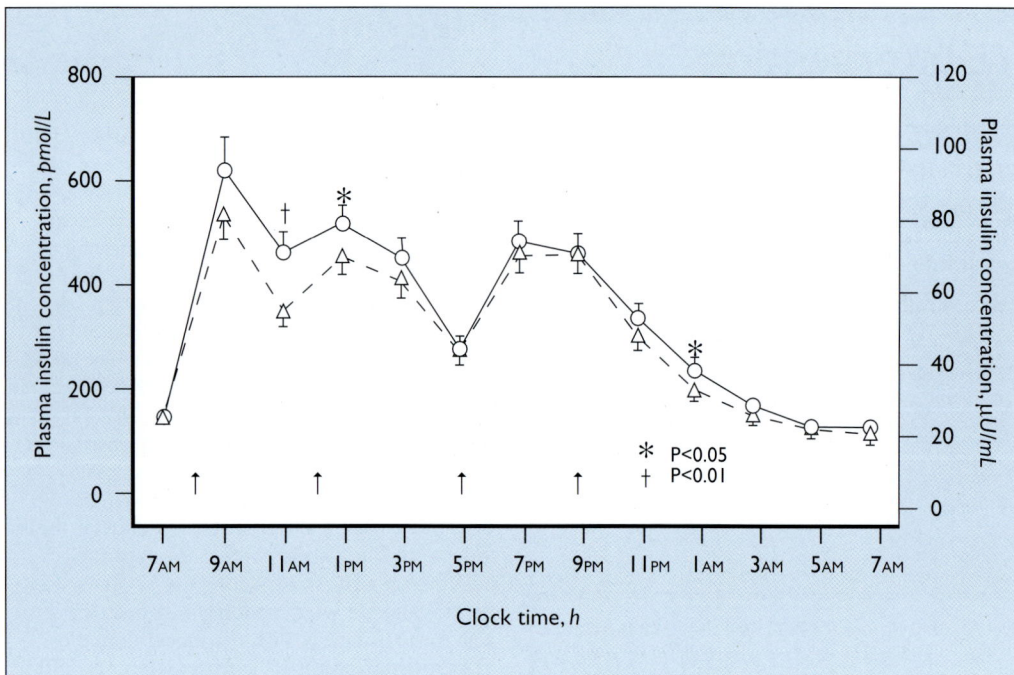

FIGURE 8-8. Plasma insulin concentrations following the two study periods described by Garg et al. [10] (see Fig. 8-6). The *circles* represent the high-carbohydrate diet period and the *triangles* the high–monounsaturated fat diet. This graph depicts the day-long plasma insulin concentration as determined on the last day of each diet period in response to the diet of that phase. Blood was sampled every 2 hours for 24 hours. *Arrows* represent meal times. Note that the patients with type 2 diabetes had ample circulating insulin, but in the face of insulin resistance the cells were not able to remove glucose normally from the blood. Again, there is no difference in the fasting insulin concentration between the two diets, but day-long insulin concentrations are higher on the high-carbohydrate diet [10]. This signifies that high-carbohydrate diets provoke greater insulin responses but not control glucose. (*Adapted from* Garg et al. [10].)

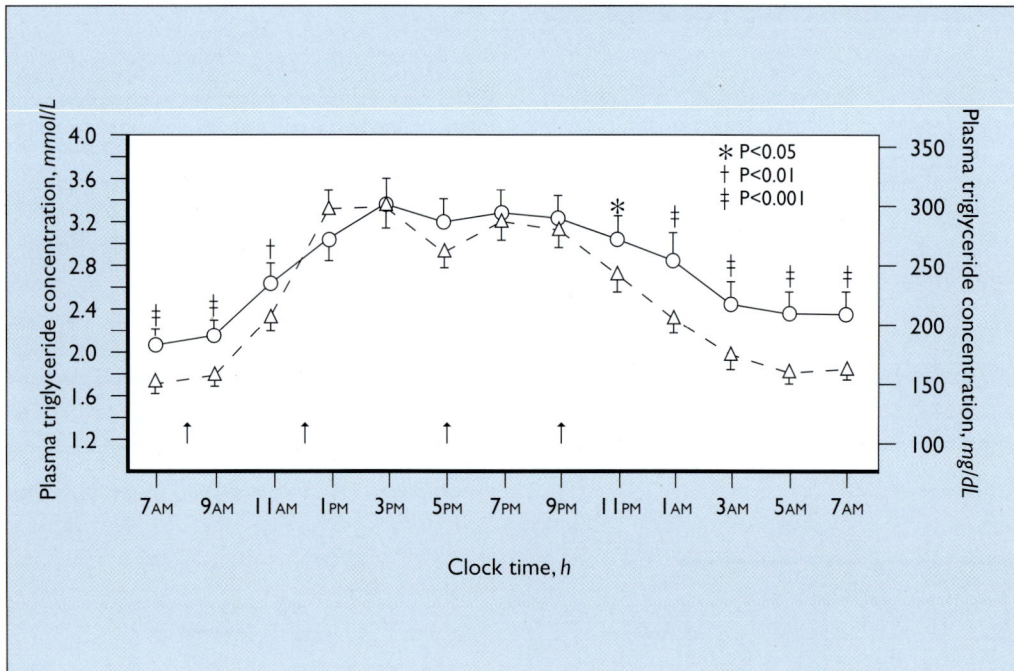

FIGURE 8-9. Plasma triglyceride concentrations following the two study periods described by Garg et al. [10] (see Fig. 8-6). The *circles* represent the high-carbohydrate diet period and the *triangles* the high–monounsaturated fat diet. This graph depicts the day-long plasma triglyceride concentration as determined on the last day of each diet period in response to the diet of that phase. Blood was sampled every 2 hours for 24 hours. *Arrows* represent meal times. The fasting plasma triglyceride concentration was significantly elevated following the high-carbohydrate diet period. Triglyceride concentrations are similar during the middle of the day, but overnight concentrations remained elevated following the high-carbohydrate diet. This pattern is typical of what has been called *carbohydrate-induced hyper-triglyceridemia*. This occurs because in patients with insulin resistance there is increased production of very-low-density lipoprotein particles in the liver and also some decrease in plasma lipid clearance [10]. (*Adapted from* Garg et al. [10].)

FASTING PLASMA LIPID AND LIPOPROTEIN CONCENTRATIONS DURING THE LAST 3 DAYS OF EACH DIET DURING PHASE 1 AND 2*

	Mean (SD)		
	High Carbohydrate Diet, Week 6	High–Monounsaturated Fat Diet, Week 6	P, ANOVA
Plasma cholesterol, mmol/L. [mg/dL]	5.07 (0.91) [196 (35)]	4.97 (0.93) [192 (36)]	0.10
Plasma triglycerides, mmol/L [mg/dL]	2.19 (0.85) [194 (75)]	1.75 (0.70) [155 (62)]	< 0.0001
VLDL cholesterol, mmol/L [mg/dL]	0.80 (0.36) [31 (14)]	0.65 (0.28) [25 (11)]	0.0001
LDL cholesterol, mmol/L [mg/dL]	3.36 (0.70) [130 (27)]	3.36 (0.78) [130 (30)]	0.94
HDL cholesterol, mmol/L [mg/dL]	0.92 (0.24) [35.4 (9.3)]	0.96 (0.27) [37.0 (10.5)]	0.27

*For each individual patient, a mean of three daily determinations for the last 3 days was calculated.

FIGURE 8-10. Fasting plasma lipid and lipoprotein concentrations following the two study periods described by Garg et al. [10] (see Fig. 8-6). The fasting lipid concentrations in this table represent the mean of the last 3 days of each diet phase. Despite an increase of 15% of calories as total fat, there were no detrimental effects on total or low-density lipoprotein (LDL) cholesterol concentrations. These data, from 42 subjects from four sites across the United States, support the findings of others [13] that the plasma cholesterol and LDL cholesterol concentrations in patients with type 2 diabetes are not out of the acceptable range. In this study, we did not see a significant change in high-density lipoprotein (HDL) cholesterol. This may be because the differences in carbohydrate and fat (only 15%) were not sufficient to show a significant change. However, these data also support the findings of others that indicate patients with type 2 diabetes tend to have low HDL cholesterol concentrations. When all of the lipid findings of this study are taken together, it is difficult to support an improvement in treatment outcomes for patients with type 2 diabetes with low-fat, high-carbohydrate nutrition guidelines [10]. ANOVA—analysis of variance; VLDL—very-low-density lipoprotein. (From Garg, et al. [10].)

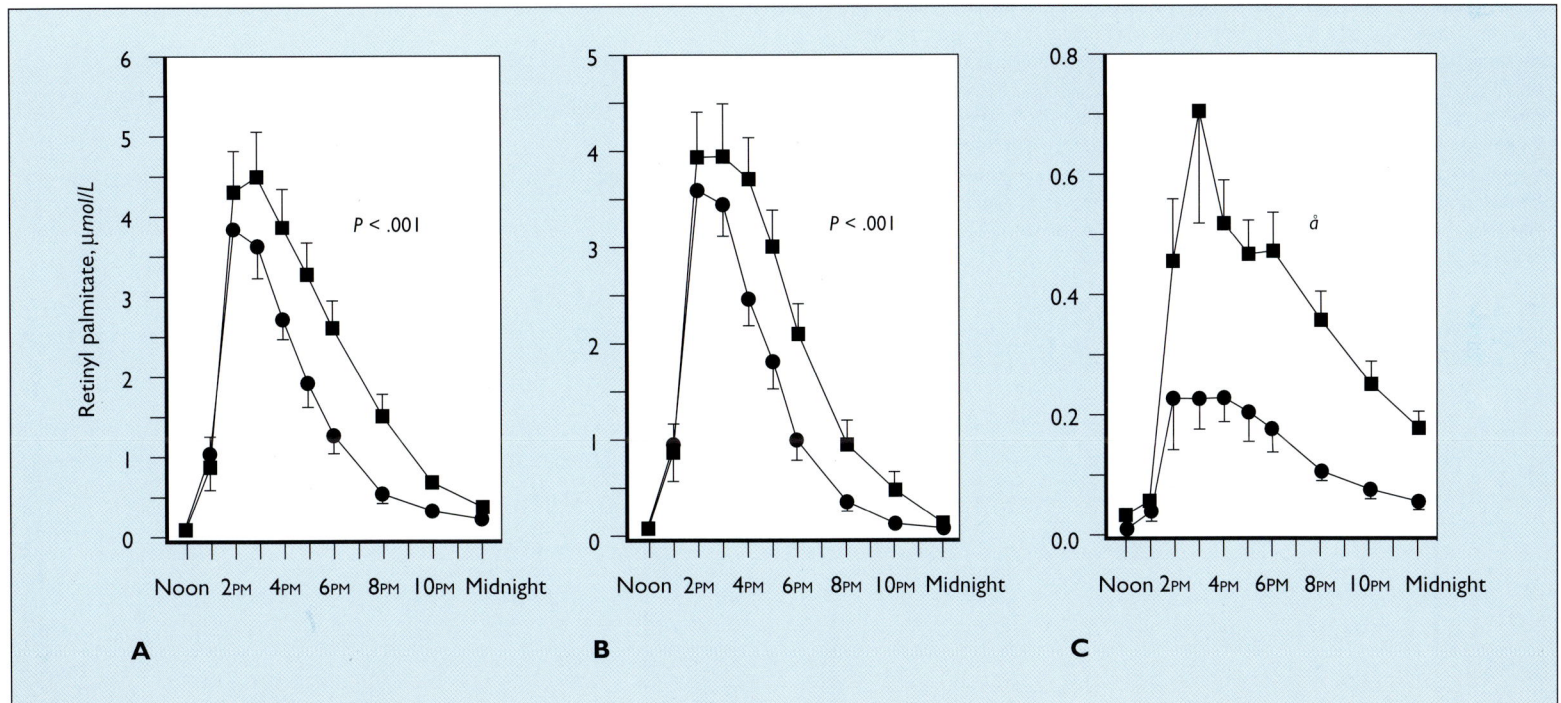

FIGURE 8-11. Plasma triglyceride clearance following high-carbohydrate, low-fat diet intervention. To examine chylomicron clearance, Chen et al. [11] added large doses of vitamin A to the midday meals of 10 patients with type 2 diabetes following the 6-week study diet described by Garg et al. [10]. Measurement of retinyl palmitate allows the study of newly synthesized triglyceride (very-low-density lipoprotein) particles in the postprandial state. Circles represent the high–monounsaturated fat diet phase (40% carbohydrates), and squares the high-carbohydrate diet phase (55% carbohydrates). These graphs represent the clearance of total triglycerides (**A**) and the density (S$_f$) fractions 400+ (**B**) and 20 to 400 (**C**) following the midday meal. Despite a reduction in total fat content of the meal, the metabolic impact of high-carbohydrate diets in patients with insulin resistance had adverse consequences on lipid clearance [11]. (Adapted from Chen et al. [11].)

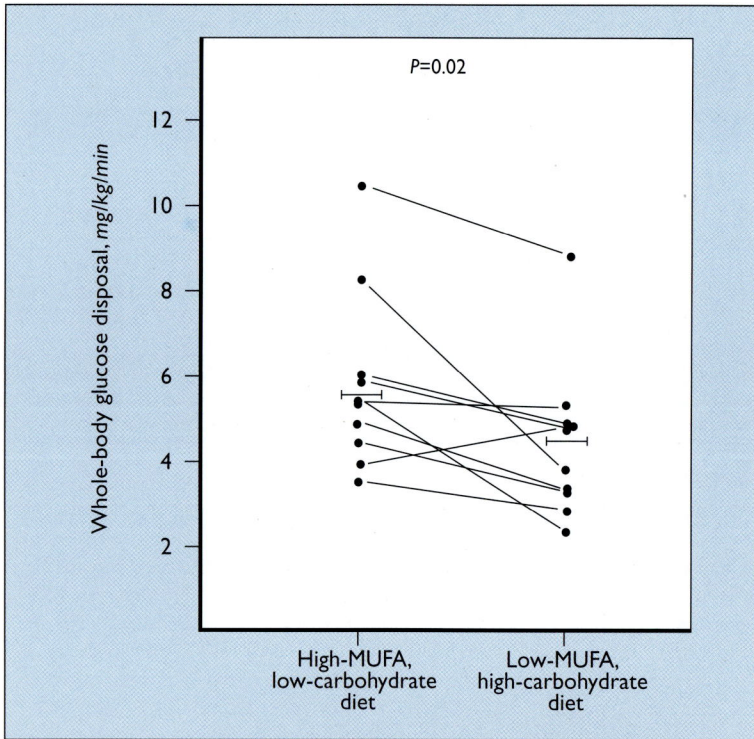

FIGURE 8-12. Improvement in insulin sensitivity or resistance. Whole-body glucose disposal was improved in patients with type 2 diabetes when a high–monounsaturated fatty acid (MUFA) diet was compared with a 10-day dietary intervention period of a high-carbohydrate diet [12]. Glucose disposal was measured using a euglycemic, hyperinsulinemic glucose-clamp technique. Insulin resistance is a genetic trait; in the environmental setting of overconsumption and decreased exercise, it can lead to type 2 diabetes. Whether alterations in insulin resistance or improvement in insulin sensitivity can be measured is a current area of much study. These data are taken from a report in which post-prandial plasma glucose and insulin concentrations were significantly elevated following the high-carbohydrate (intervention) diet phase [12]. (*Adapted from* Parillo *et al.* [11].)

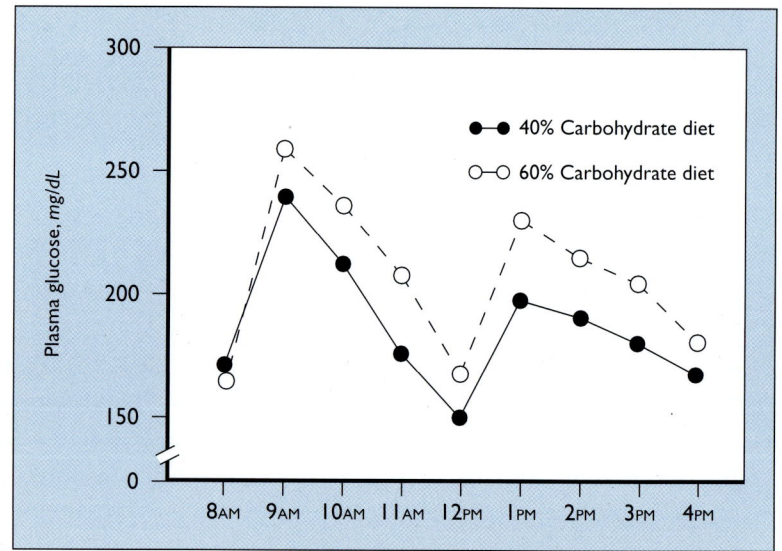

FIGURE 8-13. Impact of amount of carbohydrate on plasma glucose concentration. When caloric content is held constant and the composition of the diet is altered so that more of the calories are consumed as carbohydrates, there is no change in the fasting plasma glucose concentration but there is an increase in the postprandial plasma glucose concentration after the breakfast (8 AM) and lunch (noon) meals [13]. These data are from patients with type 2 diabetes who were randomly assigned in a crossover design for 15-day periods on a eucaloric, weight- and medication-stable diet [13]. (*Adapted from* Coulston *et al.* [13].)

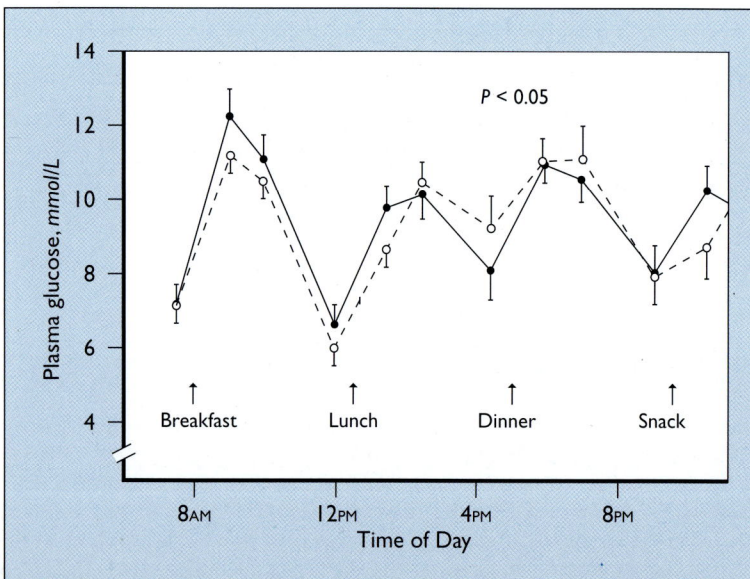

FIGURE 8-14. Impact of type of carbohydrate on plasma glucose concentration. Using a crossover design, patients with type 2 diabetes were randomly assigned to diets that contained 55% carbohydrate for 1 month [14]. In one period 3% of the calories were from sucrose (*open circles*), and in the other period 19% were from sucrose (*closed circles*). The total amount of carbohydrates eaten did not vary. There was no difference in the day-long plasma glucose concentration whether the diet contained 3% or 19% sucrose [14]. (*Adapted from* Bantle *et al.* [14].)

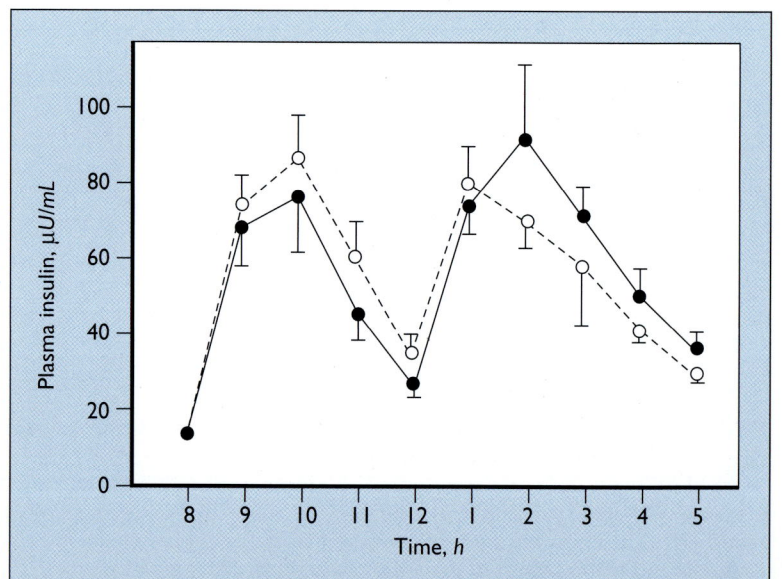

FIGURE 8-15. Impact of type of carbohydrate on plasma insulin concentration. Using a crossover design, patients with type 2 diabetes were randomly assigned to diets that contained 50% carbohydrate for 15 days [15]. In one period 1% of the calories were from sucrose (*open circles*), and in the other period 16% were from sucrose (*closed circles*). The total amount of carbohydrates eaten did not vary. There was no difference in the day-long plasma insulin concentration whether the diet contained 1% or 16% sucrose [15]. (*Adapted from* Coulston *et al.* [15].)

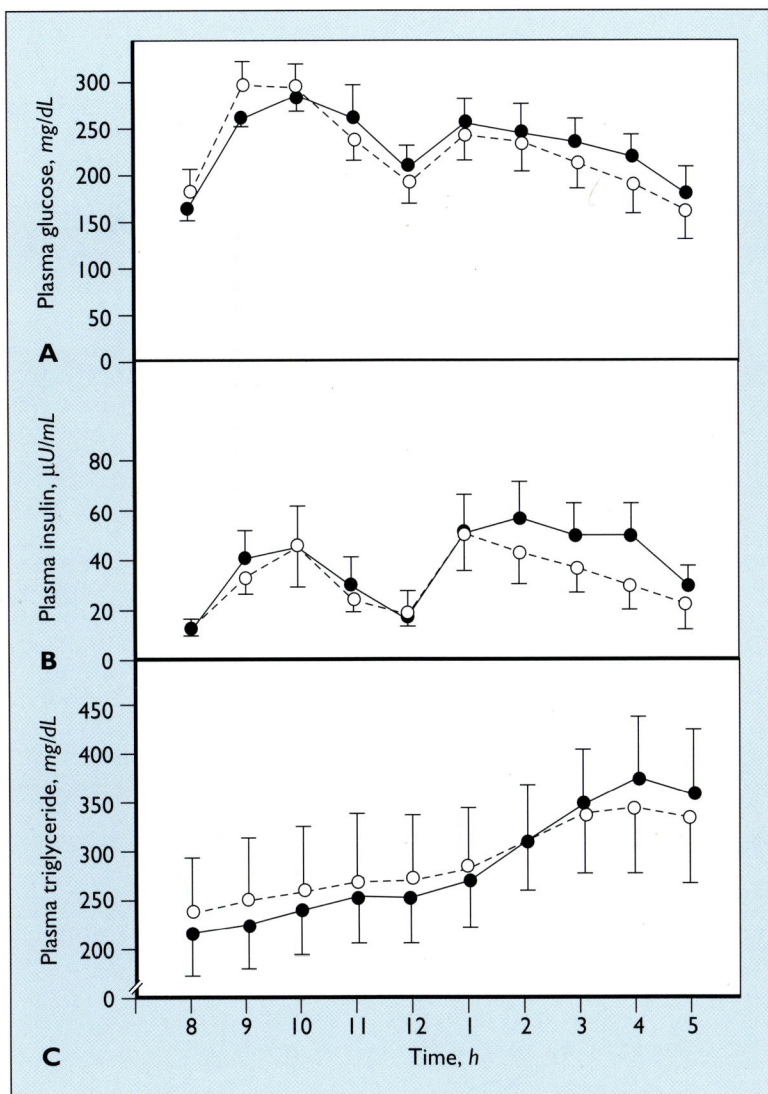

FIGURE 8-16. Impact of dietary fiber on plasma glucose (**A**), insulin (**B**), and triglyceride (**C**) concentrations [16]. Using a crossover design, patients with type 2 diabetes consumed diets that contained 11 g/1000 kcal of dietary fiber (high-carbohydrate, normal-fiber diet; *closed circles*) or 27 g/1000 kcal of mixed dietary fiber (high-carbohydrate, high-fiber diet; *open circles*) for 1 month; there was no change in the fasting or postprandial plasma glucose, insulin, or triglyceride concentrations. Whole-grain breads and cereals increased the fiber concentration of the diet over refined breads and cereals and fresh fruits and vegetables over cooked vegetables and juices [16]. (*Adapted from* Hollenbeck *et al.* [16].)

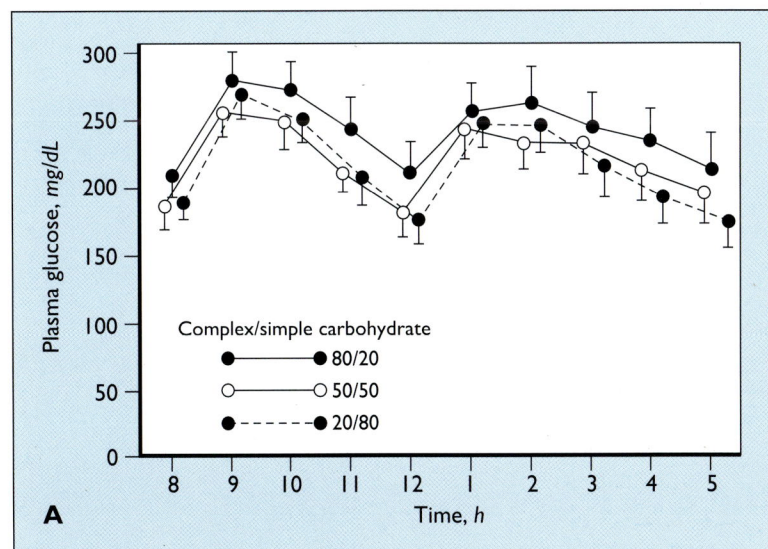

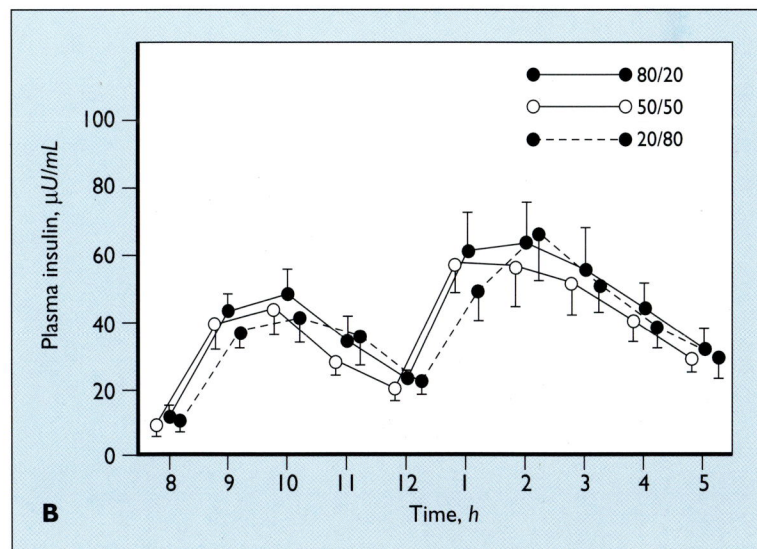

FIGURE 8-17. Plasma glucose (**A**) and insulin (**B**) response to variations in complex versus simple carbohydrates in the diet [17]. Patients with type 2 diabetes consumed 1-day test diets of a constant (50%) carbohydrate content in a randomized, crossover design (all participants received all diets). Breakfast and lunch meals were planned to contain 80% complex and 20% simple carbohydrates, 50% of each, or 80% simple and 20% complex carbohydrates. Although there was some variation in the plasma glucose and insulin concentrations in the three diets, there was no significant or clinical impact of the variation in the type of dietary carbohydrate on plasma glucose or insulin concentration. If anything, the more complex carbohydrates in the diet, the higher the postprandial plasma glucose concentration was [17]. (*Adapted from* Hollenbeck *et al.* [17].)

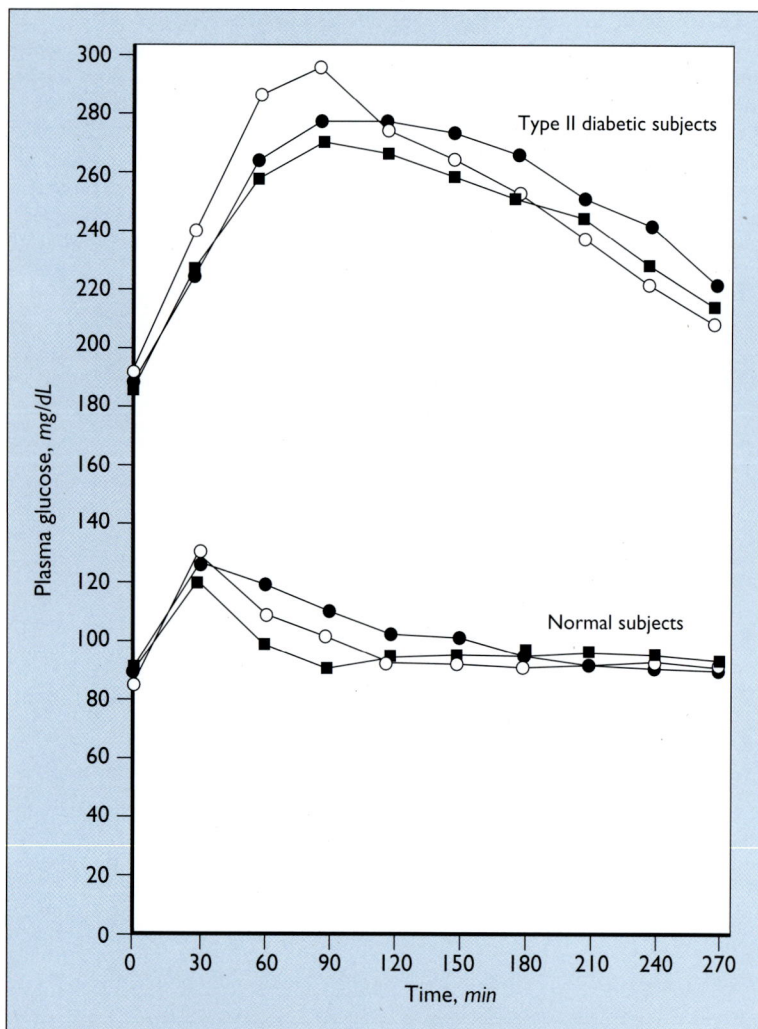

FIGURE 8-18. Plasma glucose response to meals with varying glycemic potential. When carbohydrate-rich foods are tested individually, a difference in the plasma glucose response has been noted. The plasma glucose response to a given food has been named the *glycemic index* (GI). However, when mixed meals planned to contain foods with a high (*closed circles*), intermediate (*open circles*), or low (*squares*) GI are consumed by normal glycemic patients or those with type 2 diabetes, there is no difference in the plasma glucose response to the meals [18]. (*Adapted from* Laine *et al.* [18].)

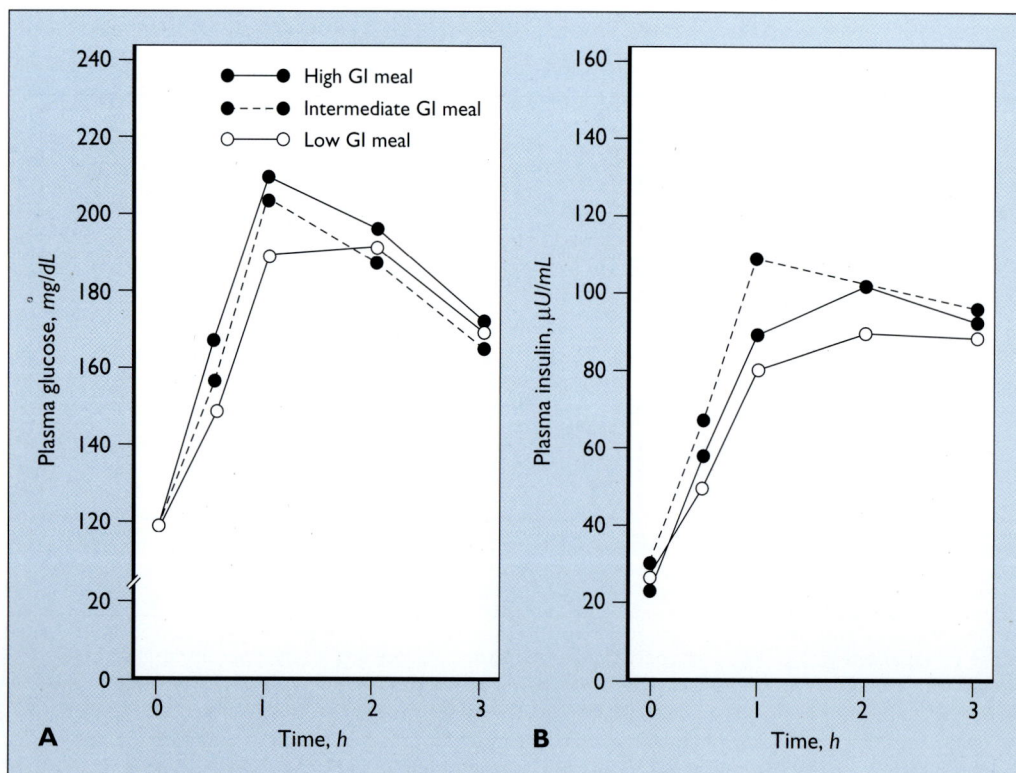

FIGURE 8-19. Plasma glucose (**A**) and insulin (**B**) response to meals with varying glycemic potential [19]. In a study similar to that by Laine *et al.* [18], plasma glucose and corresponding insulin responses did not vary to single meals provided with predicted differing glycemic potential when consumed by patients with type 2 diabetes. These meals contained 45% carbohydrate with 60% starch, 30% fruit, and 10% vegetables for the carbohydrate-rich foods [19]. (*Adapted from* Coulston *et al.* [19].)

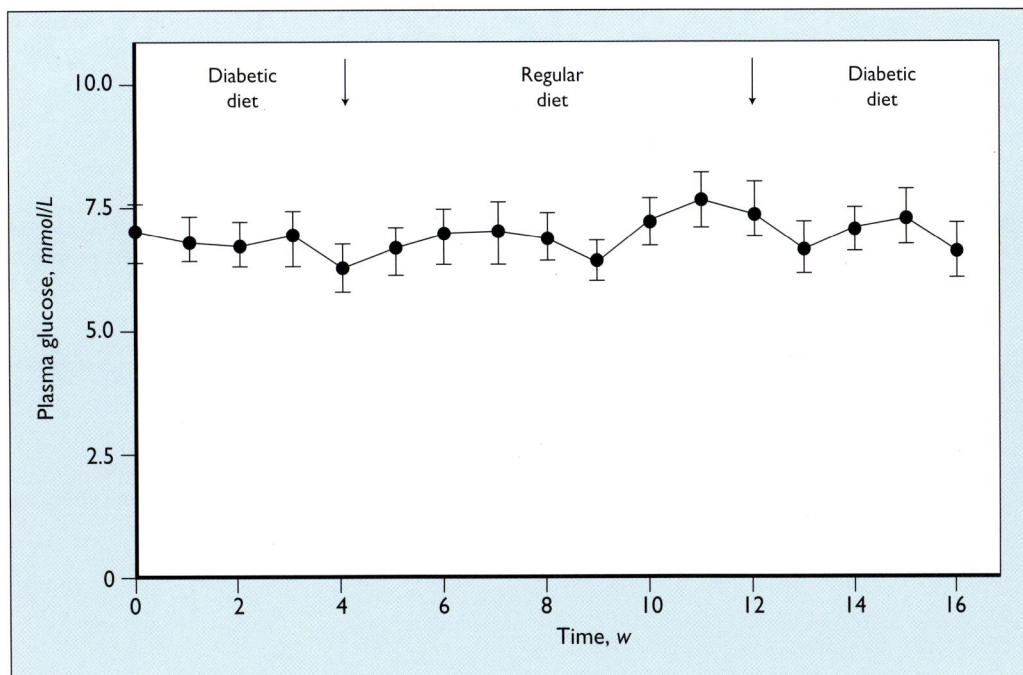

FIGURE 8-20. Fasting plasma glucose concentrations over 4 months. Patients with type 2 diabetes receiving long-term care were permitted a trial period of switching from the facility's diabetic diet to the regular diet for 1 month [20]. The types of foods served and the timing of each meal were relatively constant. Under these conditions, patients with diabetes did not experience a significant change in fasting plasma glucose concentrations whether they were served the regular or the diabetic diet. When patients are in stable metabolic control in institutional settings where most, if not all, food intake is provided by the institution, the need for "modified" diets for patients with diabetes is questionable [20]. (*Adapted from* Coulston et al. [20].)

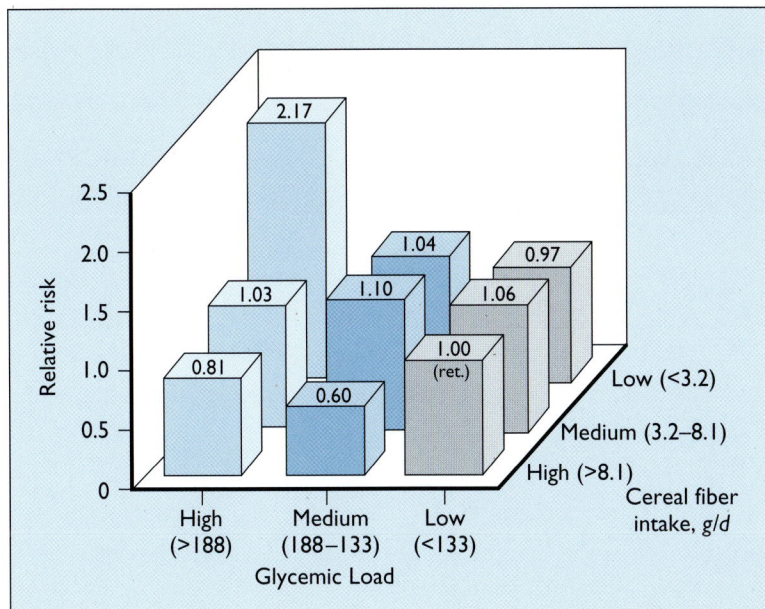

FIGURE 8-21. Relative risk of type 2 diabetes by differences of intake over time of cereal fiber and glycemic potential of the total diet. In a large study of men from the Health Professionals Follow-Up Study [21] (*n* = 42,759), dietary assessment and 6-year follow-up health assessment revealed that men whose diets were higher in glycemic potential and lower in cereal fiber had a higher relative risk for developing type 2 diabetes. Similar data were reported for women [22]. There has never before been an indication that past dietary intake (*ie*, sucrose intake) would increase the risk of diabetes. These epidemiologic findings do not correlate with those from intervention studies. Lifestyle factors related to development of type 2 diabetes, beyond genetic traits, require additional study. (*Adapted from* Salmeron [21].)

References

1. Report of the Expert Committee on the Diagnosis and Classification of Diabetes Mellitus. *Diabetes Care* 1997, 20:1183–1197.

2. Franz MJ, Horton ES, Bantle JP, et al.: Nutrition principles for the management of diabetes and related complications [technical review]. *Diabetes Care* 1994, 17:490–518.

3. Stern MP, Patterson JK, Haffner SM, et al.: Lack of awareness and treatment of hyperlipidemia in type 2 diabetes in a community survey. *JAMA* 1989, 262:360–364.

4. Reaven GM: The role of insulin resistance and hyperinsulinemia in coronary heart disease. *Metabolism* 1992, 41:16–19.

5. Reaven GM, Chen YD, Jeppesen J, et al.: Insulin resistance and hyperinsulinemia in individuals with small, dense low density lipoprotein particles. *J Clin Invest* 1993, 92:141–146.

6. Klienman JC, Donahue PR, Harris MI, et al.: Mortality among diabetics in a national sample. *Am J Epidemiol* 1988, 128:389–401.

7. Stamler J, Vaccaro O, Neaton JD, Wentworth D, for the Multiple Risk Factor Intervention Trial Research Group: Diabetes, other risk factors, and 12-yr cardiovascular mortality for men screened in the Multiple Risk Factor Intervention Trial. *Diabetes Care* 1993, 16:434–444.

8. Fontbonne A, Eschwege E, Cambien F, et al.: Hypertriglyceridemia as a risk factor of coronary heart disease mortality in subjects with impaired glucose tolerance or diabetes: results from the 11-year follow-up of the Paris Prospective Study. *Diabetologia* 1989, 32:300–304.

9. Fontbonne AM, Eschwege EM: Insulin and cardiovascular disease: Paris Prospective Study. *Diabetes Care* 1991, 14:461–469.

10. Garg A, Bantle JP, Henry RR, et al.: Effects of varying carbohydrate content of diet in patients with non-insulin-dependent diabetes mellitus. *JAMA* 1994, 271:1421–1428.

11. Chen Y-D, Coulston A, Zhou M-Y, et al.: Why do low fat, high-carbohydrate diets accentuate postprandial lipemia in patients with NIDDM? *Diabetes Care* 1995, 18:10–16.

12. Parillo M, Rivellese AA, Ciardullo AV, et al.: A high-monounsaturated fat/low-carbohydrate diet improves peripheral insulin sensitivity in non-insulin-dependent diabetic patients. Metabolism 1992, 41:1373–1378.

13. Coulston AM, Hollenbeck, CB, Swislocki ALM, et al.: Deleterious metabolic effects of high-carbohydrate, sucrose-containing diets in patients with non-insulin-dependent diabetes mellitus. Am J Med 1987, 82:213–220.

14. Bantle JP, Swanson JE, Thomas W, Laine DC: Metabolic effects of dietary sucrose in type II diabetic subjects. Diabetes Care 1993, 16:1301–1305.

15. Coulston AM, Hollenbeck CB, Donner CC, et al.: Metabolic effects of added dietary sucrose in individuals with non-insulin-dependent diabetes mellitus (NIDDM). Metabolism 1985, 34:962–966.

16. Hollenbeck CB, Coulston AM, Reaven GM: To what extent does increased dietary fiber improve glucose and lipid metabolism in patients with non-insulin-dependent diabetes mellitus (NIDDM)? Am J Clin Nutr 1986, 43:16–24.

17. Hollenbeck CB, Coulston AM, Donner CC, et al.: The effects of variations in percent of naturally occurring complex and simple carbohydrates on plasma glucose and insulin response in individuals with non-insulin-dependent diabetes mellitus. Diabetes 1985, 34:151–155.

18. Laine DC, Thomas W, Levitt MD, Bantle JP: Comparison of predictive capabilities of diabetic exchange lists and glycemic index of foods. Diabetes Care 1987, 10:387–394.

19. Coulston AM, Hollenbeck CB, Swislocki ALM, Reaven GM: Effect of source of dietary carbohydrate on plasma glucose and insulin responses to mixed meals in subjects with NIDDM. Diabetes Care 1987, 10:395–400.

20. Coulston AM, Mandelbaum D, Reaven GM: Dietary management of nursing home residents with non-insulin-dependent diabetes mellitus. Am J Clin Nutr 1990, 51:67–71.

21. Salmeron J, Ascherio A, Rimm EB, et al.: Dietary fiber, glycemic load, and risk of NIDDM in men. Diabetes Care 1997, 20:545–550.

22. Salmeron J, Manson JE, Stampfer MJ, et al.: Dietary fiber, glycemic load, and risk of non–insulin-dependant diabetes mellitus in women. JAMA 1997, 277:472–477.

NUTRITION AND ATHEROSCLEROSIS

David Kritchevsky

9

Atherosclerosis results from a gene–environment interaction mediated by a multicellular process in the arterial wall. In this process, monocytes internalize oxidized cholesterol through the actions of a scavenger receptor. Cholesterol bound to lipoproteins moves freely through the vascular wall from the circulation and, if oxidized, is taken up by monocytes, which ultimately become foam cells. These cells burst, leading to the formation of a cholesterol plaque in the vessel wall. Smooth muscle cell hyperplasia, cholesterol crystal accumulation, and calcification with the formation of bone cells in the vessel wall contribute to narrowing of the vessel lumen.

In most heart attacks, blockage of the vessel lumen is less than 50% and unstable plaques burst, triggering formation of an intraluminal clot. Many nutritional factors, including obesity, increased fat intake, reduced fiber intake, and reduced intake of fruits and vegetables, have been associated with an increased risk for heart disease. In fact, many of these factors have occurred together in modern diets, making it difficult to separately evaluate each of these nutritional entities. It is clear that cholesterol intake, when considered separately from high-fat foods, has a lesser effect on cholesterol levels than do dietary fat and calories.

Cholesterol levels correlate with risk for heart disease; patients with cholesterol levels greater than 240 mg/dL have twofold greater risk than patients with cholesterol levels less than 180 mg/dL. There are 37 million Americans with cholesterol levels greater than 240 mg/dl, and 56 million have cholesterol levels greater than 200 mg/dL. Only 3 to 4 million persons are taking cholesterol-lowering drugs, and debates on the cost-effectiveness of medication for primary prevention continue.

Despite the important effects of obesity and high-fat diets, some people exercise and eat a low-fat, high-fiber diet and still have cholesterol levels in a moderately elevated range (200–240 mg/dL). Several nutritional factors, including phytosterols, soy protein, naturally occurring inhibitors of cholesterol synthesis, and some classes of lipids (such as conjugated linoleic acid), have been shown to affect cholesterol levels. Appropriate use of dietary supplements, together with diet and exercise, offer an alternative approach to medications for the reduction of heart disease risk. The combination of population studies, experimental studies, and intervention trials suggests that nutrition plays a major role in determining the incidence of and rate of death from heart disease caused by atherosclerosis.

Atherosclerosis and Lipoproteins

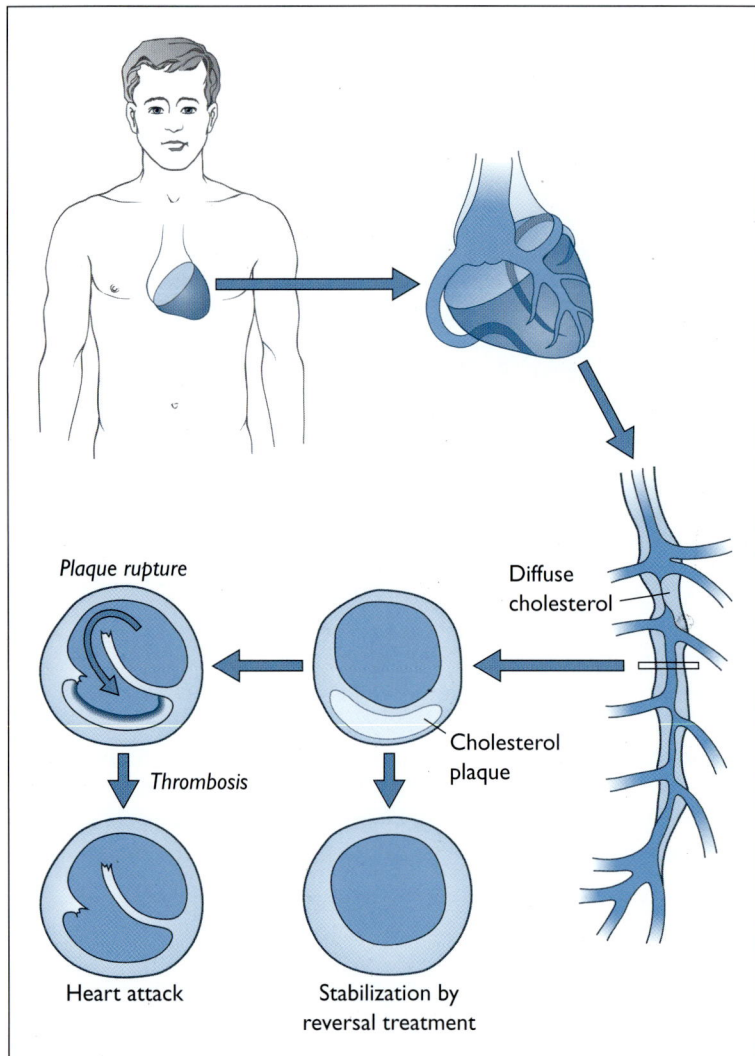

FIGURE 9-1. Results of the process of atherosclerosis. This process leads to the development of an unstable plaque in the wall of the coronary arteries that ruptures, resulting in acute thrombosis and myocardial infarction. Nutrition plays a major role in several aspects of this multicellular process through hormones that stimulate muscle cell proliferation, oxidant/antioxidant balance involved in the formation of plaque, cholesterol metabolism, and the clotting system (which mediates the arterial blockage).

CLASSIFICATION AND PROPERTIES OF PLASMA LIPOPROTEINS

Lipoprotein Class	Major Lipids	Apolipoproteins	Density, g/mL
Chylomicrons	Dietary triglycerides, cholesteryl esters	A-I, A-II, A-IV, B-48, C-I	< 0.95
Remnants	Dietary cholesteryl esters	B-48, E	< 1.006
VLDL	Endogenous triglycerides	B-100, C-I, C-II, C-III, E	< 1.006
IDL	Cholesteryl esters, triglycerides	B-100, E	1.006–1.019
Small, dense LDL	Cholesteryl esters	B-100, Lp(a)	—
LDL	Cholesteryl esters	B-100, Lp(a)	1.019–1.063
HDL2	Cholesteryl esters	A-I, A-II	1.063–1.125
HDL3	Cholesteryl esters	A-I, A-II	1.125–1.210

FIGURE 9-2. Classification and properties of plasma lipoproteins. Lipids are carried in the blood by lipoprotein particles. These include low-density lipoprotein (LDL), very-low-density-lipoprotein (VLDL), and high-density lipoprotein (HDL), which are defined by their density in a preparative ultra-centrifuge separation. It has now been shown that LDL can exist in a small dense form in which the ratio of apoprotein B-100 to cholesterol is elevated. This occurs commonly with upper-body obesity and insulin resistance (see Fig. 9-30). Lipoprotein(a) (Lp(a)) is also carried on LDL and can inhibit thrombolysis. It increases heart attack risk when it exists in the presence of other risk factors. IDL—intermediate-density lipoprotein.

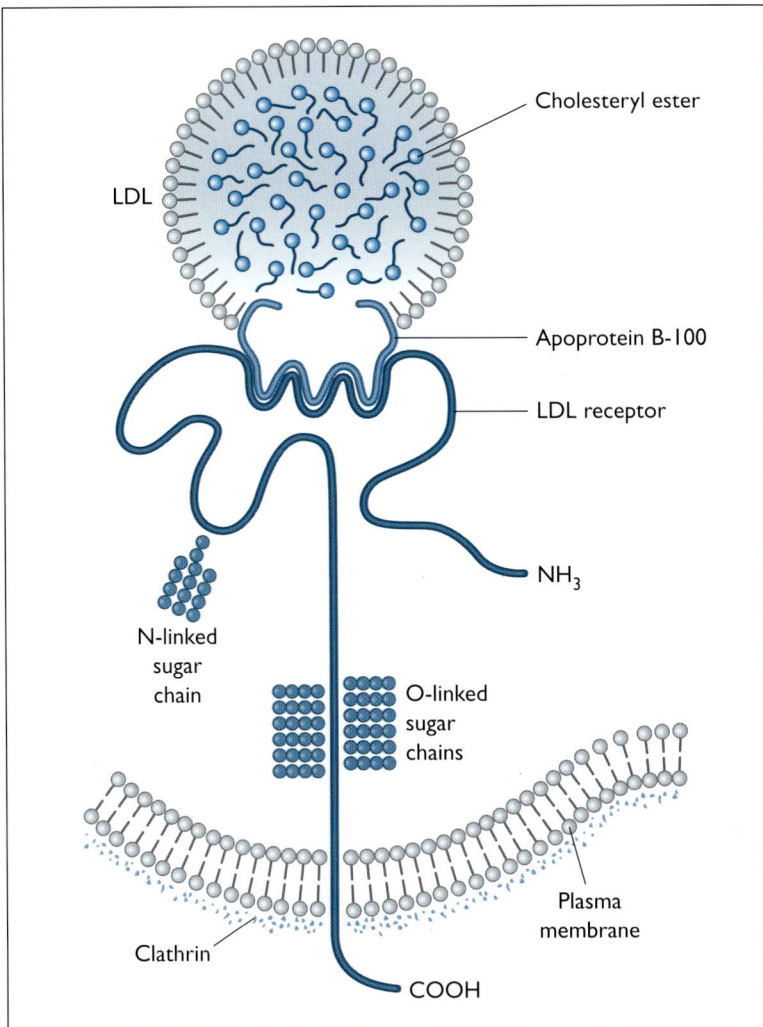

FIGURE 9-3. A low-density lipoprotein (LDL) particle with the polar heads of lipids oriented to the outside of the sphere. Triglycerides, cholesterol, and phospholipids make up the shell. An apolipoprotein B-100 cap on the particle serves as a recognition signal for the body to use in metabolizing this particle. Dietary lipids, by influencing plasma lipids, affect the lipid composition of these particles. COOH—carboxy terminal group.

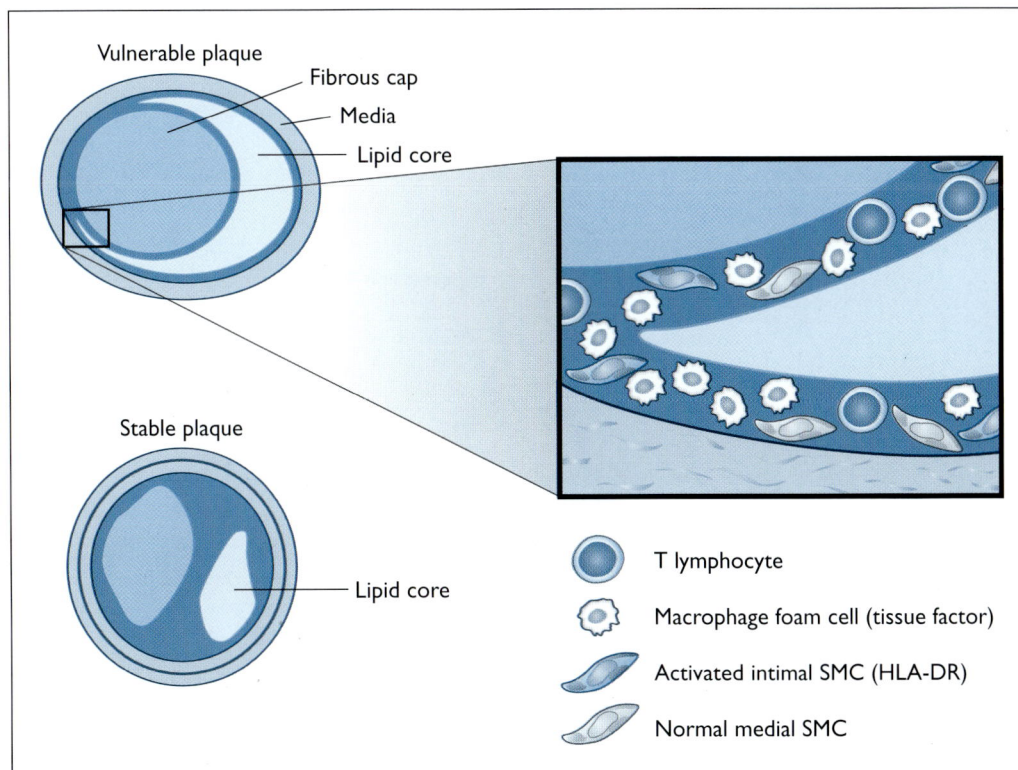

FIGURE 9-4. Plaque composition. In more than 50% of cases, blockage of the artery at the time of a heart attack is less than 50%. The yellow plaque consists of cholesterol crystals that have escaped from foam cells in the intima of the artery. These crystals are disgorged by foam cells, which are monocyte scavenger cells that take up the oxidized cholesterol in the intima. SMC—smooth muscle cells. (*From* Libby [1].)

Triglyceride Metabolism

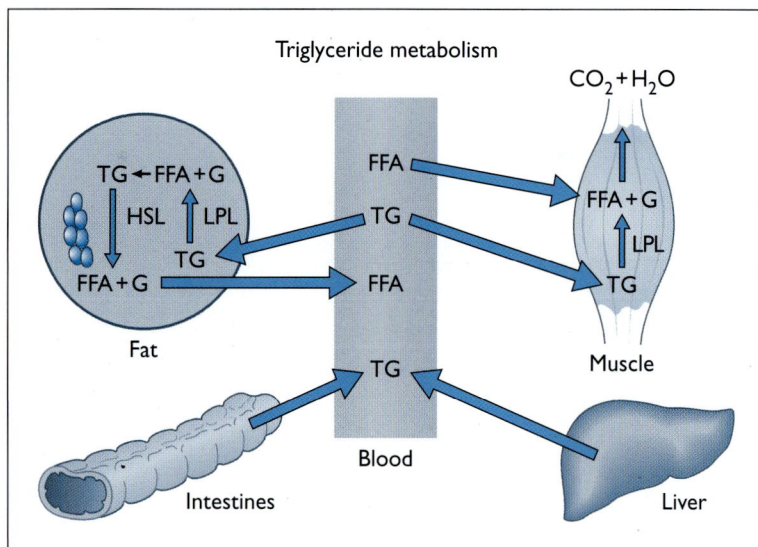

FIGURE 9-5. Triglyceride (TG) metabolism. Triglycerides make up 90% of the fats and oils in the diet. They are also produced endogenously in the liver and transported in the blood with very-low-density lipoprotein particles. Triglycerides can be burned in the muscle for energy or stored in fat cells through the action of the same enzyme, lipoprotein lipase (LPL). Triglycerides and cholesterol are increased in dietary-induced hyperlipidemias. FFA—free fatty acid; G—glucose; HSL—hormone-sensitive lipase.

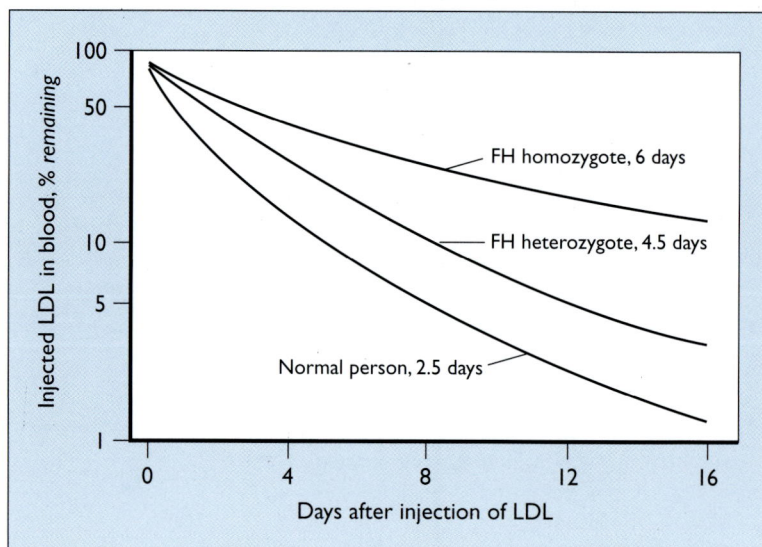

FIGURE 9-6. Clearance curves for normal persons, patients heterozygous for hypercholesterolemia, and patients with homozygous disease. In persons with familial hypercholesterolemia (FH), abnormalities of the low-density lipoprotein (LDL) receptor are reflected in reduced metabolic clearance of cholesterol-containing lipoprotein from the blood.

Atherogenesis and Cholesterol

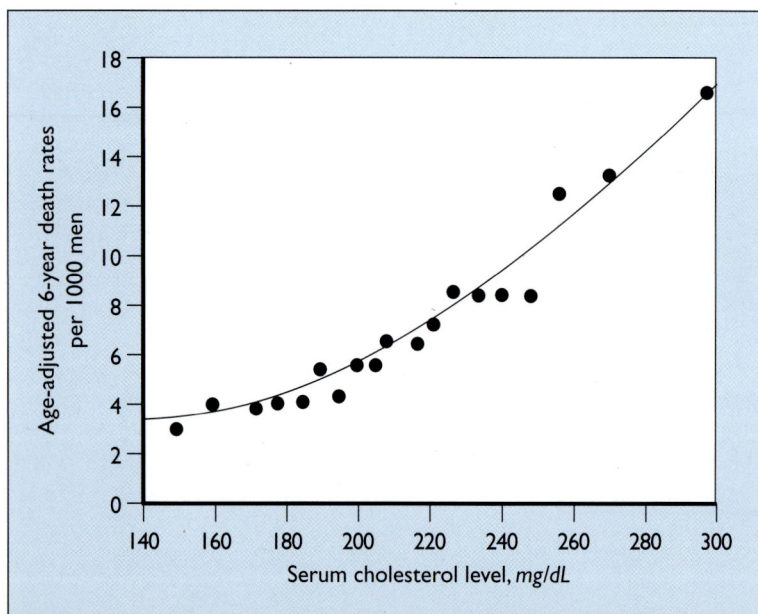

FIGURE 9-7. Data from the Multiple Risk Factor Intervention Study showing age-adjusted rates of death according to serum cholesterol levels [2]. Persons with hereditary hypercholesterolemia make up less than 5% of all individuals with heart attacks, but hypercholesterolemia due to a gene–environment interaction is a strong risk factor for heart disease. These data show that a cholesterol level of 240 mg/dL doubles the risk for heart attack compared with a cholesterol level of 180 mg/dL. It is assumed that similar risk reduction occurs whether the cholesterol level is reduced through diet or medication.

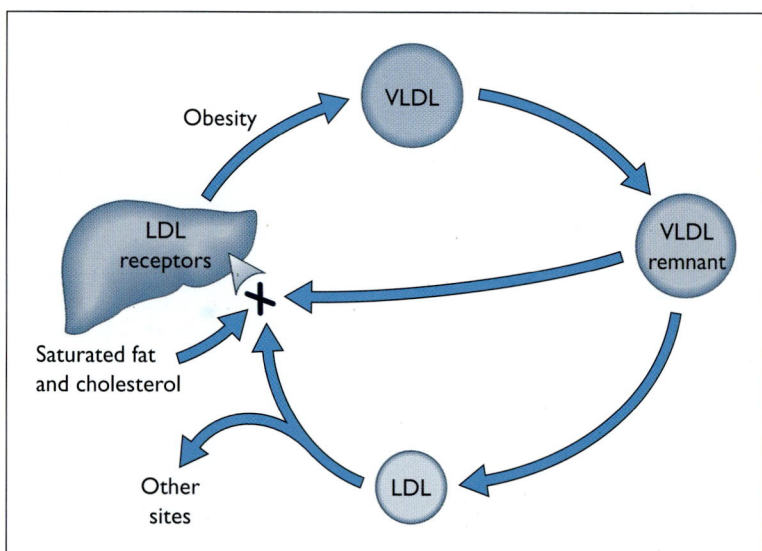

FIGURE 9-8. Gene–environment relationship in hypercholesterolemia. Obesity results in elevated insulin levels, which increase production of very-low-density lipoprotein (VLDL) particles. These particles contain 80% triglycerides and 20% cholesterol. The obesity-induced overproduction of VLDL from the liver results in increased levels of VLDL remnants and low-density lipoprotein (LDL) particles, which are atherogenic. Saturated fat and cholesterol reduce hepatic uptake of LDL particles, further increasing the levels of circulating LDL cholesterol. Therefore, hypercholesterolemia is due to a gene–environment interaction with measurable effects of obesity, saturated fat, and dietary cholesterol in susceptible individuals.

Lipid Metabolism

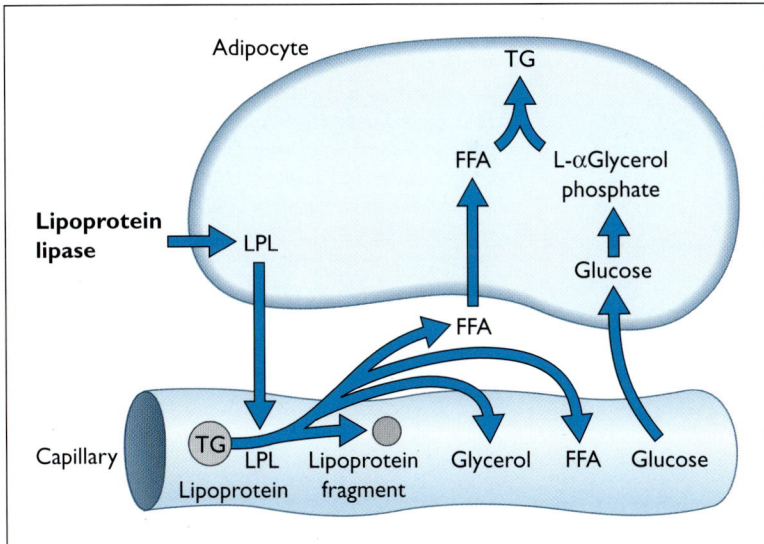

FIGURE 9-9. Mechanisms of lipogenesis. The balance between lipogenesis and lipolysis, controlled by diet, hormones, and exercise, has significant effects on lipid metabolism. Lipoprotein lipase (LPL) synthesized in the fat cell is transported to the vessel wall, where it breaks down triglycerides (TG) to glycerol and fatty acids. These are reassembled in the fat cell to be stored as triglycerides. Hormone-sensitive lipase then mediates the breakdown of stored triglycerides to fatty acids and glycerol. The fatty acids both recycle and are reused for triglyceride synthesis, but the glycerol exits the fat cell without reuptake and is metabolized. FFA—free fatty acids.

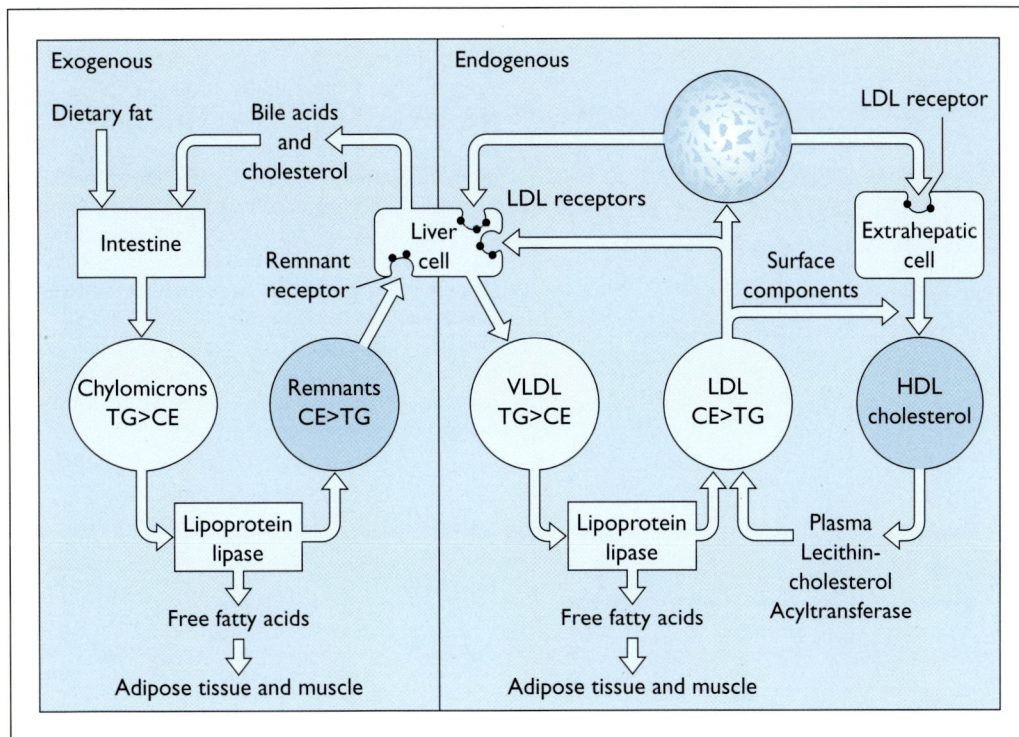

FIGURE 9-10. Pathways for exogenous and endogenous lipids. These types of lipids are metabolized differently but share common pathways. Dietary fat is taken up from the gut by chylomicrons, which are transported to the liver. Here they are metabolized and taken up in the pool for endogenous triglyceride (TG) synthesis. Endogenous triglycerides from the liver and chylomicrons carrying exogenous lipids are metabolized by lipoprotein lipase in muscle and fat cells. CE—cholesterol ester; LDL—low-density lipoprotein.

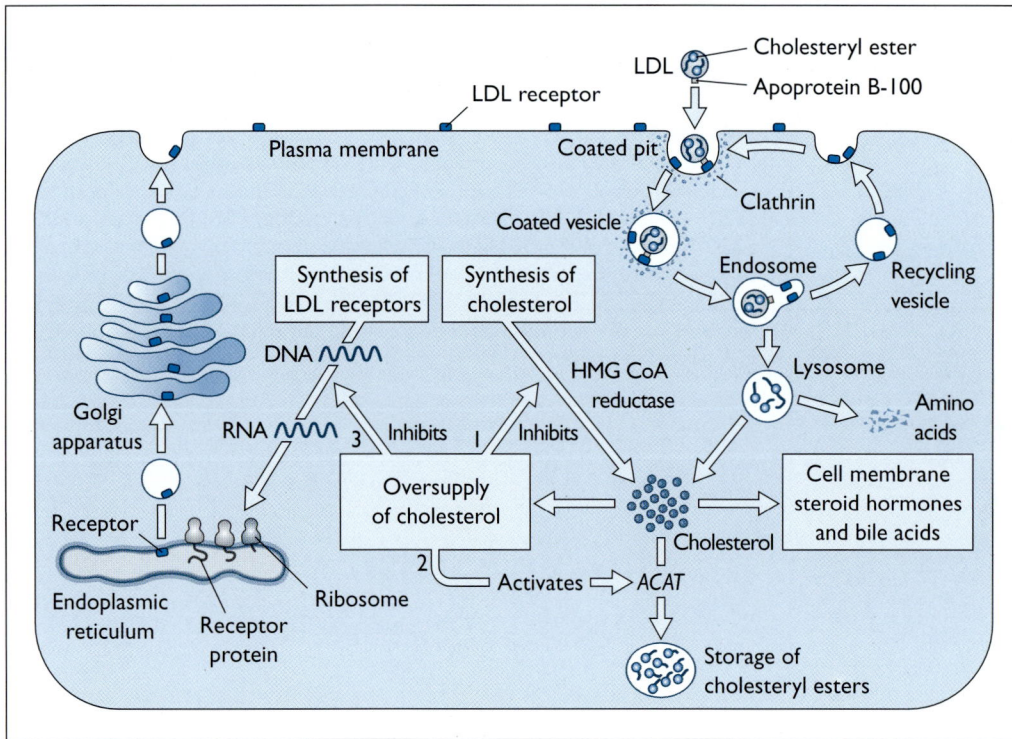

FIGURE 9-11. Regulation of cholesterol biosynthesis. At a cellular level, cholesterol biosynthesis is regulated by intracellular free cholesterol. When this pool is reduced, the number of receptors bringing cholesterol into the cell is increased and cholesterol biosynthesis is increased. When the intracellular cholesterol is increased, the number of receptors is decreased, as is cholesterol biosynthesis. Dietary fiber, by reducing cholesterol absorption in the gastrointestinal tract and removing it from the body, reduces intracellular cholesterol and triggers an increase in cholesterol biosynthesis. Therefore, the observed reduction in total cholesterol due to dietary fiber is increased when it is given in combination with an inhibitor of cholesterol biosynthesis. LDL—low-density lipoprotein.

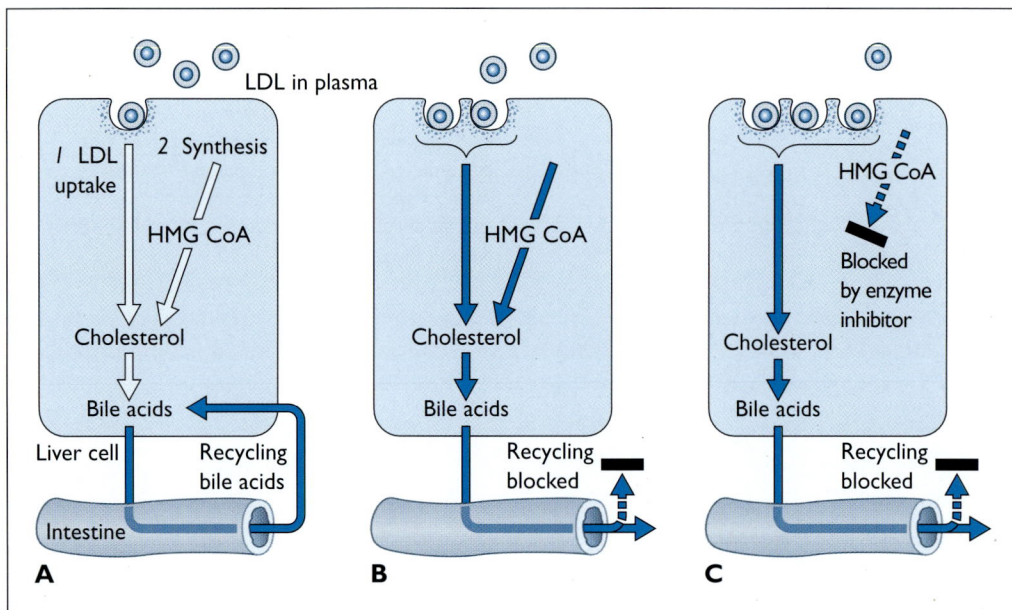

FIGURE 9-12. The synergistic effects of dietary fiber and inhibitors of cholesterol biosynthesis. Dietary substances that inhibit absorption and promote excretion include fiber and phytosterols. Naturally occurring inhibitors of cholesterol biosynthesis exist in small amounts in more than 30 species of mushrooms and fungi as monacolins. Chinese red rice yeast has been shown to reduce cholesterol levels, presumably by inhibition of cholesterol biosynthesis. **A,** Normal metabolism; **B,** after bile acid sequestrants; **C,** after HMG-CoA reductase inhibitors. HMG CoA—hepatic hydroxymethylglutaryl coenzyme A.

Dietary Fat	Cholesterol (mg/tbsp)	%	Breakdown of Fatty Acid Content (normalized to 100%), %			%
Canola oil	0	6	22	10		62
Safflower oil	0	10		77	Trace–	13
Sunflower oil	0	11		69		20
Corn oil	0	13		61	1–	25
Olive oil	0	14	8			77
Soybean oil	0	15	54		7	24
Margarine	0	17	32	–2		49
Peanut oil	0	18	33			49
Vegetable shortening	0	28	26	–2		44
Palm oil	0	49		9		37
Palm kernal oil	0	81			2–	11
Coconut oil	0	87			2–	6
Lard	12	41		11 –1		47
Beef	14	52		3– –1		44
Butter	33	66		2– –2		30

Saturated fat | Linoleic acid | Monosaturated fat

FIGURE 9-13. Fatty acid composition of common dietary fats. Among the saturated fats, coconut oil is the most atherogenic. Vegetable oils, such as corn oil, safflower oil, and soybean oil, contain large amounts of linoleic acid. Although polyunsaturated fats reduce cholesterol levels by comparison to saturated fats when calories are held constant, studies have shown that metabolites of linoleic acid may promote atherogenesis through effects on the scavenger monocytes.

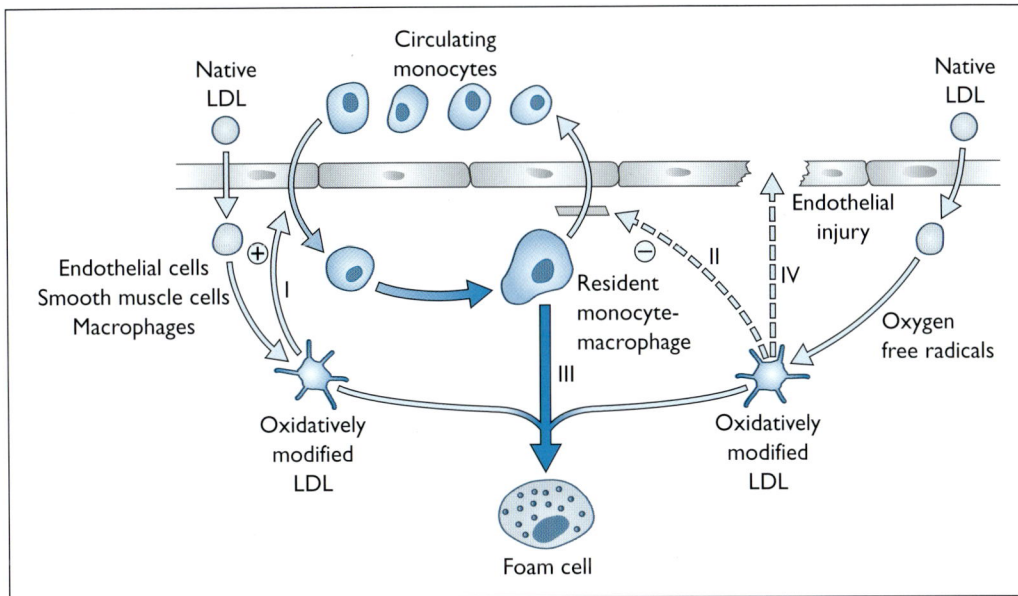

FIGURE 9-14. Linoleic acid metabolites induce the CD36 scavenger cell cholesterol receptor, which promotes atherogenesis. Oxidized cholesterol is taken up by these cells, and as the number of CD36 surface receptors is increased, the process becomes more efficient. The cellular basis of atherosclerosis involves the action of monocytes expressing a CD36 receptor that binds oxidized cholesterol. Linoleic acid increases oxidation of cholesterol and provides a stimulus to increased synthesis of the CD36 receptors. LDL—low-density lipoprotein.

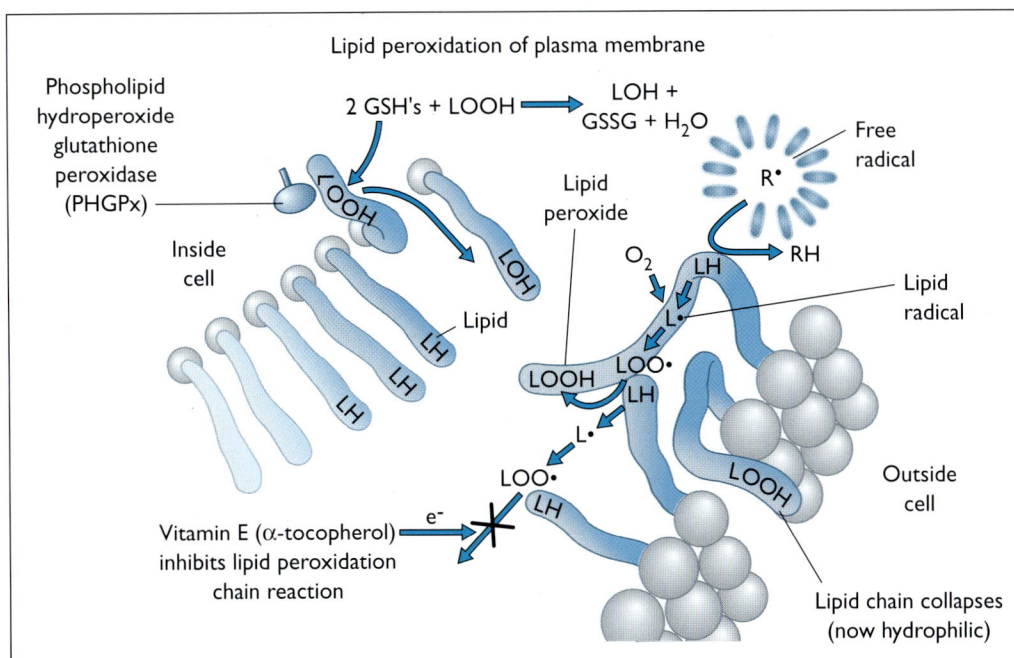

FIGURE 9-15. Lipid peroxidation of plasma membrane. Linoleic acid oxidation can lead to a chain reaction as the oxidized fatty acid itself serves as a pro-oxidant. This reaction can be seen both in the test tube and in the body. Endogenous antioxidants such as vitamin E are often removed during processing of vegetable fats and oils so that the polyunsaturated fats in the diet can contribute to oxidation processes, including oxidation of cholesterol. GSH—reduced glutathione; GSSG—oxidized glutathione; LOH—lipid hydroxide; LOO—hydroperoxide; R—free radical; RH—reduced free radical.

PHENOTYPIC EXPRESSION OF OBESITY AND HYPERCHOLESTEROLEMIA IN ADULT MEN AGES 45 TO 69 YEARS

Body Mass Index	Cholesterol Level, *mg/dL*	Triglyceride Level, *mg/dL*	HDL Cholesterol Level, *mg/dL*
≤ 21	212	141	45
21.1–23.0	222	105	49
23.1–25.0	223	140	45
25.1–27.0	235	170	45
27.1–30.0	234	204	43
> 30	230	259	38

FIGURE 9-16. Phenotypic expression of obesity and hypercholesterolemia. Obesity results in increased cholesterol and triglyceride levels through effects on very-low-density lipoprotein synthesis in the liver. These data collected from the National Health and Nutrition Examination Survey for men are typical of the association of mixed hyperlipidemia with obesity. This problem affects more than 40 million Americans and is the most common cause of elevated cholesterol levels. HDL—high-density lipoprotein. (*From* Grundy *et al.* [3].)

Diets and Treatment

AMERICAN HEART ASSOCIATION STEP 2 DIET COMPARED WITH LOVASTATIN

Group	Total Cholesterol Level	LDL Level	HDL Level	TG Level
Baseline	262	178	54	148
High Fat + Placebo	274 + 4%	182 + 2.2%	56	146
Low Fat + Placebo	257 - 5%	172 - 3.4%	53	148
High Fat + Lovastatin	219 - 27%	131 - 27%	58	123
Low Fat + Lovastatin	203 - 32%	123 - 31%	54	125

FIGURE 9-17. Comparison of the American Heart Association Step 2 diet (30% fat calories, less than 200 mg of cholesterol/d, less than 7% saturated fat) with lovastatin therapy. The step 2 diet resulted in a 5% reduction in cholesterol levels, while drug therapy accounted for a 27% reduction in cholesterol levels. LDL—low-density lipoprotein; HDL—high-density lipoprotein; TG—triglyceride. (*From* Hunninghake *et al* [4].)

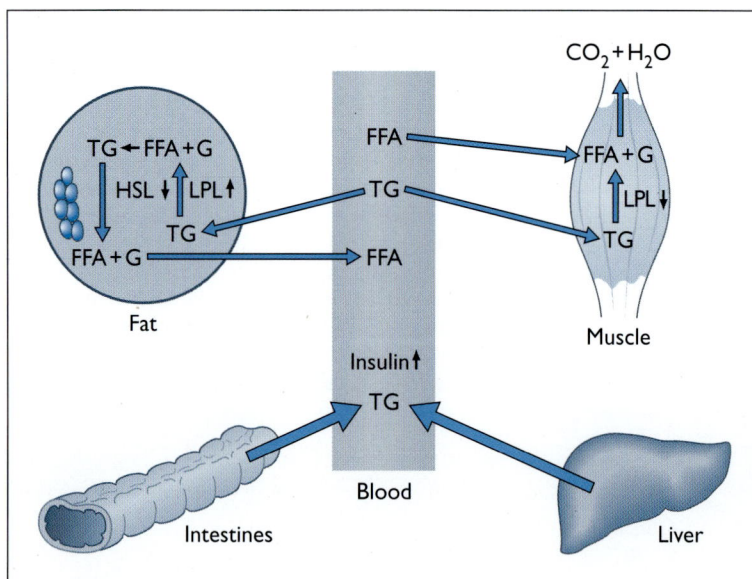

FIGURE 9-18. Effects of a high-fat, refined-sugar diet on increasing serum triglyceride (TG) and cholesterol levels. These effects are the result of both increasing insulin levels, which increase production of hepatic triglycerides, and reducing clearance by muscle lipoprotein lipase. At the same time, the deposition of triglycerides in fat depots increases, demonstrating the tissue-specific regulation of lipoprotein lipase (LPL) after changes in dietary intake. FFA—free fatty acid; G—glucose; HSL—hormone-sensitive lipase.

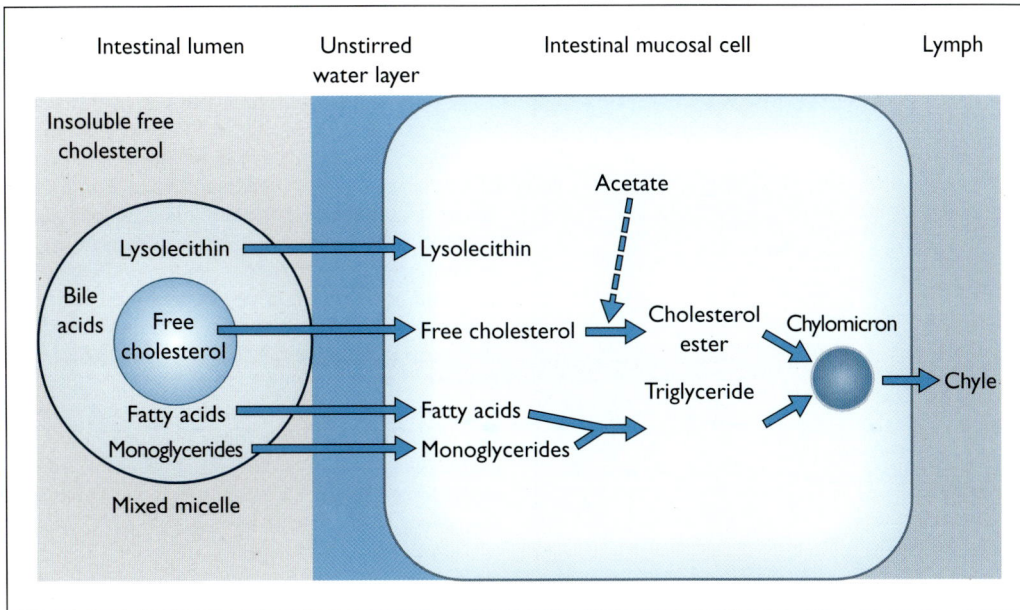

FIGURE 9-19. Absorption of dietary lipids. The process begins with the formation of a micelle. This permits the enzymes in the unstirred water layer on the intestinal mucosal cell to digest the lipids contained in the mixed micelle, releasing fatty acids, free cholesterol, lysolecithin, and monoglycerides into the intestinal cell. In this cell, they are reassembled into cholesterol esters and triglycerides. These are incorporated into chylomicrons and exported from the intestinal mucosal cell into the bloodstream.

SOURCES OF SOLUBLE AND INSOLUBLE FIBER

3.5-Ounce Serving	Fiber, g	Soluble Fiber, g
Cereals		
All Bran	30.8	5.1
Raisin Bran	13.5	2.4
Oatmeal	9.5	4.9
Shredded Wheat	12.5	1.6
Beans, peas, and nuts		
Black beans	7.1	2.8
Chick peas	5.3	1.6
Kidney beans	6.2	1.6
Walnuts	4.2	1.5
Fruits		
Apricots	7.9	4.4
Figs	8.2	4.0
Prunes	6.6	3.8
Apples	2.0	0.6
Oranges	2.0	1.0
Pears	3.5	1.3
Bananas	1.9	0.6
Vegetables		
Brussel sprouts	5.7	3.0
Broccoli	3.1	1.5
Carrots	3.2	1.5
Spinach	1.8	0.6
Asparagus	2.0	0.8
Corn	2.9	0.5
Potato	2.0	1.0

FIGURE 9-20. Sources of soluble fiber [5]. Rich sources include cereals, beans and peas, and certain fruits and vegetables. A mixture of these foods yielding a total daily intake of 25 to 35 grams of dietary fiber should assure an adequate intake of soluble fiber.

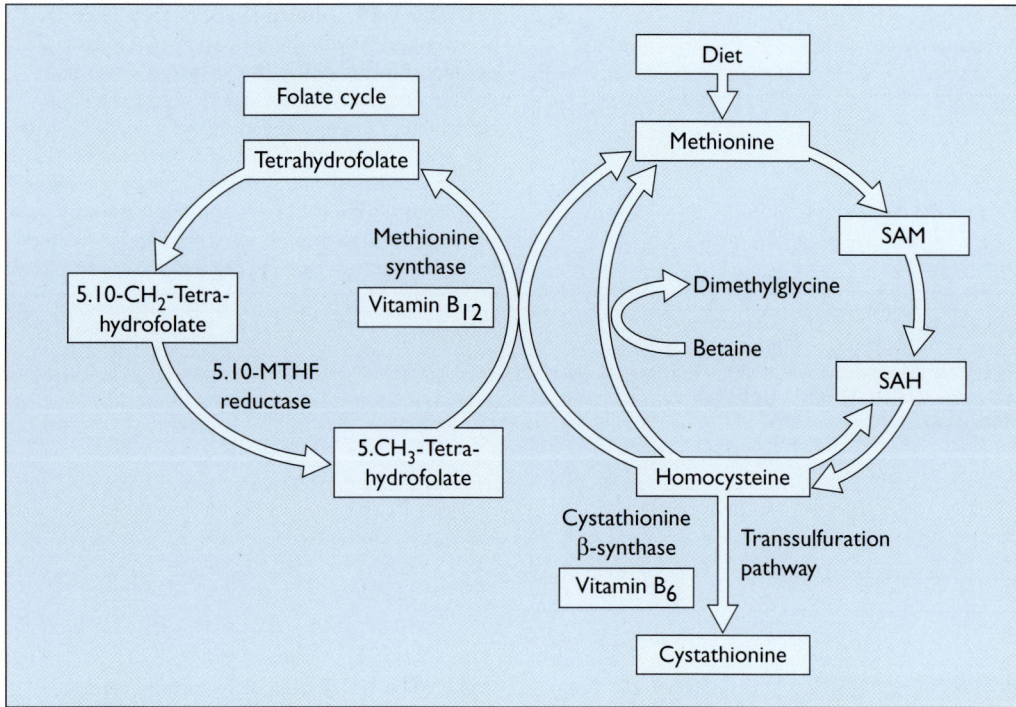

FIGURE 9-21. The folate cycle. Homocysteinuria is an inherited disease that leads to marked homocysteine elevations above the normal range and is associated with premature atherosclerosis. This can be due to any of three different inherited enzyme deficiencies. Folate is required for the conversion of homocysteine into methionine. The folate cycle demonstrates the utilization of folic acid for this purpose. Folic acid intake is often inadequate with an unsupplemented US diet. Dietary methionine, an amino acid present largely in animal protein, increases homocysteine after forming intermediates S-adenosyl methionine (SAM) and S-adenosylhomocysteine (SAH). The combination of dietary folate deficiency, increased methionine intake, and inherited metabolic changes in folate metabolism will lead to elevations in homocysteine levels. Supplementation with folic acid, vitamin B_6, and vitamin B_{12} can reduce homocysteine levels in such individuals.

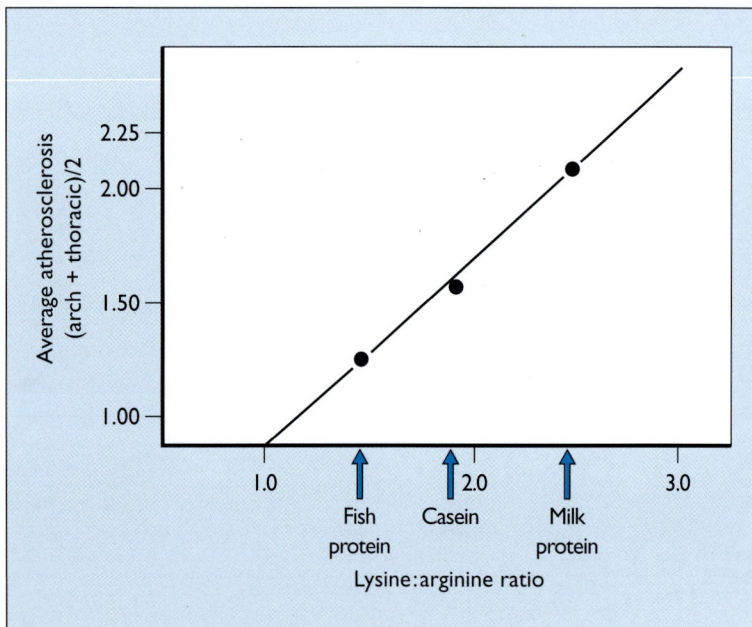

FIGURE 9-22. Severity of atherosclerosis in rabbits as a function of lysine:arginine ratio in several proteins. Effects of animal compared with vegetable protein on cholesterol levels have largely been related to the differences in the lysine-to-arginine ratio.

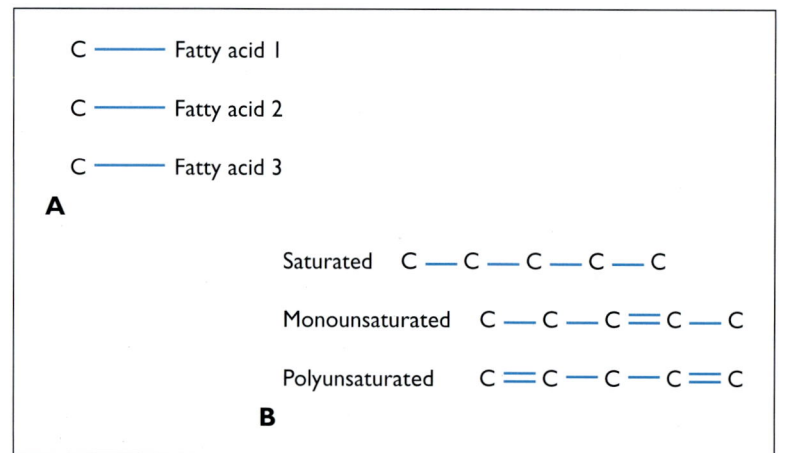

FIGURE 9-23. The structure of triglyceride and the associated fatty acids (**A**), which determine whether the triglyceride is called saturated, monounsaturated, or polyunsaturated (**B**). Both omega 6 (eg, linoleic acid) and omega 3 fatty acids (eg, linolenic acids and fish oils) are polyunsaturated fatty acids. However, the position of the double bonds in these two types of fats differs, giving them different structure-function properties in the body.

PHYTOSTEROLS

More than 50 phytosterols in nature: β-sitosterol, campesterol, stigmasterol (most abundant)

Ergosterol is nucleus for vitamin D

Phytosterols block absorption of cholesterol

FIGURE 9-24. Characteristics of phytosterols. These plant protein constituents compete with cholesterol for intestinal uptake and thus reduce the amount of cholesterol in the circulating pool. Phytosterols do not have significant effects in persons who do not eat cholesterol-containing foods.

PLANT STEROL CONTENT OF SELECTED FOODS

Food (Amount)	Plant Sterol, *mg*
Oils (1 Tbsp)	
Rice bran	167
Corn	136
Sesame	121
Safflower (≥70% linoleic acid)	62
Olive	31
Peanut	29
Soybean (hydrogenated) and cottonseed	21
Nuts and seeds (1 oz)	
Sesame seeds, dried	199
Sunflower seeds/kernels, dried	150
Peanuts, unroasted	62
Cashews, dry roasted	45
Almonds, dried	40
Pecans, dried	31
Fruit	
Orange, navel (1 orange)	45
Grapefruit, white (1/2 medium)	20
Vegetables (1/2 cup)	
Soybeans, green, boiled	45
Lettuce, shredded	11
Cauliflower, raw	9
Tomato, stewed	7

FIGURE 9-25. Plant sterol (phytosterol) content for common foods. Because many of these foods have high calorie and fat content, sterol supplements have been prepared and tested for their ability to reduce cholesterol levels.

EFFECT OF DIETARY TREATMENT WITH PLANT STANOL ESTER IN HYPERCHOLESTEROLEMIC PATIENTS

Reference	Population	Control Diet	Treatment Diet	PSE Content	Cholesterol Reduction, %	
					Total	LDL
Vanhanen et al	67 Male	37% fat 12% sat fat 270 mg chol	"Similar to controls"	3 g in 50 g mayonnaise	-7	-9
Gylling and Miettinen	11 Male, NIDDM	38% fat 324 mg chol	38% fat 357 mg chol	3 g in 30 g margarine	-6	-9
Miettinen et al	153 Male and Female	35% fat 14% sat fat 314 mg chol	36% fat 14% sat fat 340 mg chol	3 g in 24 g margarine	-10	-14
Gylling and Miettinen	8 Male, NIDDM	79 g fat 233 mg chol	"Practically unchanged"	3 g in 24 g margarine	-11	-14
Gylling et al	22 Female, PM, MI	Home diet: 36% fat 15% sat fat 247 mg chol	Fat and sat fat unchanged from home diet	3 g in 21 g margarine	-13	-20

FIGURE 9-26. Effects of dietary treatment with plant stanols, a class of phytosterols, in hypercholesterolemic patients [6]. These stanols have been sold in Europe in margarines designed to reduce cholesterol levels. Products based on stanols are now available in the United States. LDL—low-density lipoprotein; NIDDM—non–insulin-dependent diabetes mellitus; MI—myocardial infarction; PM—postmenopausal; PSE—plant stanol ester.

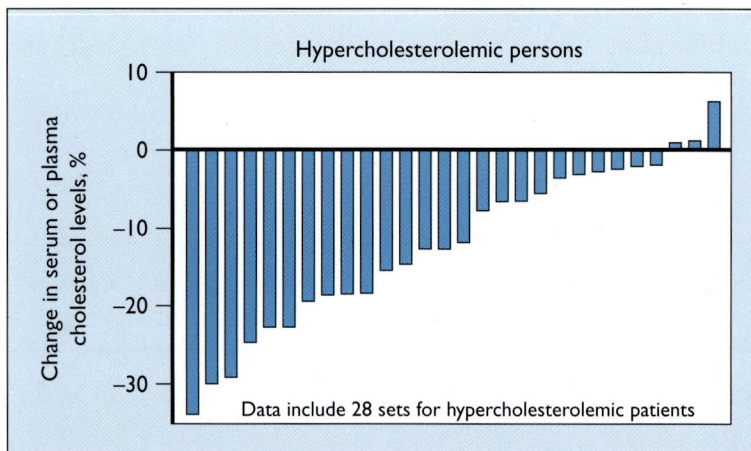

FIGURE 9-27. The effects of soy protein isolate on serum cholesterol levels when supplemented in the diet at levels of up to 47 g/d. The soy protein may contain phytosterols and exert its effect by replacing animal protein. This ability results from the protein's different lysine-to-arginine ratio. (*Adapted from Carroll [7].*)

WHEN TO INITIATE DIETARY INTERVENTION

If the patient:	Initiate dietary intervention if LDL cholesterol level is:
Is without CHD and has < 2 risk factors	≥160 mg/dL
Is without CHD and has ≥ 2 risk factors	≥130 mg/dL
Has known CHD	>100 mg/dL

FIGURE 9-28. Indications for dietary intervention. The National Cholesterol Education Program recommends that dietary intervention be instituted in patients with known coronary heart disease (CHD) who have low-density lipoprotein (LDL) cholesterol levels greater than 100 mg/dL, in patients who have two or more risk factors and have an LDL cholesterol level greater than 130 mg/dL, and in patients who have fewer than two risk factors and have an LDL cholesterol level greater than 160 mg/dL.

FIGURE 9-29. The Step 1 and Step 2 diets recommended by the National Cholesterol Education Program. Because obesity is a common cause of hypercholesterolemia, these diets have only modest effects on serum cholesterol levels. Obese patients can maintain their weight on a 30% fat diet in which calories are not restricted.

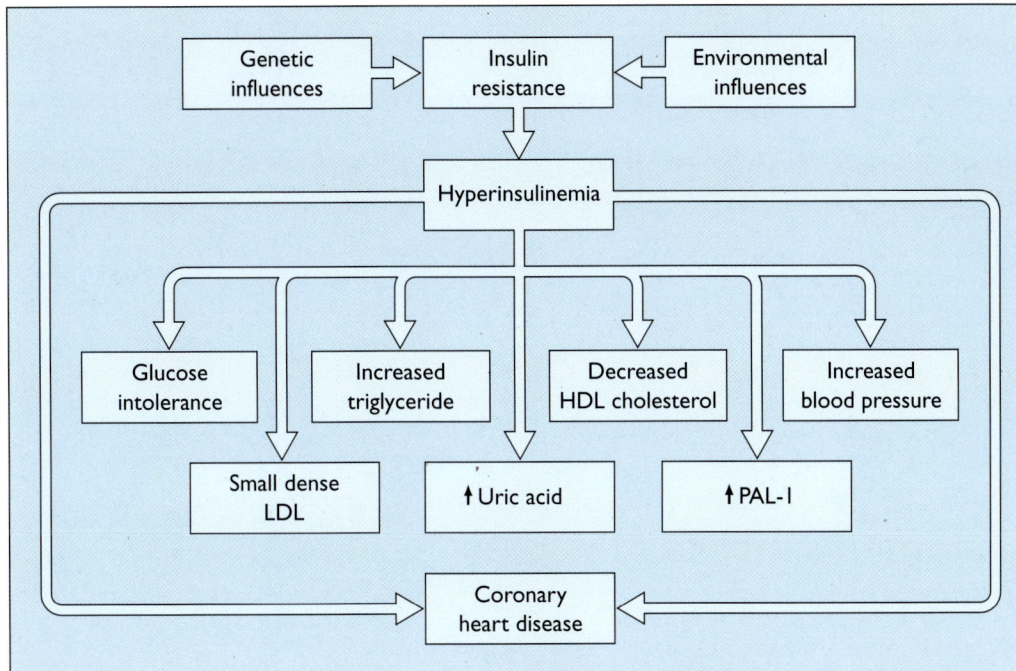

FIGURE 9-30. Effect of hyperinsulinemia on cardiovascular disease risk. Hyperinsulinemia is the result of a gene–environment interaction and leads to increased blood pressure, hyperlipidemia (small dense low-density lipoprotein [LDL] particles, increased triglyceride levels, and decreased high-density lipoprotein [HDL] cholesterol levels), glucose intolerance, hyperuricemia, and increased plasminogen activator inhibitor 1 (PAI-1). Intervention trials examining weight reduction in patients with non–insulin-dependent diabetes mellitus plan to study reduction in cardiovascular risk as the primary outcome variable.

References

1. Libby P: Molecular basis of the acute coronary syndromes. *Circulation* 1995, 91:2844–2850.
2. The Multiple Risk Factor Intervention Trial (MRFIT). A national study of primary prevention of coronary heart disease. *JAMA* 1976, 235(8):825–827.
3. Denke MA, Sempos CT, Grundy SM: Excess body weight. An under-recognized contributor to high blood cholesterol levels in white American men. *Arch Intern Med* 1993, 153:1093–1103.
4. Hunninghake DB, Stein EA, Dujovne CA, *et al.*: The efficacy of intensive dietary therapy alone or combined with lovastatin in outpatients with hypercholesterolemia. *N Engl J Med* 1993, 328:1213–1219.
5. Anderson JW: Plant fiber in foods. Lexington, KY: HCF Nutrition Research Foundation; 1990.
6. Roberts WO, ed: New Developments in the Dietary Management of High Cholesterol. Postgrad Med, Special Report. Minneapolis: McGraw-Hill Companies, Inc., 1998.
7. Carroll KK: Review of clinical studies on cholesterol-lowering response to soy protein. *J Am Diet Assoc* 1991, 91:820–827.

10

NUTRITIONAL STATUS AND REPRODUCTION

Rachelle Bross, Atam B. Singh, and Shalender Bhasin

Humans have known since antiquity that energy balance and nutritional status are intimately linked to the reproductive axis in both men and women [1–7]. The onset of puberty, the length of the reproductive period, the number of offspring, and the age of menopause have all been linked to body weight and composition, particularly the amount of body fat [3–7]. Normal reproductive function requires an optimal nutritional intake; both caloric deprivation and consequent weight loss, and excessive food intake and obesity are associated with impairment of reproductive function. Hippocrates recognized 2000 years ago that "...flabby and podgy girls... can not be prolific. The womb is unable to receive semen and they menstruate infrequently...." This may have been the earliest written description of polycystic ovary syndrome. The temporal aspects of sexual maturation are more closely associated with body growth than with chronological age [8]. In the animal kingdom, during periods of food scarcity, small animals with a short lifespan may not even achieve puberty before death. In animals with longer lifespans, sexual maturation may be substantially delayed during food deprivation. Undernutrition, caused by famine, eating disorders, and exercise, results in weight loss and changes in body composition and endocrine milieu that can impair reproductive function [1–15]. As a general rule, weight loss and body composition changes resulting from undernutrition are associated with reduced gonadotropin secretion; the decrease in follicle-stimulating hormone and luteinizing hormone levels correlates with the degree of weight loss [9–11]. However, both hypogonadotropic and hypergonadotropic hypogonadism have been described in cachexia associated with certain chronic illnesses, such as HIV-infection [12]. Collectively, these observations provide compelling evidence that energy balance is an important determinant of reproductive function in all mammals.

Biochemical Pathways

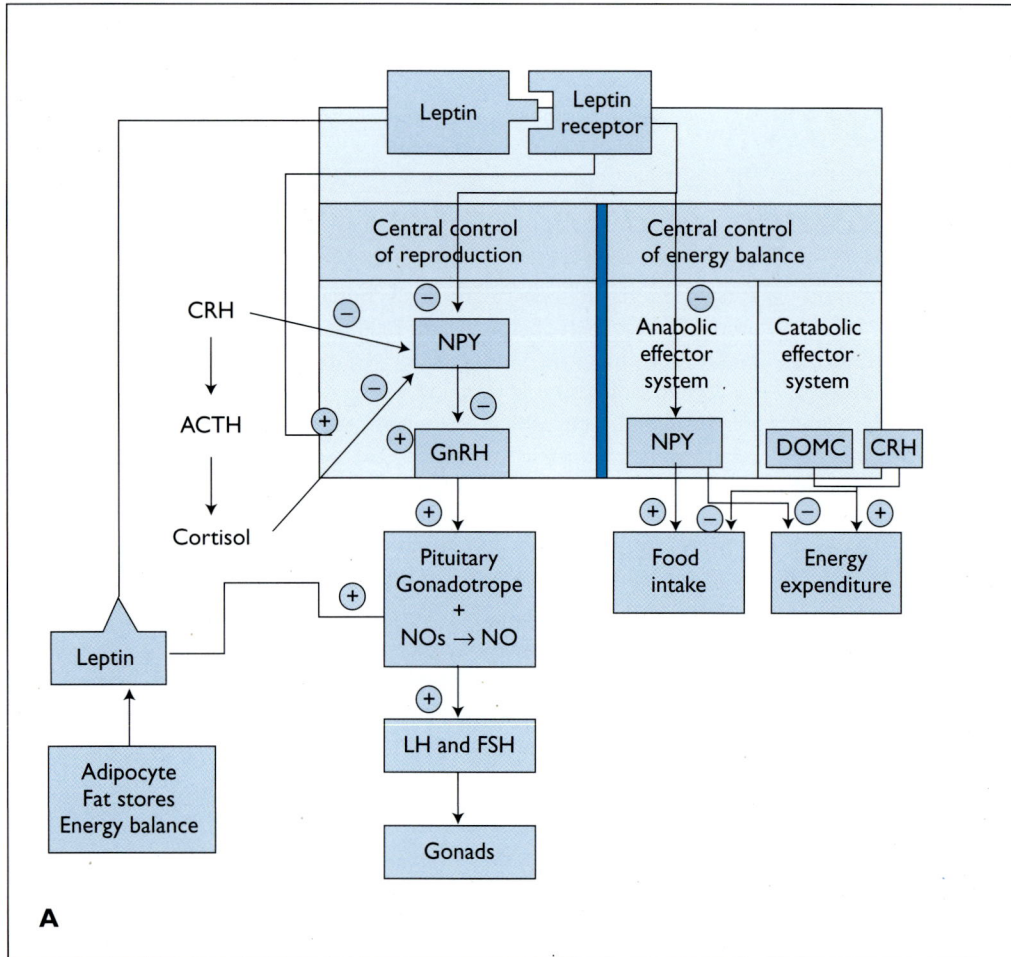

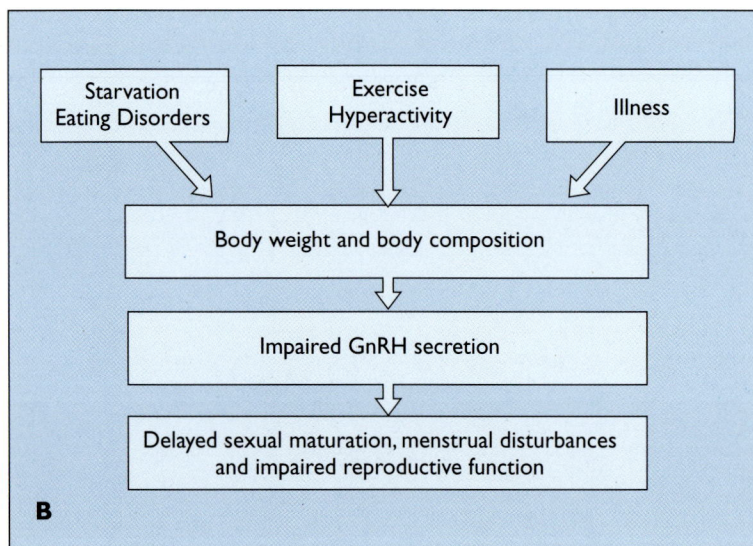

FIGURE 10-1. A, The biochemical pathways that link energy balance and reproductive axis. We do not know the precise nature of the biochemical pathways that connect these two body systems, which are essential for the survival of all species. The prevalent hypothesis is that the metabolic signals, that regulate hypothalamic secretion of gonadotropin releasing hormone (GnRH), are mediated through leptin and neuropeptide Y [8, 13–18]. Leptin, the product of the obesity (*ob*) gene, is a circulating hormone secreted by the fat cells that acts centrally to regulate the activity of central nervous system effector systems that maintain energy balance [19]. Leptin stimulates luteinizing (LH) secretion by activation of the nitric oxide (NO) synthase in the gonadotropes [18]. Leptin also inhibits neuropeptide Y secretion. Neuropeptide Y has a tonic inhibitory effect on both leptin and GnRH secretion. Leptin also stimulates NO production in the mediobasal hypothalamus; NO stimulates GnRH secretion by the hypothalamic GnRH-secreting neurons [18]. Therefore, the net effect of leptin action is stimulation of hypothalamic GnRH secretion [13–18].

Caloric deprivation in experimental animals is associated with reduced leptin levels and a concomitant reduction in circulating LH levels [14]. Leptin administration to calorically deprived mice reverses the inhibition of gonadotropin secretion that attends food restriction [14]. Similarly, genetically ob/ob mice with leptin deficiency have hypogonadotropic hypogonadism and are infertile; treatment of these mice with leptin restores gonadotropin secretion and fertility [14]. Collectively, these observations suggest energy deficit and weight loss are associated with impaired GnRH secretion (**B**), in part because of decreased leptin secretion and a reciprocal increase in neuropeptide activity. Although there is agreement that leptin is an important metabolic signal that links energy balance and reproductive axis, it remains unclear whether it is the primary trigger for the activation of the GnRH pulse generator at the onset of puberty. Emerging evidence suggests that leptin is essential but not sufficient for initiation of puberty.

Historical and Anthropological Illustrations of the Link between Nutritional Status and Fertility

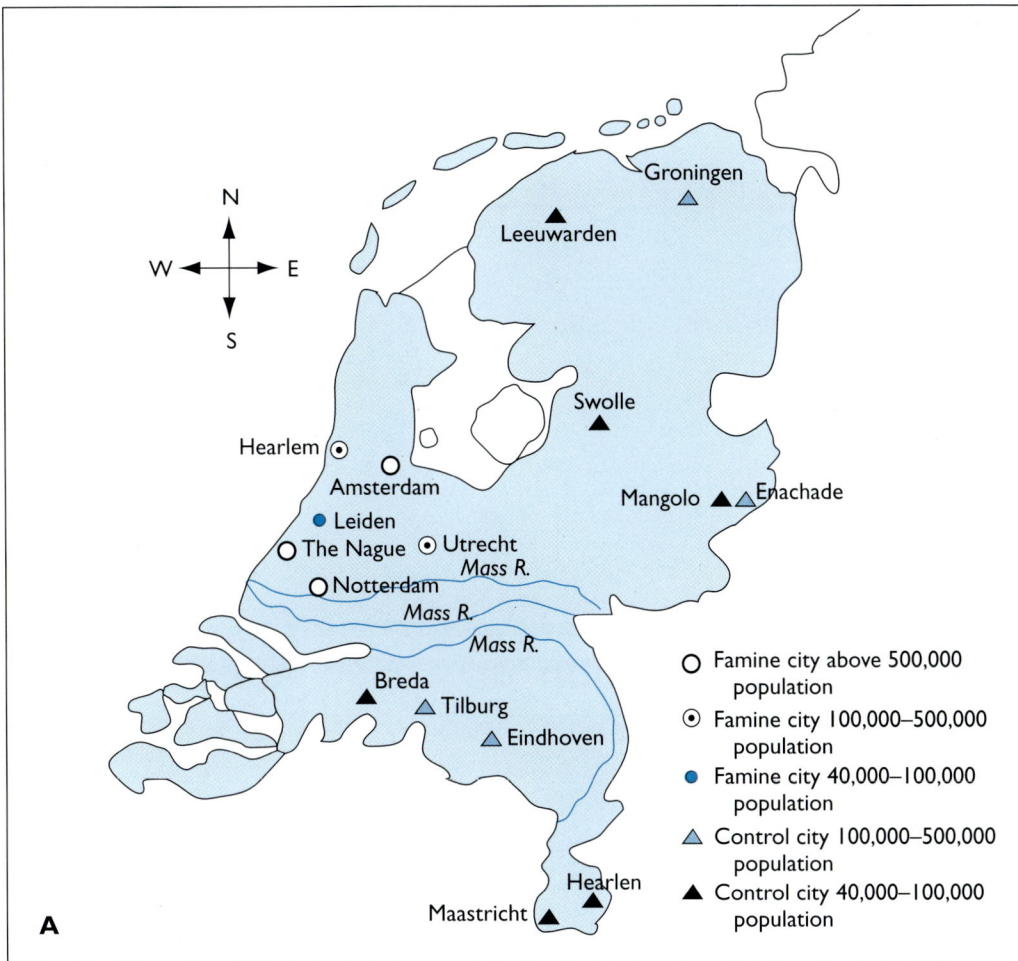

FIGURE 10-2. **A,** A map of the Netherlands showing the location of famine cities affected by the Dutch Hunger Winter and control cities [20–22]. Between October 1944 and May 1945, during the German occupation of the Netherlands, the German army restricted food supplies in certain Dutch cities; this resulted in substantial reduction in average daily energy intake to less than 1000 kcal [21,22]. Some adjacent cities, where food supplies were not curtailed by the Germans, were not affected by the famine. Susser and Stein [21,22] have reported the effects of acute food scarcity on this previously healthy and nutritionally replete population.

B, Fertility and caloric ration in famine cities. Average daily caloric intake and number of births from June 1944 through December 1946. Fifty percent of the women affected by the famine developed amenorrhea. The conception rate dropped to about 53% of that normally expected (based on control cities) and was correlated with the decreased caloric ration [21,22]. In addition to the decrease in fertility, undernutrition resulted in an increase in perinatal mortality, congenital malformations, schizophrenia, and obesity [22]. These observations indicate that optimal caloric intake is essential for normal fertility and prenatal growth. (*From* Susser and Stein [20–22].)

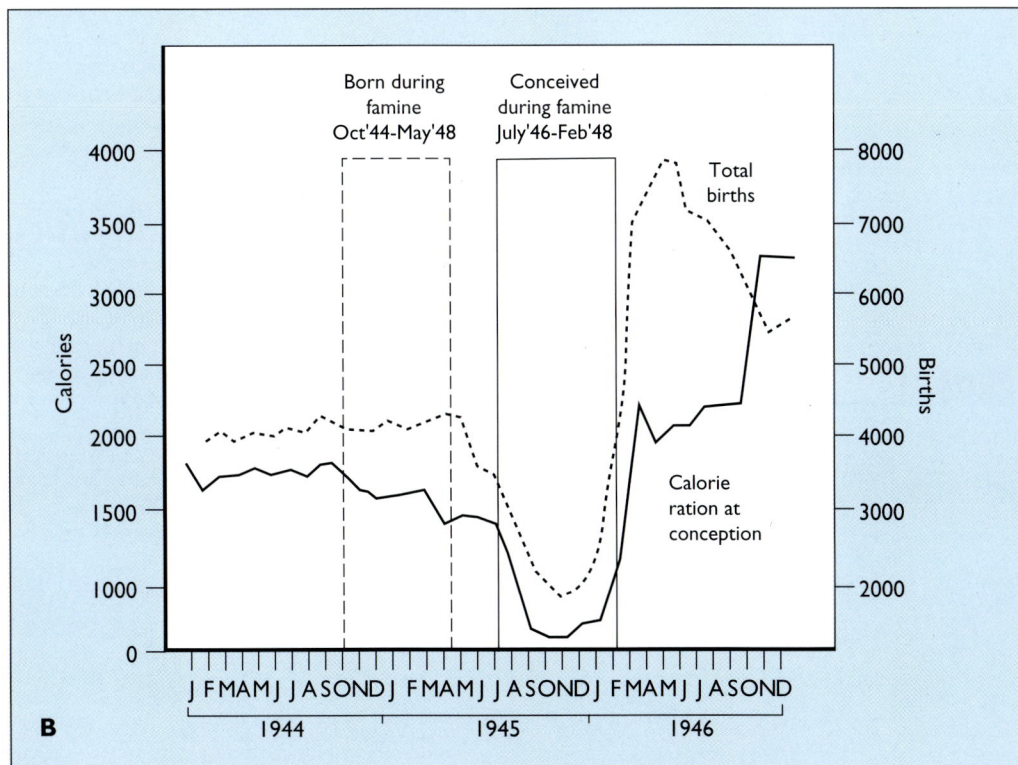

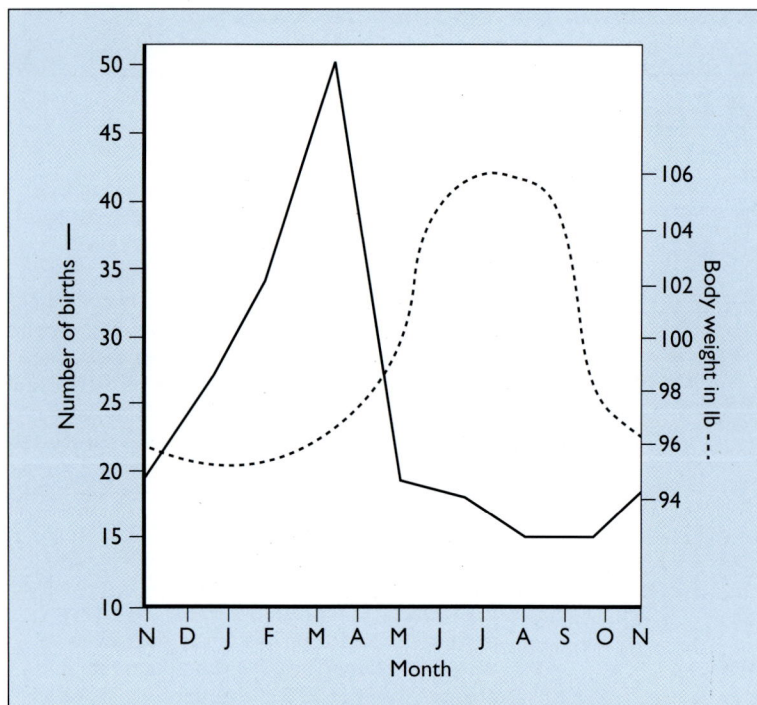

FIGURE 10-3. Weight change and fertility in !Kung San of Botswana. The !Kung San of Botswana were a tribe of hunter-gatherers until about 20 years ago [23] . The body weight of the men and women in the tribe varied substantially throughout the year depending on the availability of food. In the summer months, the food supply was more abundant and body weight increased, and the nadir of body weight was achieved in winter months. The number of births in the tribe peaked about 9 months after the peak of body weight [23]. This is another example of how the availability of food can affect fertility patterns in nature. (*From* Van Der Walt *et al.* [23]).

Clinical Paradigms of Chronic Undernutrition Associated with Reproductive Dysfunction

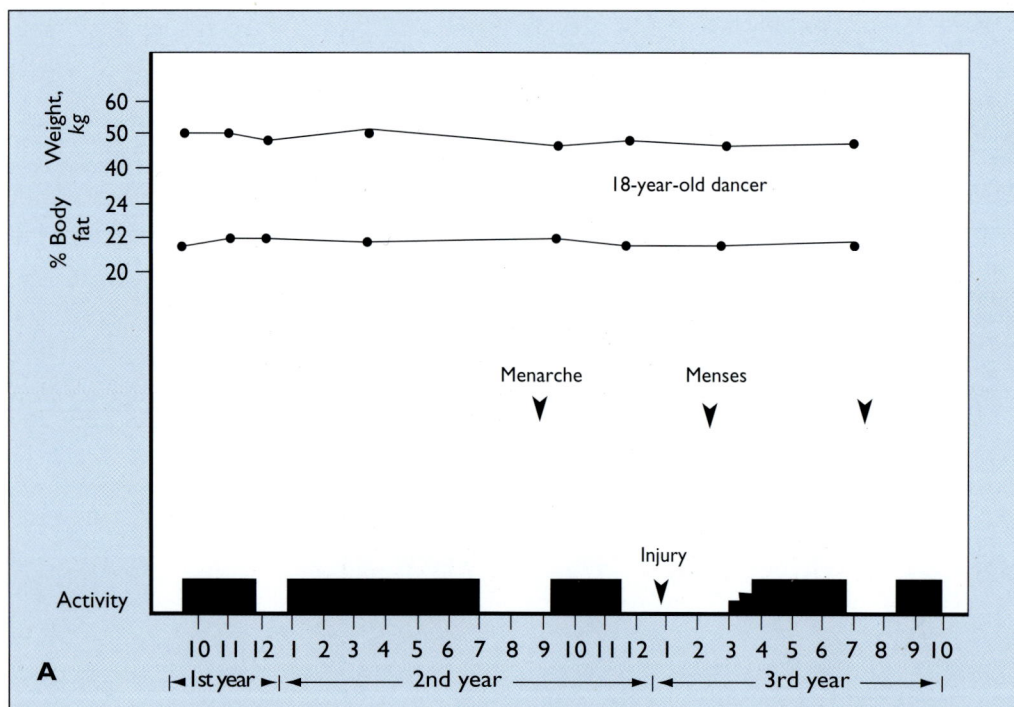

FIGURE 10-4. Delayed onset of menses in ballet dancers (**A** and **B**). The onset and progression of puberty in girls are markedly affected by intense exercise training and energy drain. Studies of ballet dancers in the peripubertal age range demonstrate that menarche is substantially delayed in these girls compared with normal controls (onset of menarche, 15.4 years in ballet dancers *vs* 12.6 years in normal controls [5–7, 24,25]. Periods of rest or reduction in exercise intensity due to injury are associated with rapid sexual development and the occurrence of menses [24]. Although breast development and menarche are delayed in ballet dancers, the development of pubic hair is not affected; this is consistent with the proposal that separate control mechanisms exist for the regulation of adrenarche and menarche [25]. Ballet dancers have lower body weight and body fat than age-matched controls, but we do not know whether the resetting of the hypothalamic gonadotropin-releasing hormone (GnRH) pulse generator in ballet dancers is due to energy drain, low body weight, or low body fat [24,25].

(Continued on next page)

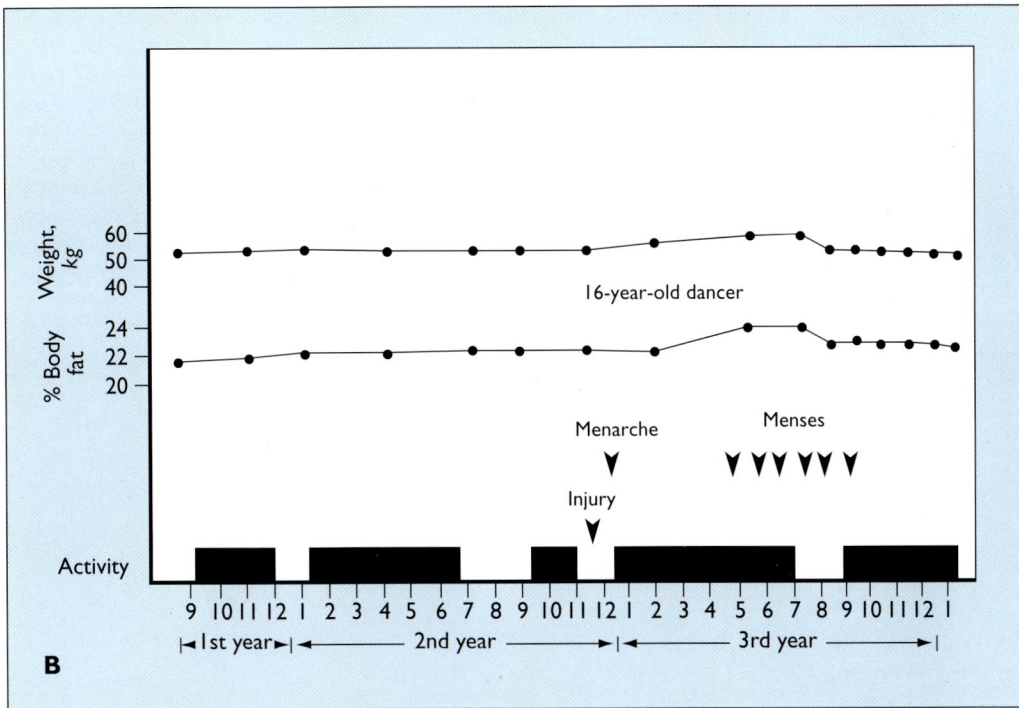

FIGURE 10-4. (*Continued*) Frisch [3–7] has proposed that achievement of a minimum fat-to-body mass ratio (approximately 17% fat/body mass) is necessary for triggering the onset of menarche. This hypothesis is supported by studies showing a correlation between increased GnRH secretion and percentage of body fat in pubertal girls [7]. However, some investigators have questioned whether low body fat important is the sole critical determinant of the onset of puberty [26,27]. (*From* Warren [24].)

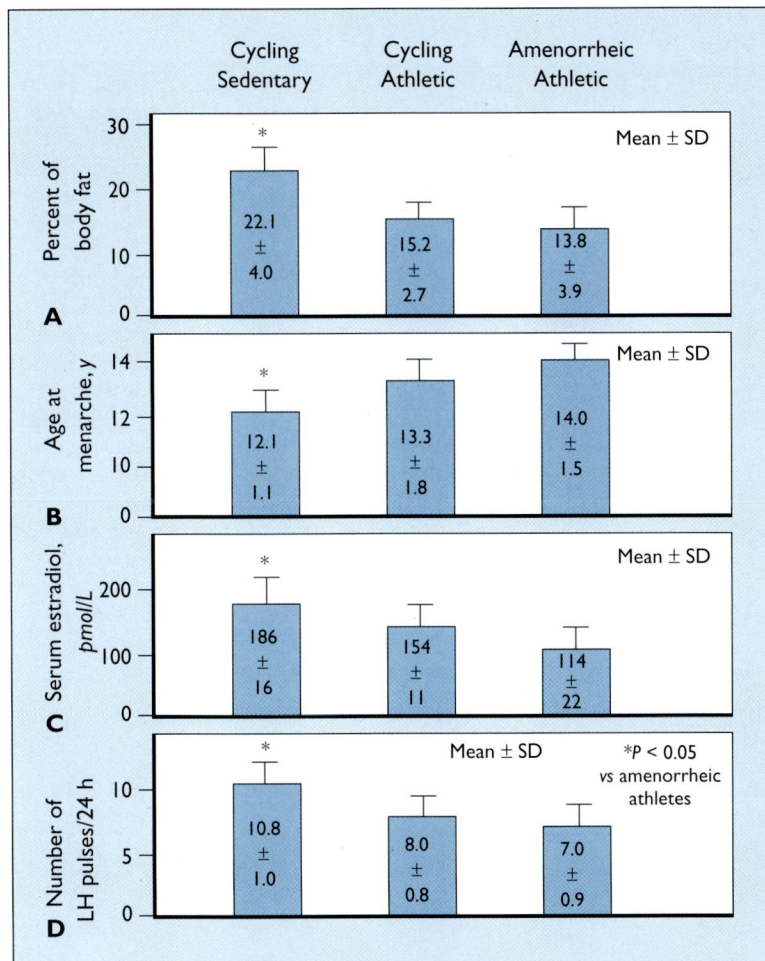

FIGURE 10-5. Percentage of body fat, age at menarche, and hormone levels in cyclic and amenorrheic female athletes. There is a high prevalence of amenorrhea, anovulatory cycles, and other menstrual irregularities in adult female athletes, particularly long-distance runners, dancers, and swimmers [28–30]. The athletes tend to weigh less, have a lower percentage of body fat (**A**), and a later onset of menarche than age-matched healthy controls [28,29] (**B**). In long-distance runners, the number of miles run each week tends to correlate with the degree of menstrual dysfunction. Female athletes typically exhibit hypogonadotropic hypogonadism, presumably caused by an acquired hypothalamic gonadotropin-releasing hormone (GnRH) deficiency. Serum estradiol levels (**C**) and the frequency of luteinizing hormone (LH) pulses (**D**) are lower in athletes who are amenorrheic than in nonexercising controls [28]. Some, but not all, female athletes with hypothalamic amenorrhea will respond to pulsatile GnRH administration, suggesting that additional pathophysiologic mechanisms may be operative. The bone mineral content of amenorrheic athletes is lower than that in age-matched controls, presumably because of the cumulative effects of estrogen deficiency [29]. Female athletes have a lower prevalence of breast cancer and other estrogen-dependent reproductive neoplasms than nonathletic controls because of decreased estrogen exposure [3–7].

Frisch [3–7] has hypothesized that maintenance of normal reproductive function in women requires a minimum fat-to-body mass ratio of 22%. Body fat plays an important role in estrogen production and metabolism. Testosterone and androstenedione are converted to estrogens by aromatase enzyme in adipocytes. Excessively lean women, such as marathon runners or those with anorexia nervosa, produce more catechol estrogens than women with a greater percentage of body fat. Catechol estrogens tend to have less estrogenic activity than non-catechol estrogens, such as estradiol. In addition, there is an inverse relationship between percentage of body fat and sex hormone–binding globulin concentrations. Therefore, alterations in sex hormone–binding globulin concentrations may affect estrogen metabolism and clearance in lean women.

Women with exercise-induced amenorrhea also have abnormalities of their hypothalamic-pituitary-adrenal axis, including higher cortisol levels in early morning and blunted cortisol and adrenocorticotropin response to corticotropin-releasing hormone in comparison to healthy controls, leading to speculation that alterations in the cortisol axis may play a role in the pathophysiology of gonadal dysfunction [28,29]. (*From* Loucks et al. [28].)

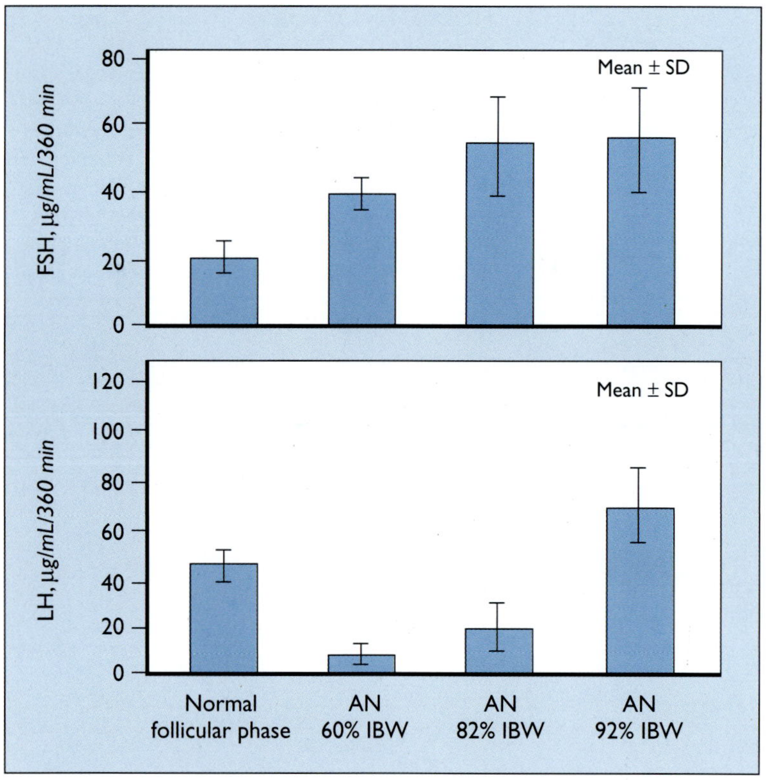

FIGURES 10-6. Hypogonadotropic hypogonadism in patients with anorexia nervosa [31,32]. Anorexia nervosa is a psychiatric disorder characterized by distortion of body image and self-induced weight loss [32]. Loss of body weight is associated with prepubertal patterns of luteinizing hormone (LH) and follicle-stimulating hormone (FSH) secretion, in which levels of both LH and FSH are low and respond poorly to gonadotropin-releasing hormone stimulation [31]. Refeeding and restoration of body weight are associated with normalization of pulsatile LH and FSH secretion, illustrating the correlation among energy balance, body weight, and reproductive function. Variants of eating disorders, such as bulimia and mild forms of self-induced dieting, are common in young women and may be missed unless the physician maintains a high index of suspicion. AN—anorexia nervosa; IBW—ideal body weight. (Part A *from* Sherman *et al* [31]; part B *from* Comerci [32].)

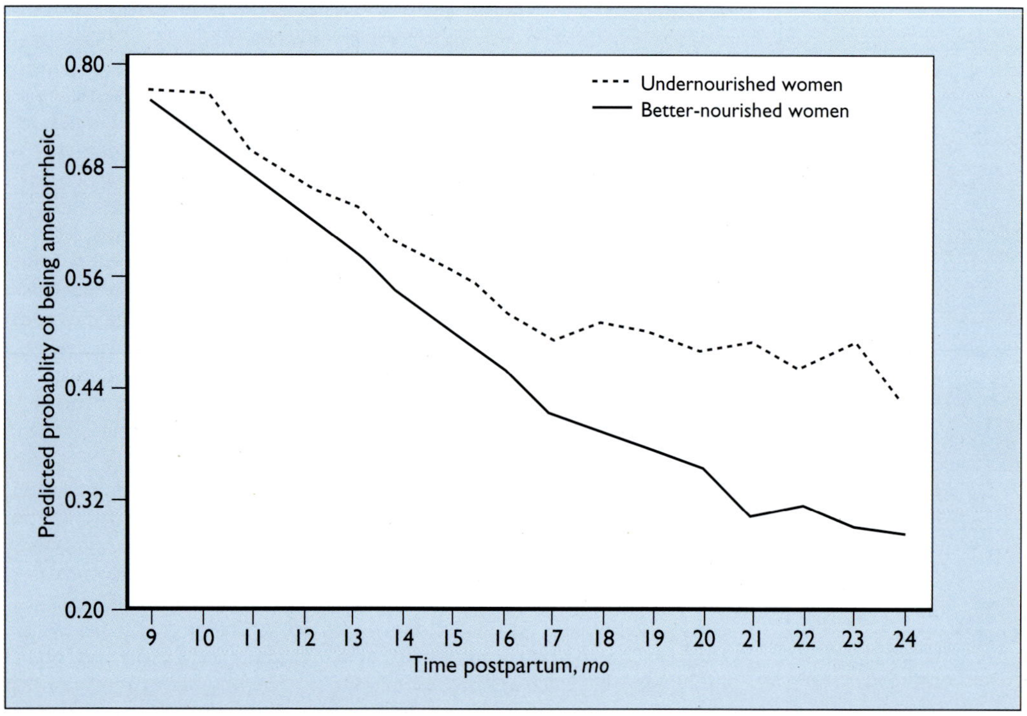

FIGURE 10-7. Maternal undernutrition and lactational amenorrhea: results from demographic and health surveys in Sub-Saharan Africa. A survey of postpartum women in seven Sub-Saharan countries found maternal nutritional status to be inversely associated with the duration of lactational amenorrhea. Undernourished woman (body mass index less than 18.5 kg/m^2) had a higher probability of remaining amenorrheic (odds ratio, 1.6 [95% confidence interval, 1.2 to 2.3]) than better-nourished women [33]. Overall, lactational amenorrhea lasted 1.4 months longer in undernourished women than in better-nourished women. This finding suggests that maternal nutritional status may independently affect the return of ovulation after childbirth. Because breast feeding and the associated lactation amenorrhea are important determinants of fertility in countries where effective contraceptive methods are not widely available, these data indicate that undernutrition may play a role in limiting family size by extending the duration of amenorrhea after child birth. (*From* Peng *et al.* [33].)

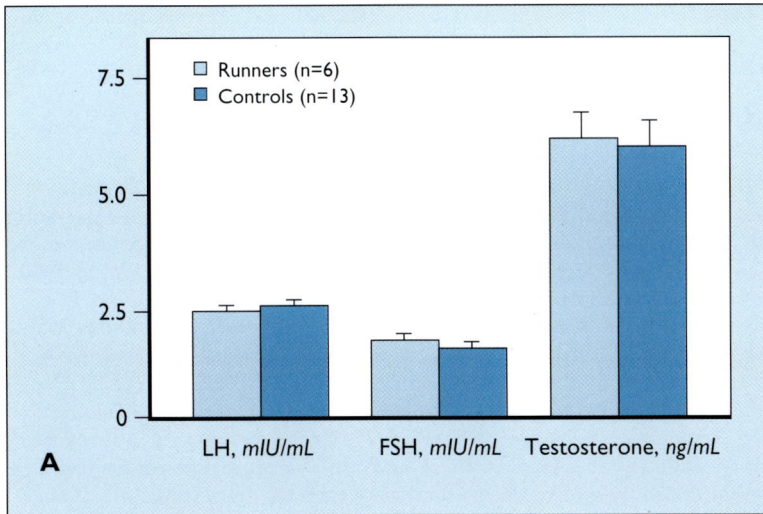

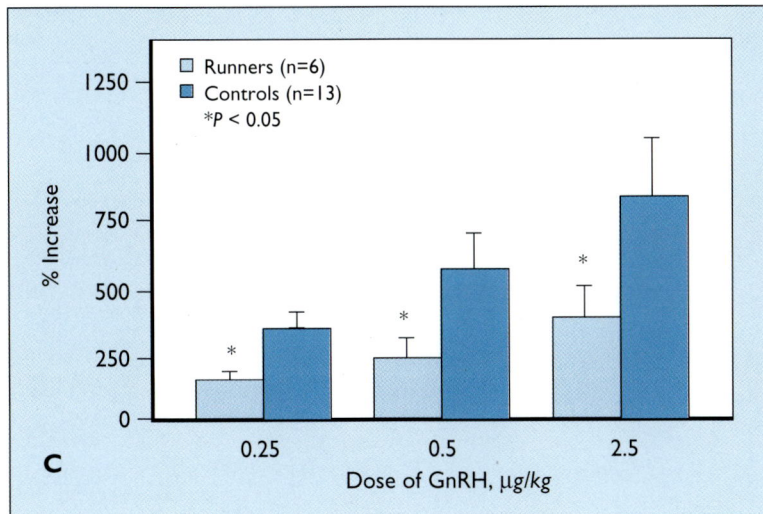

FIGURE 10-8. Long-term effects of running on the hypothalamic-pituitary-gonadal axis in men. Whereas abnormalities of gonadotropin-releasing hormone (GnRH) secretion and menstrual function are well documented in female athletes, similar reproductive abnormalities have not been widely reported in male athletes [34,35]. Although the signs and symptoms of androgen deficiency in men may be subtle and therefore remain undetected, clinically important hypogonadism does not appear to be common in male endurance athletes. Serum testosterone and luteinizing hormone (LH) concentrations are usually normal or low to normal in these athletes [34,35]. In one such study, MacConnie et al. [34] examined the hypothalamic-pituitary-gonadal axis in six highly trained marathon runners who were running 125 to 250 km every week. The frequency and amplitude of LH pulses were significantly lower in runners than in age-matched controls, even though mean plasma LH, follicle-stimulating hormone (FSH), and testosterone concentrations were not significantly different between the two groups (**A** and **B**). **C** shows the acute response of LH to increasing doses of GnRH in terms of the percentage increase in the concentration of the hormone above mean baseline levels. At all doses of GnRH, the response of LH was lower in runners than in controls [34]. The finding of pituitary hyposensitivity to GnRH serves as indirect evidence of impaired hypothalamic-GnRH secretion in male marathon runners. These data indicate that male marathon runners, in a manner similar to the female runners, also exhibit perturbations of hypothalamic GnRH pulse generator; however, clinically overt androgen-deficiency is less common in male runners than in their female counterparts [34]. (*Adapted from* MacConnie et al. [34].)

Effects of Experimental Caloric Deprivation on Reproductive Function in Young Men: The Minnesota Experiment

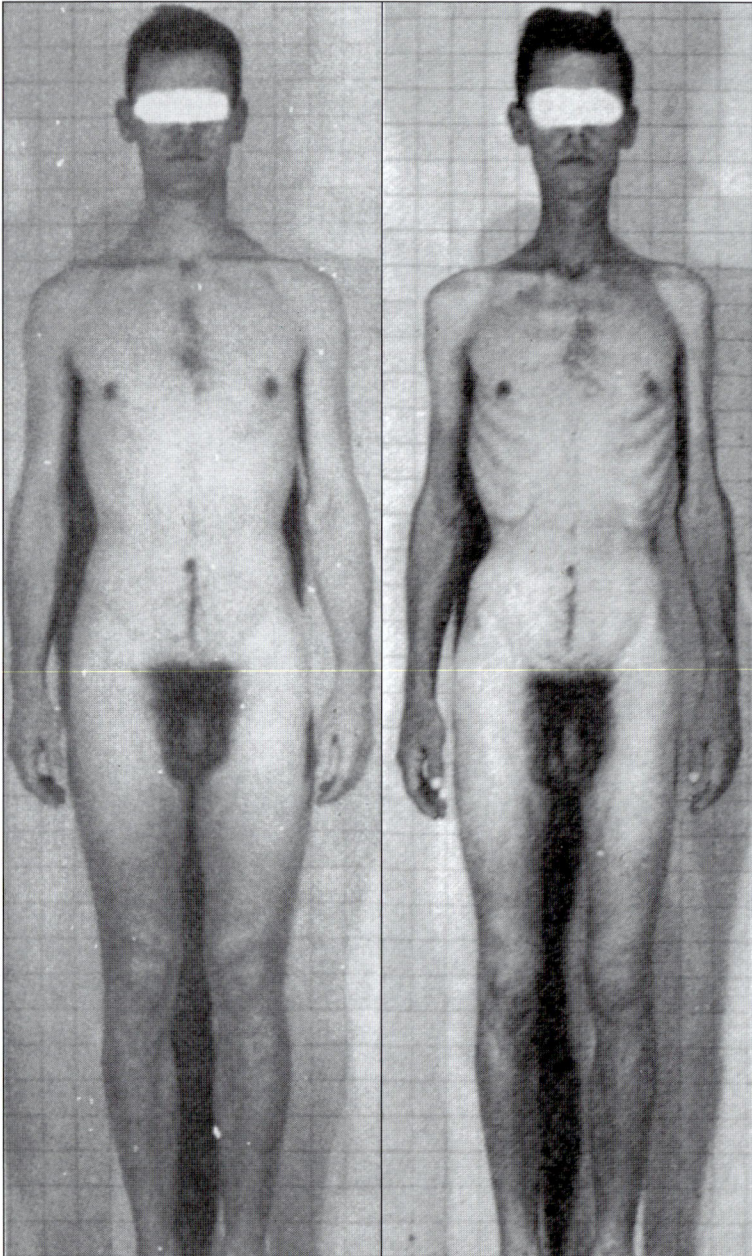

FIGURE 10-9. Two views of a man before (*left*) and after (*right*) 24 weeks of semi-starvation. In the late 1940s, Keys and coworkers studied human starvation in an experiment in which 32 young men volunteered to live on the campus of the University of Minnesota and consume a diet providing approximately 1600 kcal per day, about two thirds of their normal energy requirement [36]. The volunteers lost an average of 23% of their initial body weight; more than 70% of body fat and 24% of lean tissue were lost in the process. Keys *et al.* found that a decrease in caloric intake and subsequent weight loss first caused a loss of libido. Continued weight loss resulted in a reduction of prostate fluid and lessened motility and longevity of sperm; the production of sperm was reduced when men weighed approximately 25% less than the normal weight for their height. Weight gain restored reproductive function in these volunteers. (*From Keys et al* [36]; with permission.)

Reproductive Dysfunction and Endocrine Abnormalities of Obesity

SUMMARY OF ENDOCRINE ABNORMALITIES OF OBESITY

Tissue	Abnormalities Associated With Obesity
Hypothalamus-pituitary	
Adrenal	Increased cortisol turnover
	Increased cortisol in central obesity
	Increased cortisol response to stress in women with central obesity
Thyroid	Normal levels in obesity
	Possible association between T3 and resting energy expenditure
Gonadal	Decreased SHBG with increased BMI
Men	Increased aromatization of adrenal androgens into estrogens
	Decreased free testosterone
	Pattern of hypogonadotrophic hypogonadism with severe obesity
Women	Increased aromatization of adrenal androgens into estrogens
	Increased free testosterone
Prolactin	Normal basal levels
	Decreased stimulated levels
GH-IGF	Decreased GH secretion
	Decreased IGF-1 (total)
	Decreased IGFBP-1
	Increased IGF-1 (free)
Endocrine pancreas	
Insulin	Increased fasting levels
	Peripheral tissues insulin-resistant
	Altered β-cell pulsatility
Adipose tissue	Increased TNF-α
	Leptin levels correlate with fat mass

FIGURE 10-10. Summary of endocrine abnormalities of obesity. Obesity is associated with a spectrum of endocrine alterations, including changes in the plasma levels, secretion patterns, and clearance rates of circulating hormones. BMI—body mass index; IGF—insulin-like growth factor; IGFBP—insulin-like growth factor–binding protein-1; SHBG—sex hormone—binding globulin; T3—triiodothyronine. (*From* Smith [37].)

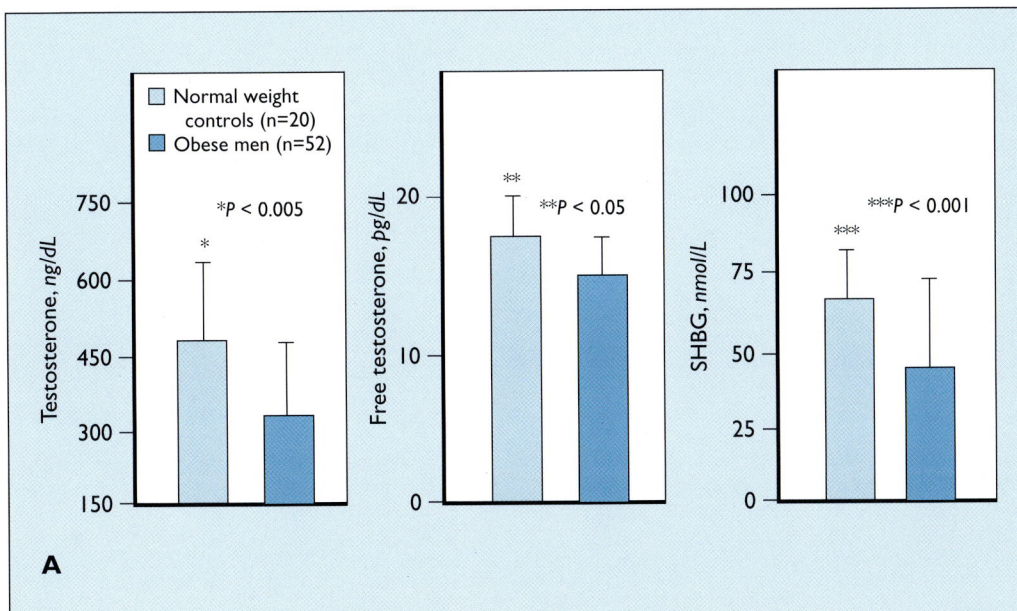

FIGURE 10-11. Obesity and androgens in men. In a majority of obese men with mild to moderate obesity, the alterations in total testosterone levels are due to changes in circulating levels of sex hormone– binding globulin (SHBG). Because SHBG levels decrease in inverse proportion to the degree of obesity, serum total testosterone levels decrease as body weight increases (**A**) [38,39]. Serum free testosterone levels, measured by equilibrium dialysis or as non-SHBG–bound testosterone, however, remain within the normal range in many men with mild to moderate obesity or may be slightly reduced [38,39]. In severe obesity, even the non-SHBG– bound testosterone level is reduced.

(Continued on next page)

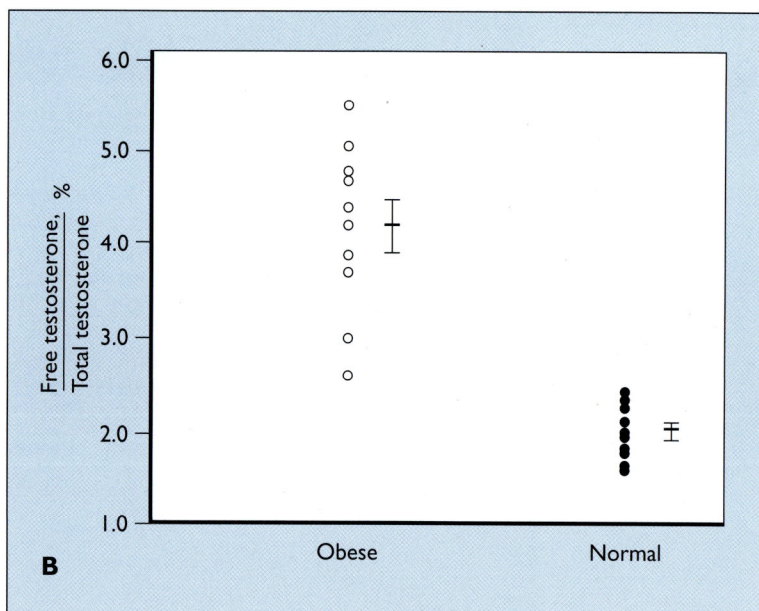

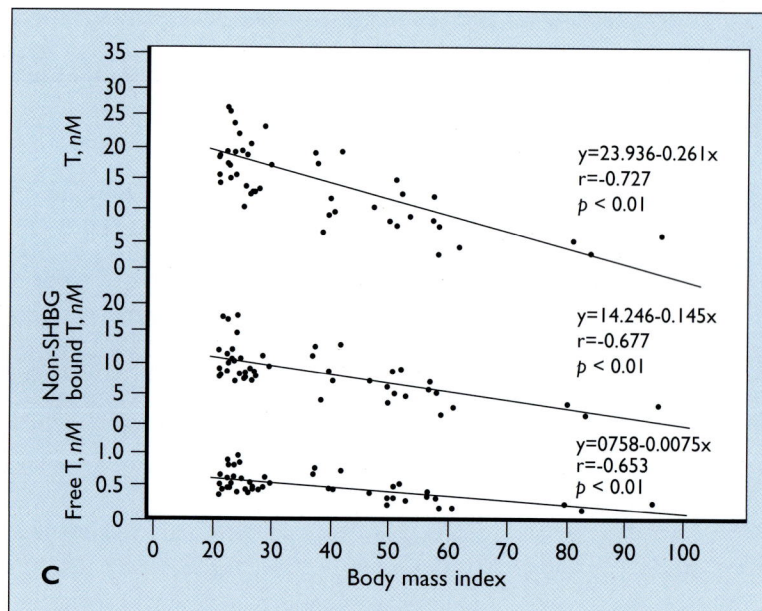

FIGURE 10-11. (*Continued*) The ratio of free to total testosterone levels is, therefore, higher in obese men than in nonobese men (**B**) [40]. Serum total, non-SHBG– bound, and free testosterone levels are inversely correlated with body mass index (**C**).

Serum estradiol levels may be higher in obese men than in healthy, nonobese controls because of aromatization of testosterone to estradiol in the fat cells. Weight loss is associated with a reversal of many of these abnormalities, including an increase in serum total and free testosterone levels and a decrease in estradiol levels; the most rapid change is an increase in SHBG levels.

The decrease in SHBG levels in obese men is believed to be due, in part, to the increase in circulating insulin concentrations that attends weight gain. Insulin is an inhibitor of SHBG production, and plasma insulin levels are inversely correlated with SHBG levels. A subpopulation of massively obese men may have a defect in the hypothalamic-pituitary axis, as suggested by low free testosterone in the absence of elevated gonadotrophins or hyper-response to luteinizing hormone– releasing hormone [39,40]. These individuals have low total and free testosterone levels and low or inappropriately "normal" luteinizing hormone (LH) and follicle-stimulating hormone levels. It has been speculated that very high estrogen levels in massively obese men may suppress GnRH and gonadotropin secretion. Testosterone response to human chorionic gonadotropin stimulation, an LH-like hormone, is normal in most obese men, indicating normal testicular reserve and function [39].

Several congenital hypothalamic syndromes, such as the multiple lentigenes syndrome, Laurence-Moon and Bardet-Biedl syndromes, Cohen syndrome, Borjeson-Forssman-Lehmann syndrome, congenital ichthyosis, Rud syndrome, cerebellar ataxia, optico-septal dysplasia, and Möbius syndrome [41] are associated with obesity and hypogonadotropic hypogonadism. The pathophysiology of hypogonadotropic hypogonadism in these disorders is not known, and the diagnosis is made by recognizing the specific somatic abnormalities associated with these syndromes. These somatic features are described in detail in a monograph by Rimoin and Schimke [41].

Prader-Willi syndrome, a disorder of genomic imprinting, most commonly results from deletions of the proximal portion of paternally derived chromosome 15q [42–44]. It is associated with constitutional obesity, mental retardation, and hypogonadotropic hypogonadism. The maternally derived copies of genes responsible for this syndrome in proximal 15q are normally silent [42,43]. Therefore, deletion of the paternally derived copy of the normally active genes produces the disease. The Prader-Willi syndrome can also occur if both copies of the gene are derived from the mother because the maternal copies are inactivated, presumably by DNA methylation [42,43]. This condition is known as uniparental disomy. Structural abnormalities of the imprinting center can also produce the Prader-Willi syndrome. The genes responsible for the syndrome have not been identified. Allele-specific methylation at locus D15S63 can be detected by a polymerase chain reaction method and has been used as a diagnostic test for this syndrome [43]. (Parts A and B *from* Glass *et al.* [39]; part C *from* Zumoff *et al.* [40].)

Hormonal Abnormalities in Obese Women

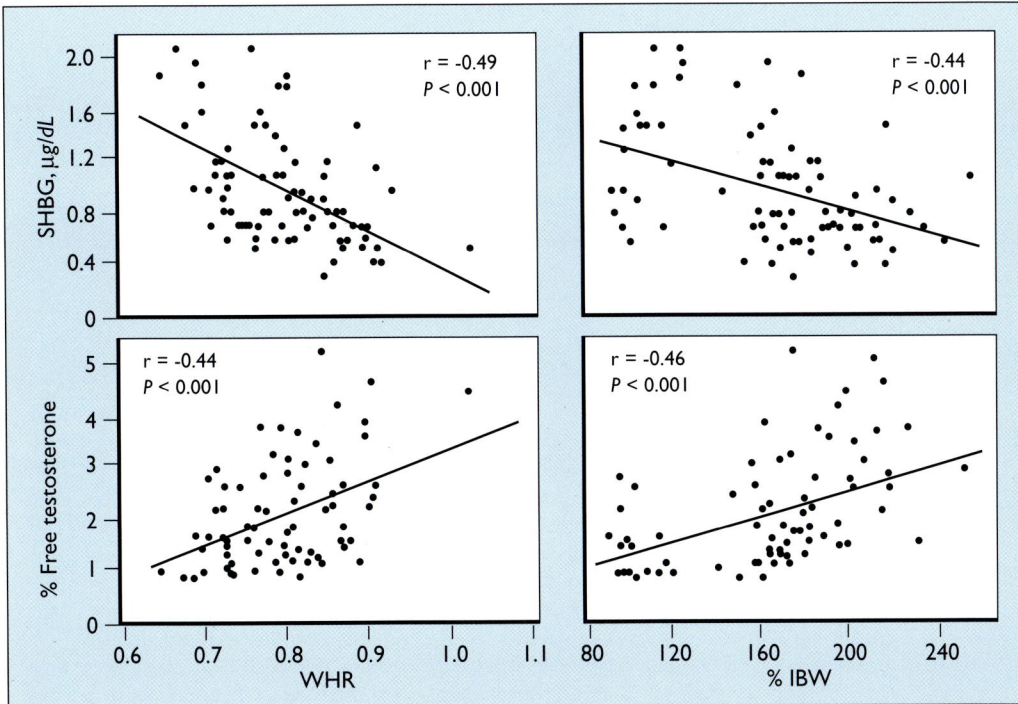

FIGURE 10-12. Relationship of sex hormone–binding globulin (SHBG) and percentage of free testosterone levels with waist-to-hip ratio and body mass index in women. Obese adolescent girls have an earlier onset of puberty [3–7]. It has been speculated that attainment of a critical amount of body fat and weight is essential for triggering the onset of puberty. Because obese girls cross this critical threshold earlier than lean girls, menses develops at an earlier age in obese girls than in their lean counterparts.

Excess body fat has been associated with an increased risk for oligoovulation or anovulation [45]. Obesity is related to an increased risk for hyperandrogenism and anovulatory cycles in women [46,47]. The unbound fraction of testosterone is increased in overweight women who have predominantly upper-body fat deposition (ie, a high waist-to-hip ratio). Androgen metabolism is also accelerated in obesity [47]. This increased clearance of androgens may result from an obesity-associated reduction in SHBG levels. Serum SHBG and percentage of free testosterone levels are negatively correlated with waist-to-hip ratio and weight expressed as a percentage of ideal body weight [47]. (*Adapted from* Erans, *et al.* [47a].)

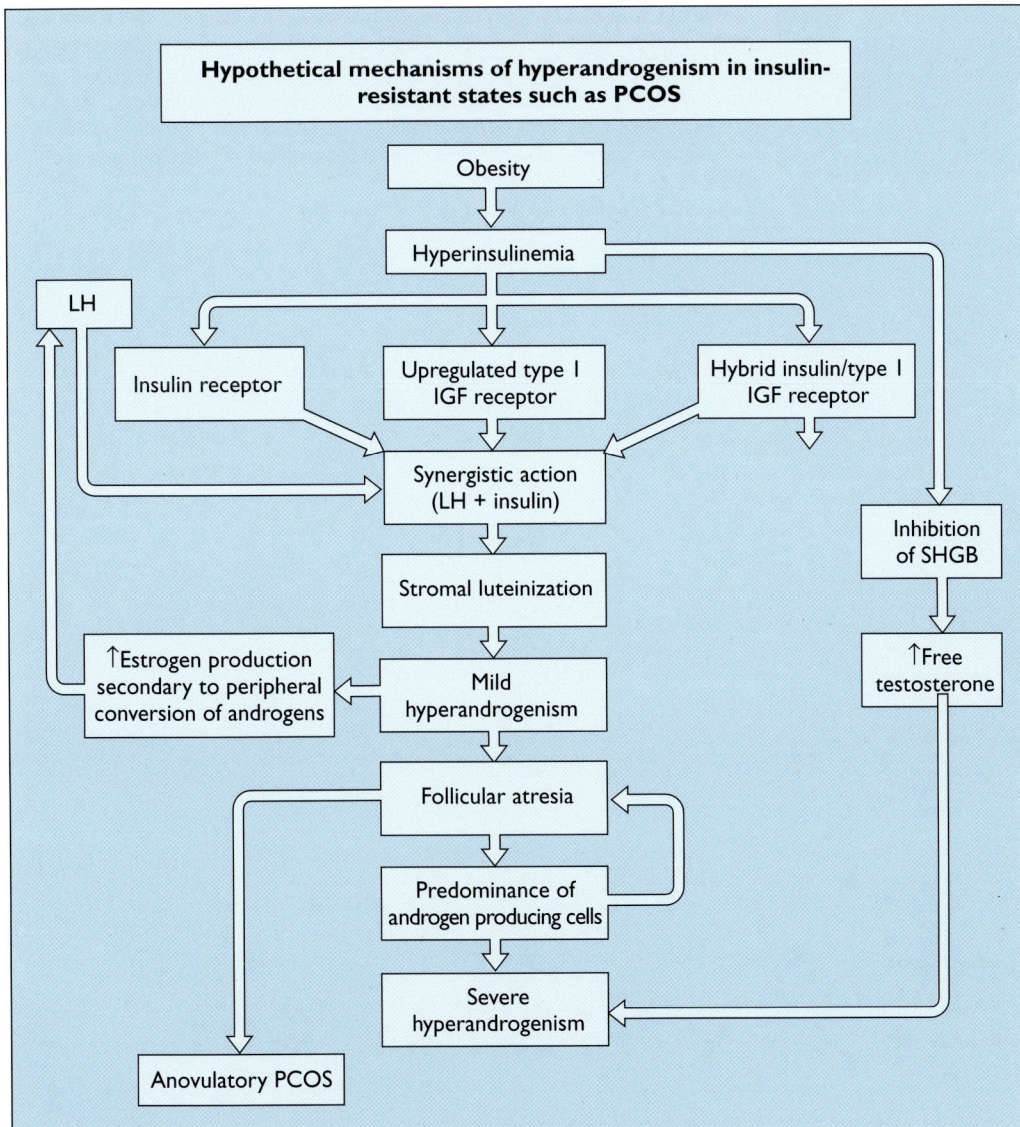

FIGURE 10-13. Hypothetical mechanisms of hyperandrogenism in insulin-resistant states: hyperandrogenemia, metabolic abnormalities and body composition changes in polycystic ovarian syndrome (PCOS). This syndrome, a common disorder in premenopausal women, is characterized by increased androgen secretion, chronic anovulation, obesity, and insulin resistance [46–51]. The syndrome is often associated with significant defects of insulin secretion and action [46]. In these patients, obesity is frequently related to increased waist-to-hip ratio, consistent with the intra-abdominal accumulation of fat. Increases in lean and fat mass contribute to the overall increase in body weight.

The pathophysiologic basis of PCOS is unknown. Several studies have demonstrated that insulin stimulates ovarian synthesis of androgens, estrogens, and progesterone [46]. Insulin acts synergistically with luteinizing hormone (LH) in stimulating ovarian androgen production and also up-regulates LH receptors; thus, ovarian responsiveness to circulating LH is increased [46,47]. Increased estrogen levels enhance pituitary sensitivity to gonadotropin-releasing hormone, resulting in increased LH secretion. Insulin and LH act synergistically to produce thecal luteinization. This initially causes mild overproduction of androgens, which is sufficient to induce follicular atresia [47]; continued stimulation of stromal and thecal cells by LH and insulin leads to further increase in circulating androgens. IGF—insulin-like growth factor; SHBG—sex hormone–binding globulin. (*Adapted from* Poretsky [45] and Bates and Whitworth [46].)

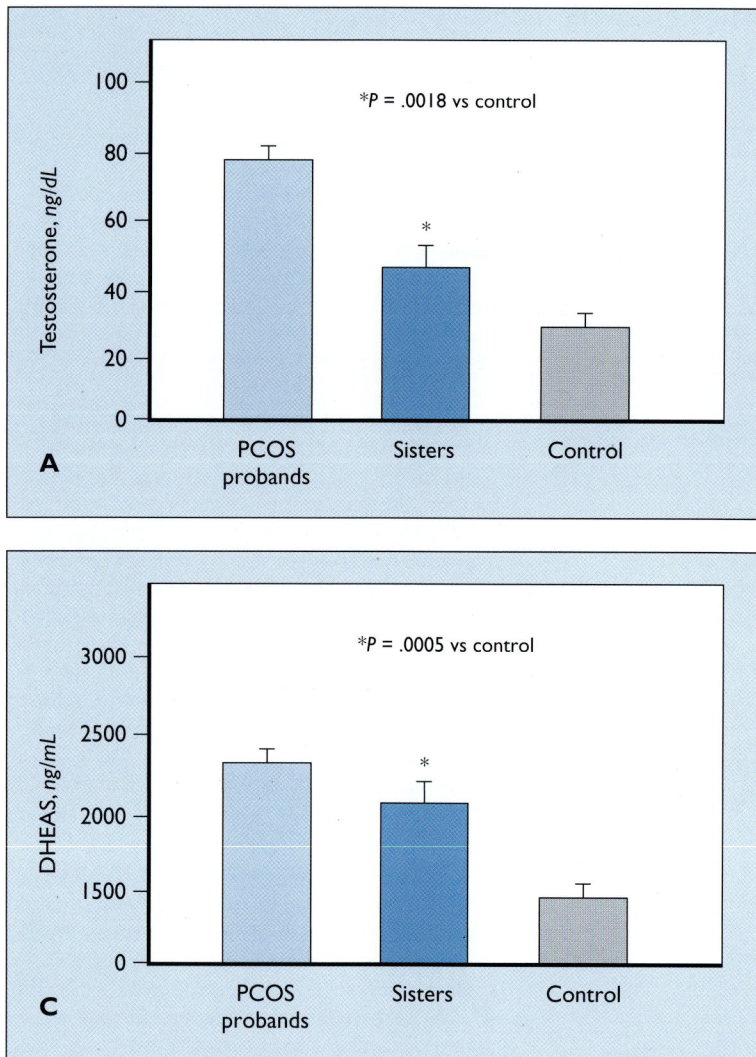

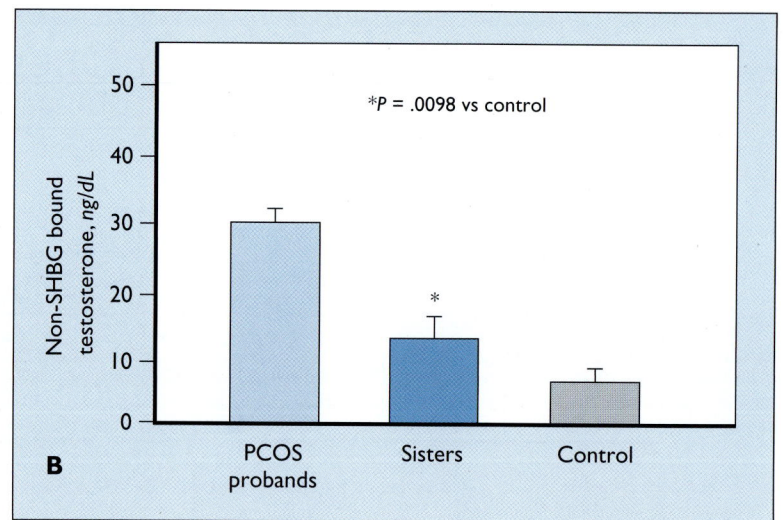

FIGURE 10-14. Serum androgen levels in probands with polycystic ovary syndrome (PCOS), sisters of patients with the syndrome, and controls (**A–C**). Both PCOS and the insulin resistance that accompanies it appear to have major genetic components [49–51]. Familial clustering has been described, and the mode of inheritance is dominant type. A recent study [49,50] of the sisters of women with PCOS has established that there is familial aggregation of hyperandrogenemia in kindreds. In this study, 24% of sisters of PCOS probands had the syndrome. Total testosterone, testosterone that was not –sex hormone–binding globulin (SHBG)–bound, and dehydroepiandrosterone (DHEAS) were all significantly increased not only in probands but also in their sisters. Many of the sisters of patients with this clinical disorder had high androgen levels but normal menstrual cycles; these patients presumably had a milder form or an early stage of the disease.

Women with PCOS are often insulin resistant, have insulin secretory defects, and are at significantly increased risk for non–insulin-dependent diabetes mellitus and impaired glucose tolerance [51]. A significant proportion of women with this clinical disorder have been found to have a defect in insulin-mediated receptor autophosphorylation. Fifty percent of first-degree relatives of patients with this disorder have non–insulin-dependent diabetes mellitus or impaired glucose tolerance by the oral glucose tolerance test, indicating that glucose intolerance in this disorder may also have a genetic basis. (*From* Legro *et al.* [49,50].)

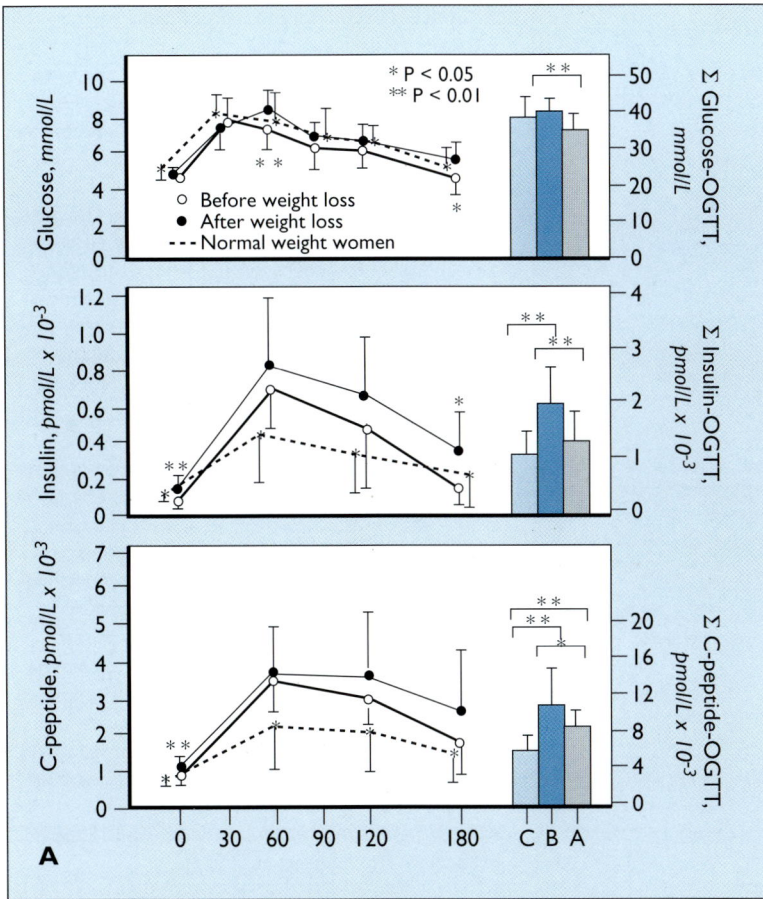

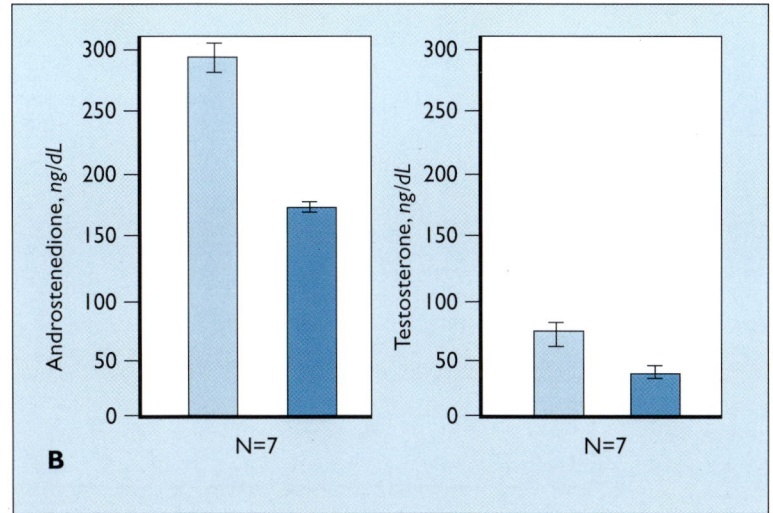

FIGURE 10-15. Effects of weight loss on insulin sensitivity and reproductive function in obese, hyperandrogenic women. **A,** Weight loss improves glucose and insulin profiles. Weight loss results in a significant decrease in the mean fasting and post-glucose plasma insulin and C-peptide values in obese, amenorrheic hyperandrogenic women [51]. After weight reduction, the sum of insulin, C-peptide, and glucose values after a standardized oral glucose load was lower than that before treatment and was similar to that in normal-weight women. **B,** Weight reduction decreases serum androgen levels in infertile, obese women. The *light blue bars* indicate the plasma levels before weight loss; the *dark blue bars* indicate the plasma levels after weight loss. With weight loss, plasma androgens are reduced and ovulation is restored in 85% of women who lost at least 15% of their body weight [48]. This is due to a reduction in extraglandular aromatization found in association with obesity.

The data in *panels A* and *B* demonstrate that with weight loss, both hyperinsulinemia and androgen levels improve and menstrual cycles are restored in many patients. (Part A *from* Pasquali *et al.* [51]; part B *from* Bates and Whitworth [46].)

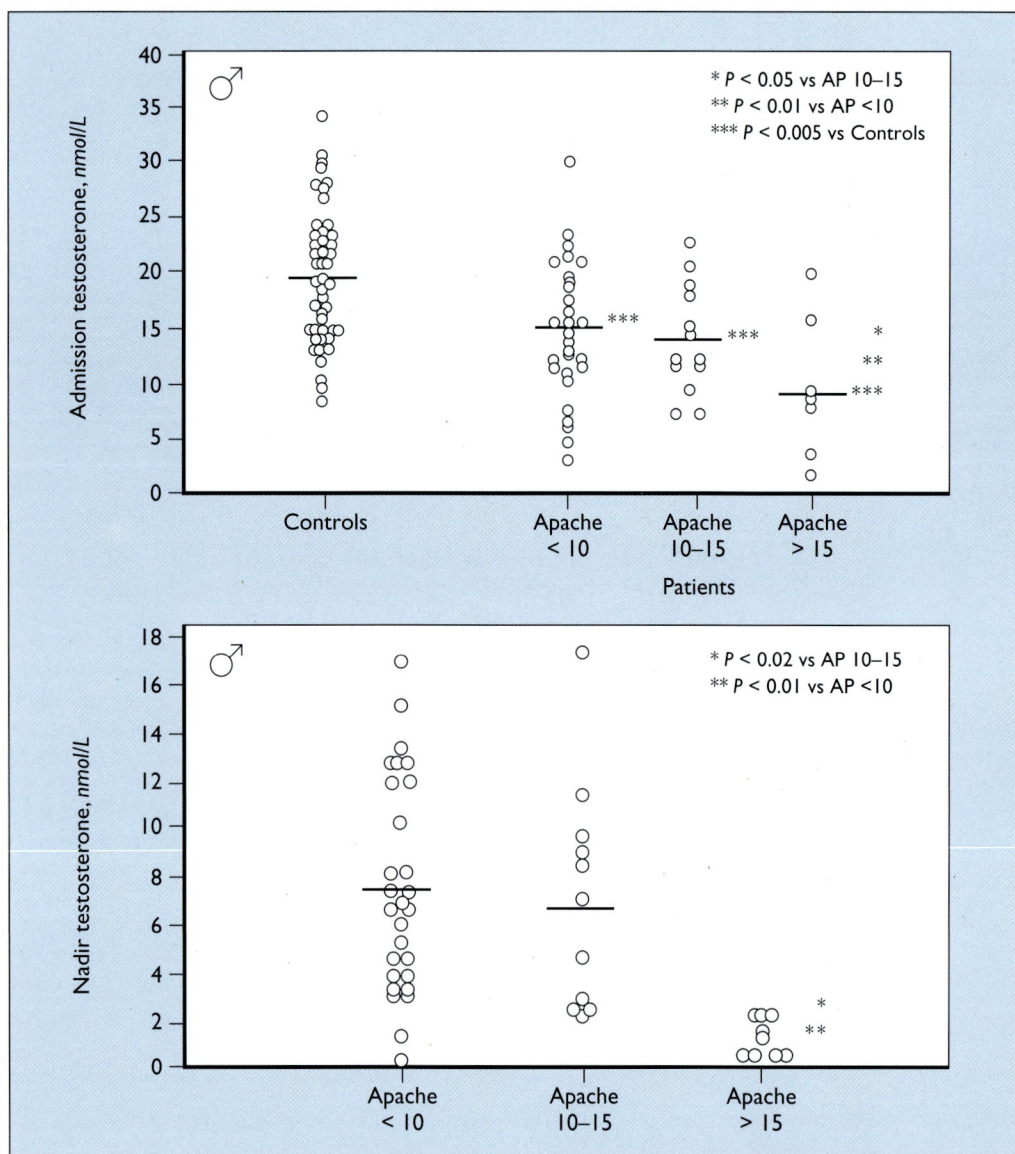

FIGURE 10-16. Suppression of hypothalamic-pituitary gonadal axis during an acute illness: serum testosterone levels at hospital admission and at nadir in a group of hospitalized, acutely ill men. Hypogonadism in critical illness is well documented. The degree of suppression of the hypothalamic-pituitary-gonadal axis correlates with the severity of illness [52]. Serum testosterone levels decrease at the onset of illness and recover during recuperation, suggesting a relationship to progression of illness. Although a majority of acutely ill patients have hypogonadotropic hypogonadism, a subset of patients may have increased luteinizing hormone (LH) and follicle-stimulating hormone (FSH) levels consistent with primary testicular dysfunction [52].

Although the magnitude of gonadotropin suppression is generally correlated to the severity of illness, there is considerable heterogeneity in serum gonadotropin profiles in acutely ill patients. Although a majority of patients with acute illness have hypogonadotropic hypogonadism, others may have elevated levels of LH and FSH, suggestive of primary gonadal dysfunction.

The pathophysiology of reproductive dysfunction that attends the course of acute illness is unknown. Malnutrition, cytokines, and other mediators and products of systemic inflammatory response, as well as drugs, may all contribute to the suppression at multiple levels of the reproductive axis [52]. APACHE—Acute Physiology and Chronic Health Evaluation. (*From* Spratt *et al.* [52].)

References

1. Van Der Spruy ZM: Nutrition and reproduction. *Clin Obstet Gynaecol* 1985, 12:579–604.

2. Knuth VA, Hull MGR, Jacobs HS: Amenorrhea and loss of weight. *Br J Obstet Gynaecol* 1977, 84:801–807.

3. Frisch RE: Fatness and fertility. *Sci Am* 1988, 258:88–95.

4. Frisch RE: Body weight and reproduction. *Science* 1989, 246:432.

5. Frisch RE: The right weight:body fat, menarche and fertility. *Proc Nutr Soc* 1994, 53:113–129.

6. Frisch RE, McArthur JW: Menstrual cycles: fatness as a determinant of minimum weight for height necessary for their maintenance or onset. *Science* 1974, 185:949–995.

7. Frisch RE: Body fat, menarche, fitness, and fertility. *Hum Reprod* 1987, 2:521–533.

8. Foster DL, Nagatani S: Physiological perspectives on leptin as a regulator of reproduction: role in timing puberty. *Biol Reprod* 1999, 60:205–215.

9. Penny R, Goldstein IP, Frasier SD: Gonadotropin excretion and body composition. *Pediatrics* 1978, 61:294–300.

10. Rock CL, Gorenflo DW, Drewnowski A, *et al.*: Nutritional characteristics, eating pathology, and hormonal status in young women. *Am J Clin Nutr* 1996, 64:566–571.

11. Bates GW, Bates SR, Whitworth NS: Reproductive failure in women who practice weight control. *Fertil Steril* 1982, 37:373–378.

12. Arver SA, Sinha-Hikim-I, Beall G, *et al.* Dihydrotestosterone and testosterone levels in HIV-infected men. *J Androl* 1999 (In press.)

13. Macut D, Micic D, Pralong FP, *et al.*: Is there a role for leptin in human reproduction? *Gynecol Endocrinol* 1998, 12:321–326.

14. Cunningham MJ, Clifton DK, Steiner RA: Leptin's actions on the reproductive axis: perspectives and mechanisms. *Biol Reprod* 1999, 60:216–222.

15. Aubert ML, Pierroz DD, Gruaz NM, *et al.*: Metabolic control of sexual function and growth: role of neuropeptide Y and leptin. *Mol Cell Endocrinol* 1998, 140:107–113.

16. Clarke IJ, Henry BA: Leptin and reproduction. *Biol Reprod* 1999, 4:48–55.

17. Mohamed-Ali V, Pinkney JH, Coppack SW: Adipose tissue as an endocrine and paracrine organ. *Int J Obes Rel Metab Disord* 1998, 22:1145–1158.

18. McCann SM, Kimura M, Walczewska A, *et al.*: Hypothalamic control of FSH and LH by FSH-EF, LHRH, cytokines, leptin and nitric oxide. *Neuroimmunomodulation* 1998, 5:193–202.

19. Schwartz MW, Baskin DG, Kaiyala KJ, *et al.*: Model for the regulation of energy balance and adiposity by the central nervous system. *Am J Clin Nutr* 1999, 69:584–596.

20. Susser M, Stein Z: Timing in prenatal nutrition: a reprise of the Dutch Famine Study. *Nutr Rev* 1994, 52:84–94.

21. Stein Z, Susser M: Famine and fertility. In: *Nutrition and Human Reproduction.* Edited by Mosley WH. New York: Plenum Press; 1978:123–145.

22. Stein Z, Susser M, Saenger G, et al.: *Famine and Human Development: The Dutch Hunger Winter of 1944-1945.* New York: Oxford University Press; 1975

23. Van Der Walt LA, Wilmsen EN, Jenkins T: Unusual sex hormone patterns among desert-dwelling hunter gatherers. *J Clin Endocrinol Metab* 1978, 46:658–663.

24. Warren MP: Effects of exercise on pubertal progression and reproductive function in girls. *J Clin Endocrinol Metab* 1980, 51:1150.

25. Warren MP: Effects of undernutrition on reproductive function in the human. *Endocrin Rev* 1983, 4:363–377.

26. Bronson FH, Manning JM: The energetic regulation of ovulation: a realistic role for body fat (minireview). *Biol Reprod* 1991, 44:945–950.

27. Pirke KM, Schweiger U, Strowitzki T: Dieting causes menstrual irregularities in normal weight young women through impairment of episodic luteinizing hormone secretion. *Fertil Steril* 1989, 51:263–268.

28. Loucks AB, Mortola JF, Girton L, et al.: Alterations in the hypothalamic-pituitary-ovarian and the hypothalamic-pituitary-adrenal axes in athletic women. *J Clin Endocrinol Metab* 1989, 68:402–411.

29. Drinkwater BL, Nilson K, Chestnut CH, et al.: Bone mineral content of amenorrheic and eumenorrheic athletes. *N Engl J Med* 1984, 311:277–292.

30. Chrousos GP, Torpy DJ, Gold PW: Interactions between the hypothalamic-pituitary-adrenal axis and the female reproductive system: clinical implications. *Ann Intern Med* 1998, 129:229–240.

31. Sherman BM, Halmi KA, Zamudio R: LH and FSH response to gonado-tropin-releasing hormone in anorexia nervosa: effect of nutritional rehabilitation. *J Clin Endocrinol Metab* 1975, 41:135–142.

32. Comerci GD: Medical complications of anorexia nervosa and bulimia nervosa. *Med Clin North Am* 1990, 74:1293–1309.

33. Peng YK, Hight-Laukaran V, Peterson AE, et al.: Maternal nutritional status is inversely associated with lactational amenorrhea in Sub-Saharan Africa: results from demographic and health surveys II and III. *J Nutr* 1998, 128:1672–1680.

34. MacConnie SE, Barkan A, Lampman RM, et al.: Decreased hypothalamic gonadotropin-releasing hormone secretion in male marathon runners. *N Engl J Med* 1986, 315:411–417.

35. Skarda ST, Burge MR: Prospective evaluation of risk factors for exercise-induced hypogonadism in male runners. *West J Med* 1998, 169:9–12.

36. Keys A, Brozek J, Henschel A, et al.: *The Biology of Human Starvation.* Minneapolis: University of Minnesota Press; 1950.

37. Smith SR: The endocrinology of obesity. *Endocrinol Metab Clin North Am* 1996, 25:921–942.

38. Pasquali R, Casimirri F, Melchionda N, et al.: Effects of obesity and body fat distribution on sex hormones and insulin in men. *Metabolism* 1991, 40:101–104.

39. Glass AR, Swerdloff RS, Bray GA, et al.: Low serum testosterone and sex-hormone-binding-globulin in massively obese men. *J Clin Endocrinol Metab* 1977, 45:1211–1219.

40. Zumoff B, Strain G, Miller L, et al.: Plasma free and non-sex-hormone-binding-globulin-bound testosterone are decreased in obese men in proportion to their degree of obesity. *J Clin Endocrinol Metab* 1990, 71:929–931.

41. Rimoin DL, Schimke RN: The gonads. In: *Genetic Disorders of the Endocrine Glands.* Edited by Rimoin DL, Schimke RN. St. Louis: Mosby, 1971:258–356.

42. Cassidy SB, Schwartz S: Prader-Willi and Angelman syndromes. Disorders of genomic imprinting. *Medicine* 1998, 77:140–51.

43. LaSalle JM, Ritchie RJ, Glatt H, et al.: Clonal heterogeneity at allelic methylation sites diagnostic for Prader-Willi and Angelman syndromes. *Proc Natl Acad Sci U S A* 1998, 95:1675–80.

44. Kaufman ED, Mosman J, Sutton M, et al.: Characterization of basal estrogen and androgen levels and gonadotropin release patterns in the obese adolescent female. *J Pediatr* 1981, 98:990–993.

45. Poretsky L: On the paradox of insulin-induced hyperandrogenism in insulin-resistant states. *Endocr Rev* 1991, 12:3–13.

46. Bates GW, Whitworth NS: Effect of body weight reduction on plasma androgens in obese, infertile women. *Fertil Steril* 1982, 38:406–409.

47. Legro RS, Spielman R, Urbanek M, et al.: Phenotype and penotype in polycystic ovary syndrome. *Rec Progr Hormone Res* 1998, 53:217–256.

47a. Evans DJ, Hoffman RG, Kalkhoff RK, Kissebah AH: Relationship of andro-genic activity to body-fat tomography, fat-cell morphology, and metabolic aberrations in premenopausal women. *J Clin Endo Metab* 1983, 57:304–310.

48. Azziz R: Reproductive endocrinologic alterations in female asymptomatic obesity. *Fertil Steril* 1989, 52:703–725.

49. Legro RS, Driscoll D, Strauss JF 3rd, et al.: Evidence for a genetic basis for hyperandrogenemia in polycystic ovary syndrome. *Proc Natl Acad Sci U S A* 1998, 95:14956–14960.

50. Legro RS, Kunselman AR, Dodson WC, et al.: Prevalence and predictors of risk for type 2 diabetes mellitus and impaired glucose tolerance in polycystic ovary syndrome: a prospective, controlled study in 254 affected women. *J Clin Endocrinol Metab* 1999, 84:165–169.

51. Pasquali R, Antenucci D, Casimirri F, et al.: Clinical and hormonal charac-teristics of obese amenorrheic hyperandrogenic women before and after weight loss. *J Clin Endocrinol Metab* 1989, 68:173–179.

52. Spratt D, Cox P, Orav J, et al.: Reproductive axis suppression in acute illness is related to disease severity. *J Clin Endocrinol Metab* 1993, 76:1548–1554.

NUTRITION AND GASTROINTESTINAL DISEASES

Charles H. Halsted and V. L. W. Go

The gastrointestinal system plays an integral role in the assimilation of all nutrients from the diet. The major nutrients—fat, carbohydrate, and protein—undergo digestion within the intestinal lumen or on the brush-border surface of the absorbing enterocytes, followed by intestinal mucosal uptake and transport of the digestive products. Gastrointestinal hormones, enzymes, and transport proteins closely regulate each process. Fat-soluble vitamins are integrated into processes of dietary lipid absorption, whereas water-soluble vitamins typically have their own mechanisms for transport across the intestinal membrane. Understanding these processes and their perturbations by disease first requires a general overview of the functional anatomy of the stomach and intestines.

Functional Gastrointestinal Anatomy

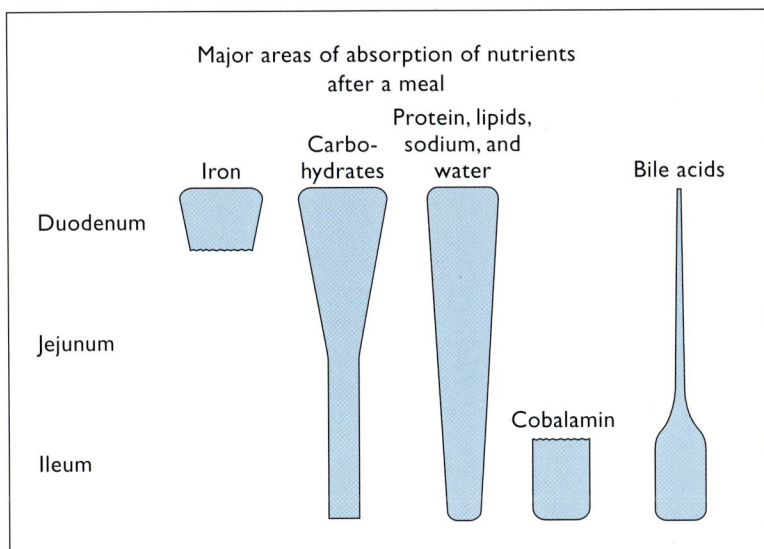

FIGURE 11-1. Regional functions of the small intestine. The various regions of the small intestine perform different absorptive functions. The duodenum (first 30 cm beyond the stomach) is the site of initial fat digestion by pancreatic enzymes, micellar solubilization of fat, and absorption of iron across the intestinal mucosa. The duodenum and jejunum are the major sites of digestion and absorption of carbohydrates, proteins, and fats; absorption of most vitamins and minerals; and osmotic equilibrium of intestinal contents following ingestion of a meal. The ileum, roughly the distal half of the small intestine, is the major site of absorption of water and electrolytes, and the last 100 cm is the obligate site of absorption of vitamin B_{12} and bile acids. Following surgical resection of the jejunum, the more distal ileal small bowel is capable of adaptively assuming the functions of the proximal jejunal small bowel. The reverse situation does not occur, however, because the jejunum does not contain specific transport mechanisms for bile acids and vitamin B_{12}. The colon is the principal site of absorption of electrolytes such as sodium chloride and water. In addition, colonic bacteria are the main source of such short-chain fatty acids as butyrate and acetate, which have localized nutritional value to the colonic absorbing cells. (*Adapted from* the American Gastroenterological Association Undergraduate Teaching Project [1]; with permission.)

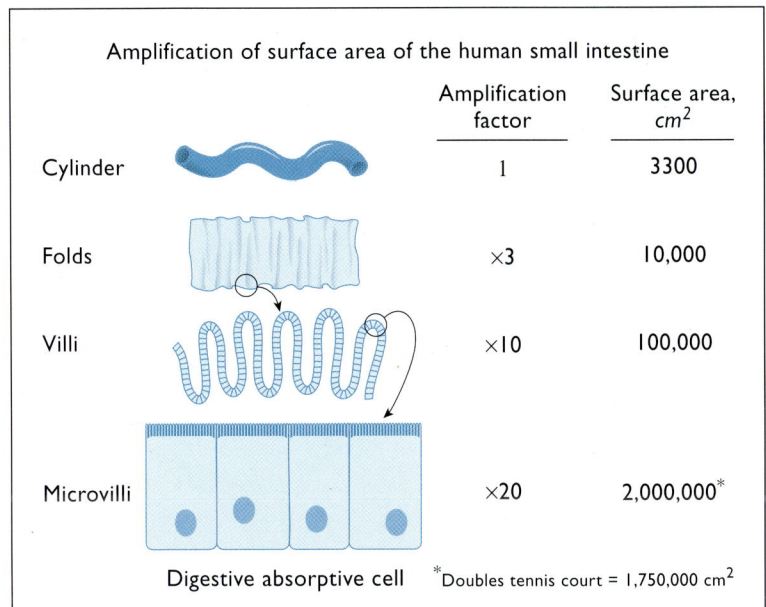

FIGURE 11-2. Functional anatomy of the small intestine. The normal human small intestine is about 600 cm in length, of which the first 30 cm is the duodenum, the next 250 cm is the jejunum, and the last half is the ileum. Although the small intestine is commonly viewed as a cylinder, its mucosal surface is actually represented by folds on which the surface is represented by villi of 300 μm in length, each villus lined with absorbing enterocytes with their own brush-border microvilli. The net effect is a magnification of the surface area to the size of a doubles tennis court. (*Adapted from* the American Gastroenterological Association Undergraduate Teaching Project [1]; with permission.)

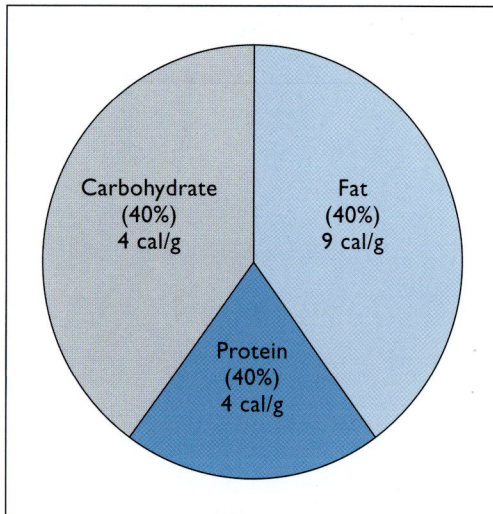

FIGURE 11-3. Distribution of major nutrients in the American diet. The distribution of fat, carbohydrate, and protein in the typical American diet is represented in this chart. At about 40% of calories consumed, dietary fat is composed almost entirely of triglycerides, with a small amount of cholesterol and phospholipid, and is ingested at about 100 g/d. Carbohydrates represent 40% to 50% of dietary energy and are consumed at 200 to 300 g/d. Protein represents 15% to 20% of dietary calories and is ingested at about 1.2 g/kg body weight per day, to which is added approximately 65 g of protein from intestinal secretions and sloughed intestinal cells. (*Adapted from* the American Gastroenterological Association Undergraduate Teaching Project [2].)

Regulatory Mechanisms of Gut Function

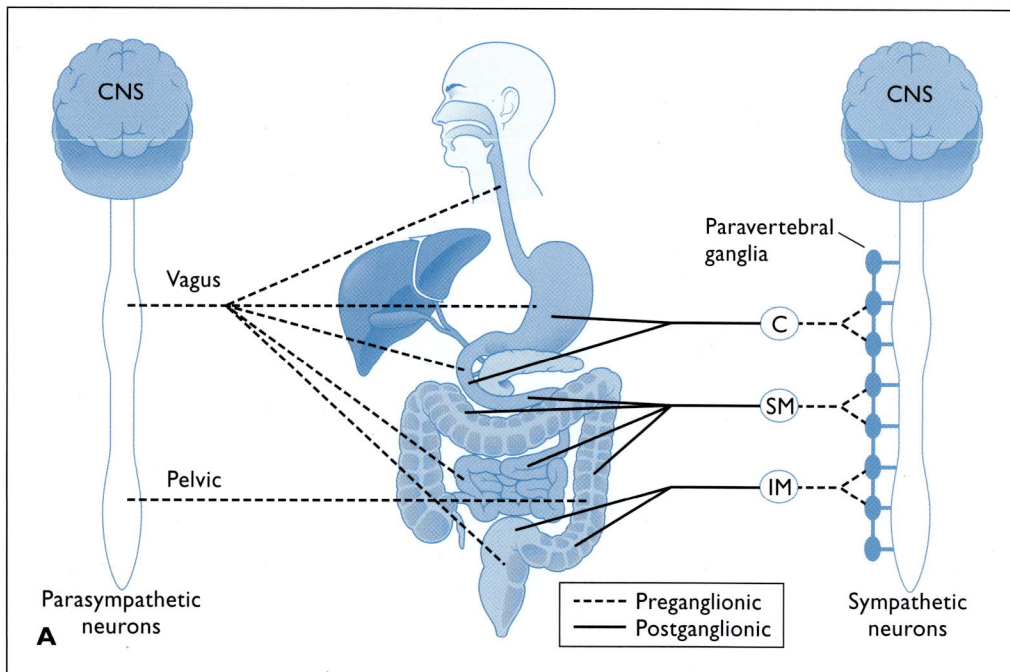

FIGURE 11-4. Neural innervation of the gut (**A** and **B**). The gastrointestinal tract is the largest neurally innervated organ system in the body, and it contains numerous hormones as well as paracrine, autocrine, and neurocrine pathways. The functions of the gut (secretion, digestion, motor, and absorption) are modulated by the central nervous system (CNS), the ingested food, and nutrients. The gut receives its autonomic nervous system innervation from the extrinsic sympathetic innervation from the spinal cord and its parasympathetic innervation from the vagus nerve. Both extrinsic innervations contain both afferent and efferent pathways that synapse with the intrinsic enteric nervous system at the intestinal wall ganglia and plexus.

(Continued on next page)

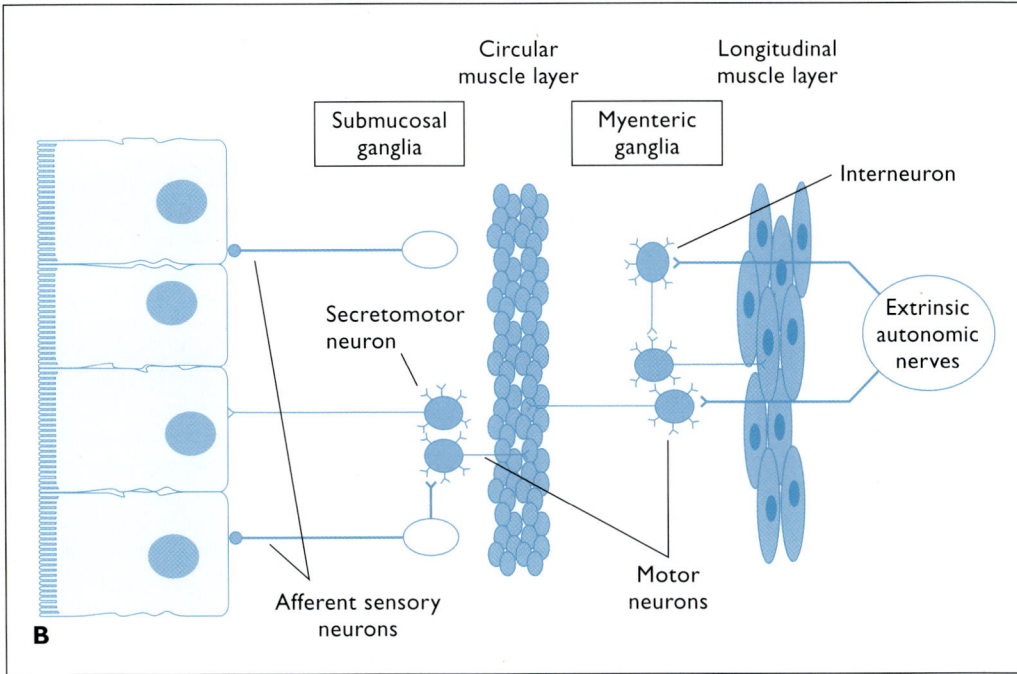

Circular muscle layer

Longitudinal muscle layer

Submucosal ganglia

Myenteric ganglia

Interneuron

Secretomotor neuron

Extrinsic autonomic nerves

Afferent sensory neurons

Motor neurons

B

FIGURE 11-4. (*Continued*) The gut can function independently of the CNS because of an overlapping regulatory intrinsic system that responds reflexively to the luminal contents and metabolic needs of the body. **C,** Peptide and nonpeptide neurotransmitters. A large number of neuropeptide and nonpeptide neurotransmitters are expressed by myenteric plexus neurons. C—celiac plexus; IM—inferior mesenteric plexus; SM—superior mesenteric plexus. (Parts A and B *adapted from* Chang *et al.* [3].)

C. PEPTIDE AND NONPEPTIDE NEUROTRANSMITTERS

Peptides	Nonpeptides
Secretin	Acetylcholine
Gastrin	Norepinephrine
Gastric inhibitory polypeptide	Serotonin
Neurotensin	Nitric oxide
Peptide YY	Dopamine
Substance P	Purinergic agonist
Cholecystokinin	(Adenosine, ATP)
Somatostatin	
Vasoactive intestinal peptide	
Gastrin releasing peptide	
Enkephalin	
Calcitonin gene-related peptide	
Neuropeptide Y	

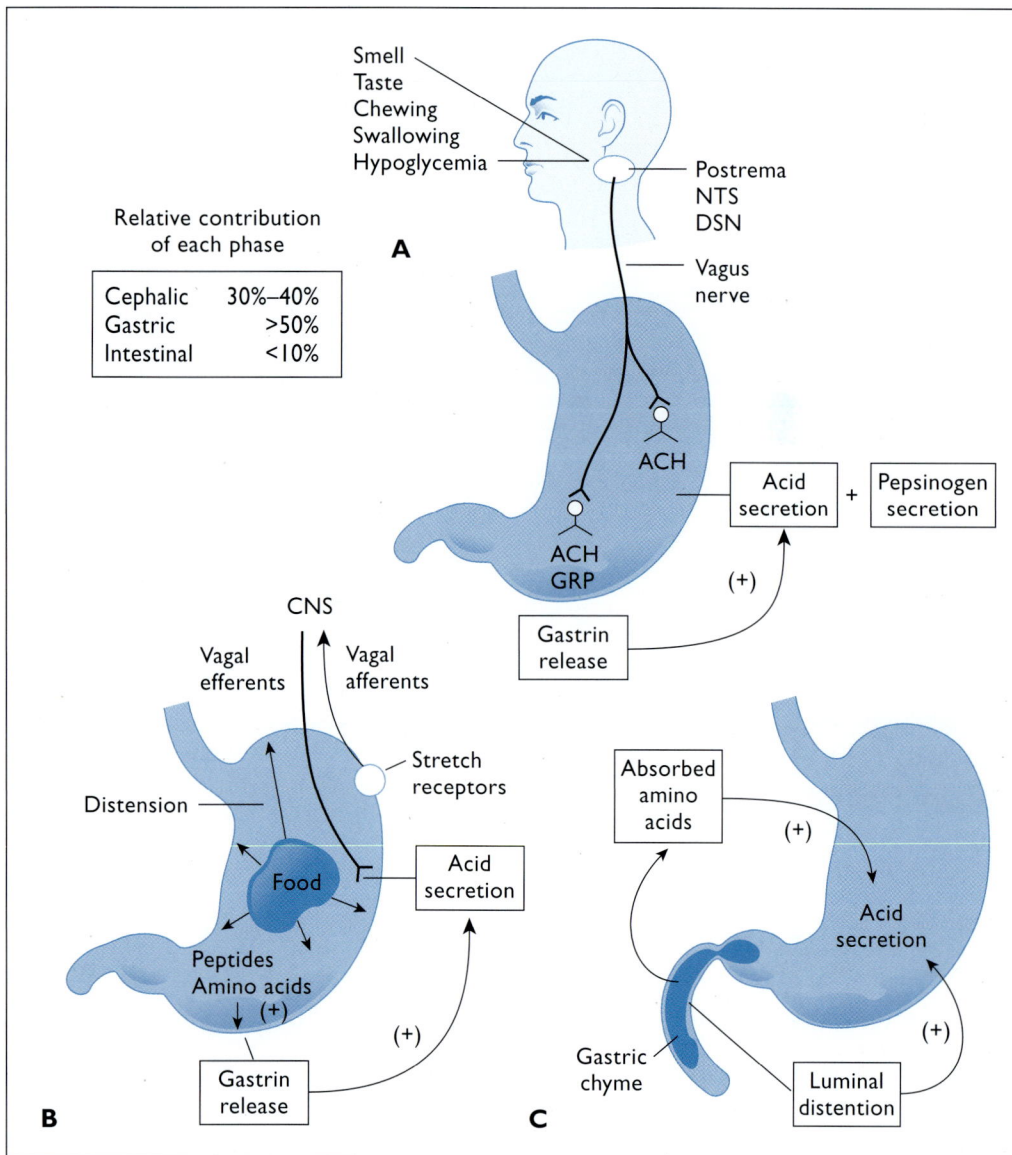

FIGURE 11-5. Regulation of gastric secretion after a meal. Three phases are important in the regulation of meal-stimulated gastric secretion of acid and enzymes. **A,** The cephalic phase is initiated by the sight, smell, taste, chewing, and swallowing of food and is mediated by three areas in the brainstem: the area postrema, the nucleus tractus solitarius (NTS), and the dorsal motor nucleus (DSN). **B,** The gastric phase, which occurs when food or fluid is present in the gastric lumen, accounts for 50% of total acid secretion stimulated by a meal. The greater the gastric distention, the greater the acid secretion will be. Vagal nerve fibers and local intrinsic factors mediate this phase. Gastrin is also released in this phase. **C,** The intestinal phase accounts for less than 10% of gastric acid secretion. Distention and digestion products of protein are the initiators of this phase and activate hormonal (eg, cholecystokinin) and neural pathways. ACH—acetylcholine; GRP—gastrin-releasing peptide. (*Adapted from Chang et al. [3].*)

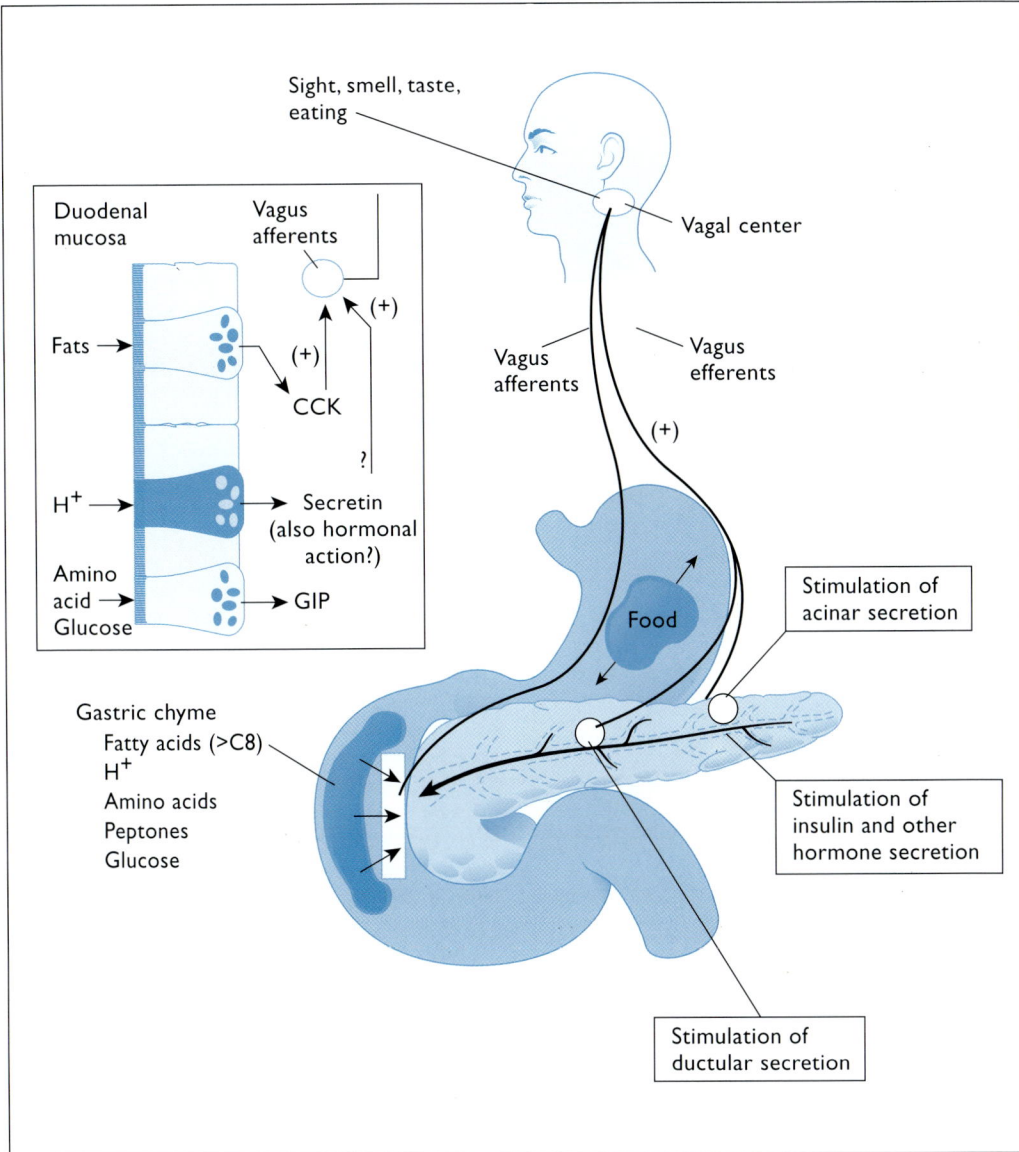

FIGURE 11-6. Regulation of pancreatic secretion after a meal. The pancreas releases both exocrine and endocrine secretions in response to meal ingestion. Exocrine secretions consist of water, electrolytes, and digestive enzymes for carbohydrates, proteins, and fats, respectively. The endocrine secretions are insulin, glucagon, somatostatin, and pancreatic polypeptides, which affect the metabolism of ingested nutrients and modulate gut function.

The postprandial physiologic regulation of pancreatic exocrine functions can also be classified into cephalic, gastric, and intestinal phases. The cephalic phase is the response to the central integration of sight, smell, taste, and eating of food and activates efferent vagal impulses that stimulate pancreatic acinar and ductal secretion. The gastric phase is initiated by gastric distention, by food, and by the presence of amino acids and peptides in the gastric lumen that activate vagovagal reflexes and gastrin release. The intestinal phase, which is quantitatively the most important, is initiated by the entry of gastric chyme into the duodenum and the upper small intestine. This phase is primarily mediated by activating cholinergic reflexes and the release of gastrointestinal hormones, cholecystokinin (CCK), secretin, and gastric inhibitory polypeptide (GIP). The intestinal phase of pancreatic exocrine regulation also stimulates endocrine secretions of the pancreas. (*Adapted from* Chang *et al.* [3].)

Digestion and Absorption of Nutrients

Triglycerides, Carbohydrates, and Protein

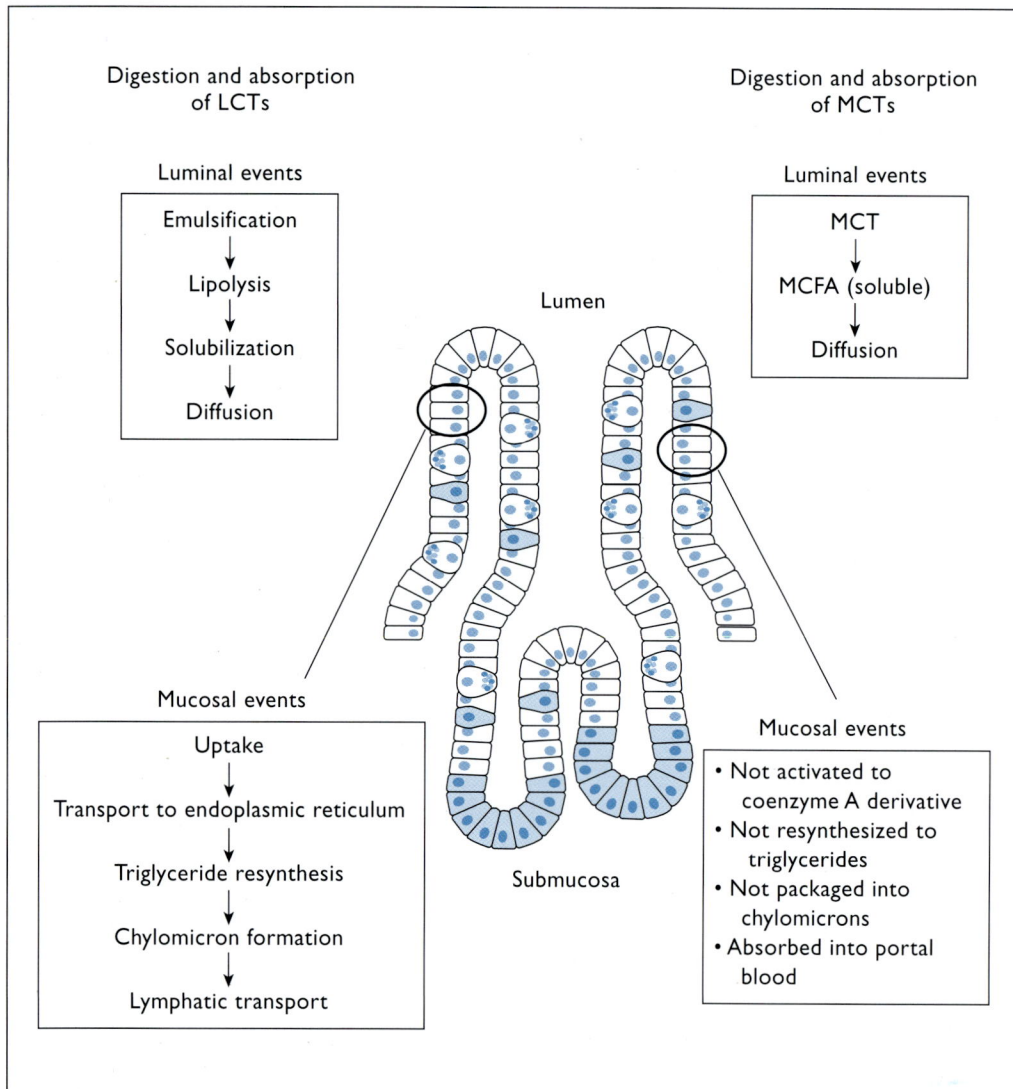

Digestion and absorption
of LCTs

Luminal events

Emulsification
↓
Lipolysis
↓
Solubilization
↓
Diffusion

Lumen

Digestion and absorption
of MCTs

Luminal events

MCT
↓
MCFA (soluble)
↓
Diffusion

Mucosal events

Uptake
↓
Transport to endoplasmic reticulum
↓
Triglyceride resynthesis
↓
Chylomicron formation
↓
Lymphatic transport

Submucosa

Mucosal events

• Not activated to coenzyme A derivative
• Not resynthesized to triglycerides
• Not packaged into chylomicrons
• Absorbed into portal blood

FIGURE 11-7. Digestion and absorption of long-chain triglycerides (LCT) and medium-chain triglycerides (MCT). Triglycerides consist of three fatty acids attached by ester linkage to a glycerol backbone. Most dietary triglycerides are composed of various long-chain (C_{14} to C_{22}) saturated or unsaturated fatty acids. Very few triglycerides are medium chain (C_6 to C_{12}) and short chain ($<C_6$). Ingested triglycerides are emulsified and hydrolyzed by pancreatic lipase to fatty acids, which are ingested with bile salts into micelles. The uptake of fatty acids has traditionally been thought to be through passive diffusion. Recent research shows that a carrier-dependent mechanism most likely plays an important role. Within the endoplasmic reticulum of the enterocyte, fatty acids and monoglycerides are resynthesized into triglycerides. The triglycerides are then packaged into chylomicrons and transported into the lymph. MCTs are hydrolyzed by lipase and are efficiently taken up by the enterocyte even in the absence of bile salts because they are much more water soluble. Some MCTs can be absorbed intact by the small intestine without digestion. The MCTs are released into the portal circulation and taken to the liver and other tissues to be used as an energy source. MCFA—medium-chain fatty acid. (*Adapted from* Chang et al. [3].)

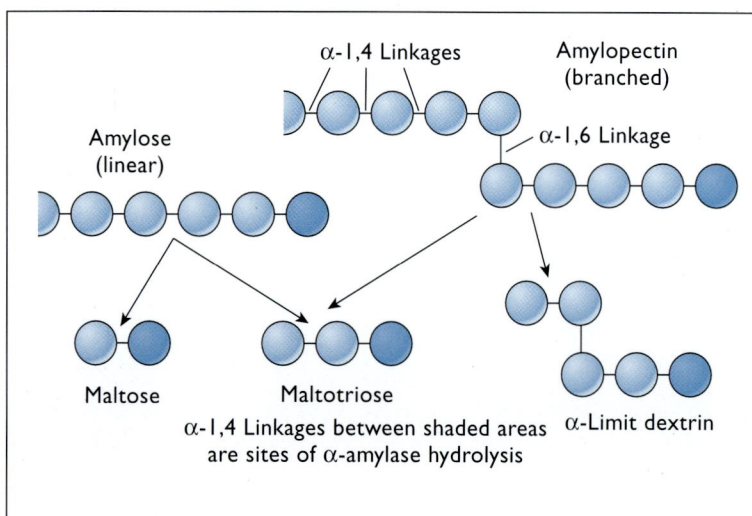

α-1,4 Linkages

Amylose
(linear)

Amylopectin
(branched)

α-1,6 Linkage

Maltose   Maltotriose   α-Limit dextrin

α-1,4 Linkages between shaded areas
are sites of α-amylase hydrolysis

FIGURE 11-8. Structure and initial digestion of starch. Starches consist of amylose or α-1,4–linked chains of glucose and amylopectin or α-1,4–linked straight chains with α-1,6–linked branching chains. Amylose and amylopectin are digested in the mouth and in the lumen of the small intestine by salivary and pancreatic amylase to maltose, maltotriose, and α-limit dextrins.

In general, carbohydrates are composed of 60% complex starches and 40% disaccharides, including 30% sucrose and 10% lactose. Whereas starch requires complex intraluminal and brush-border digestion followed by intestinal monosaccharide transport, sucrose is digested to glucose and fructose by brush-border sucrase and lactose is digested to glucose and galactose by brush-border lactase. (*Adapted from* Chang et al. [3].)

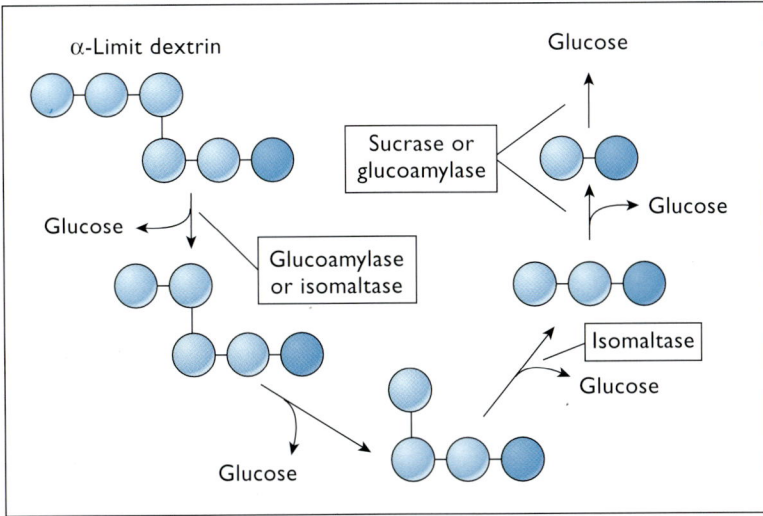

FIGURE 11-9. Final digestion of starch by brush-border enzymes. The final digestion of starch requires two enzymes in the enterocyte brush-border membrane. Glucoamylase continues to remove glucose residues from the α-1,4 chain. Sucrase isomaltase exists in its two components at the intestinal surface. Isomaltase cleaves the α-1,6 bond from a-limit dextrins, whereas sucrase cleaves the remaining α-1,4 bonds yielding glucose as the final product. (*Adapted from Chang et al.* [3].)

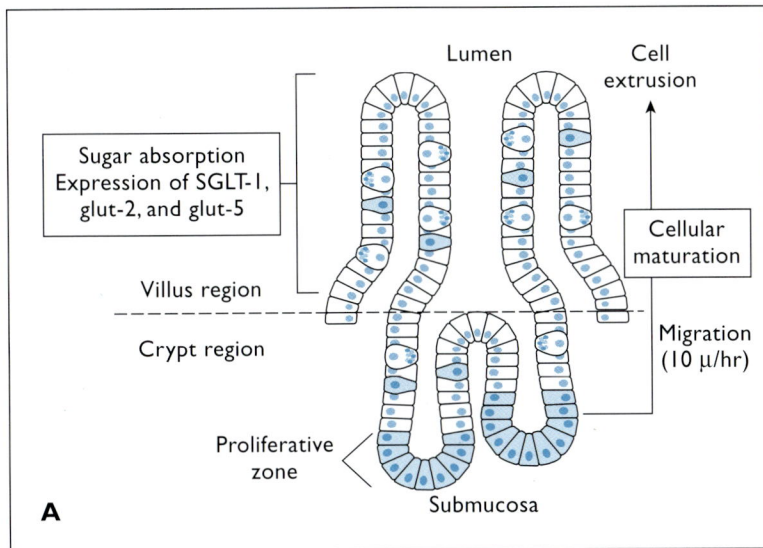

FIGURE 11-10. A, Transport of monosaccharides across absorbing cells. Specific proteins and mechanisms transport the monosaccharides glucose, galactose, and fructose across the enterocyte. Glucose and galactose are transported across the enterocyte brush-border membrane by sodium-dependent glucose transporter (SGLT-1) using a secondary active transport system in which energy is provided by Na^+,K^+-ATPase at the basolateral membrane. Fructose is transported across the brush-border membrane by facilitated diffusion using the glut-5 transporter. Both glucose and fructose use glut-2 for transport across the basolateral membrane.

B, Prevalence of late-onset lactose malabsorption among various ethnic and racial groups. Lactose malabsorption or intolerance is present in increased amounts in all nonwhite races due to relative postweaning decreases in the persistence of intestinal brush-border lactase. The symptoms of lactose intolerance typically include increased abdominal gas, cramps, and stool production following ingestion of variable amounts of lactose from milk and other dairy products in the diet. (Part A *adapted from* Chang et al. [3].)

B. PREVALENCE OF LATE-ONSET LACTOSE MALABSORPTION AMONG VARIOUS ETHNIC AND RACIAL GROUPS

Group	Prevalence of Lactose Malabsorption, %
Asian-Americans in the United States	100
American Indians (Oklahoma)	95
Ibo and Yoruba (Nigeria)	89
Black Americans	81
Italians	71
Aborigines (Australia)	67
Mexican Americans	56
Greeks	53
White Americans	24
Danes	3
Dutch	0

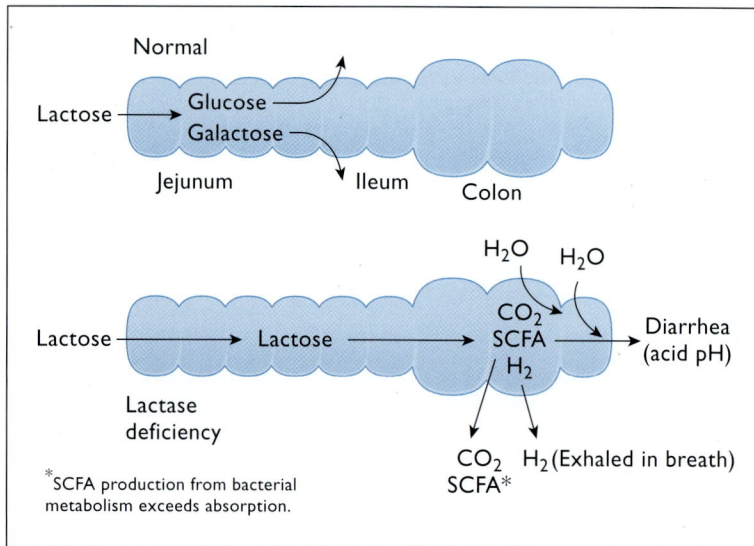

FIGURE 11-11. Mechanism of lactose intolerance. In contrast to individuals with high postweaning levels of lactase who are able to digest lactose completely to the absorbed products glucose and galactose, dietary lactose passes through the small bowel to the colon in lactase-deficient patients, where it is fermented to CO_2, short-chain fatty acids (SCFAs), and hydrogen. The production of hydrogen is the basis of the hydrogen breath test for lactose intolerance, whereas unabsorbed fatty acids and other fermentation products stimulate water secretion into the colon and diarrhea at a low pH. (*Adapted from* Chang et al. [3].)

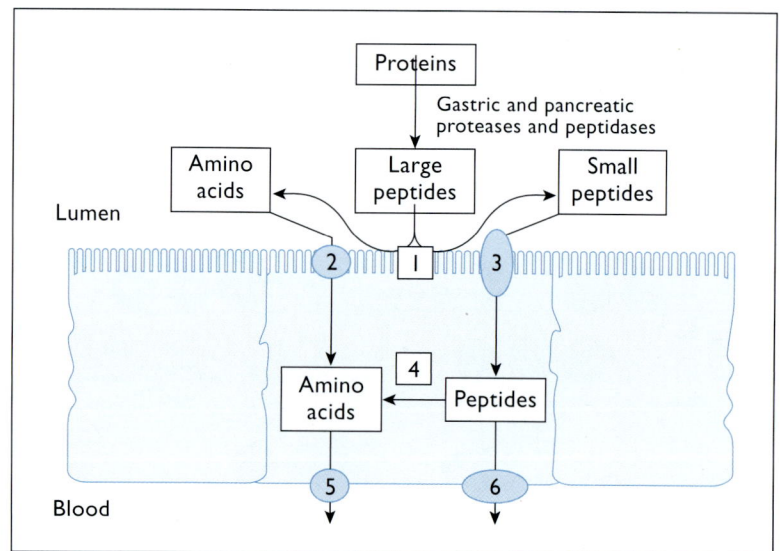

FIGURE 11-12. Brush-border digestion and transport of protein.

Proteins exist in the diet as polypeptides, which are first digested by proteolytic enzymes in gastric juice (pepsins A and C) and then by pancreatic proteases. Within the duodenal lumen, the pancreatic proenzyme trypsinogen is activated by intestinal brush-border enterokinase to trypsin, which then activates the other pancreatic proenzymes. The proteases trypsin, chymotrypsin, elastase (endopeptidases), and carboxypeptidases A and B (exopeptidases) cleave various portions of protein polypeptide chains within the duodenal lumen, resulting in a mixture of 40% amino acids and 60% short-chain polypeptides.

Following intraluminal digestion by proteases, oligopeptides are further digested by brush-border peptidases (*1*) to produce a mixture of amino acids and smaller (di- and tri-) peptides, all of which are actively transported across the brush-border membrane by specific transport mechanisms (*2,3*). Most transported small peptides are completely digested by intracellular peptidases (*4*). Subsequently, specific basolateral membrane transporters take amino acids and undigested dipeptides and tripeptides into the portal blood system (*5,6*). Each of these transport systems is specific for groups of amino acids and peptides (eg, neutral amino acids, basic amino acids and cystine, and proline and hydroxyproline). (*Adapted from* Chang et al. [3].)

Vitamin B_{12}

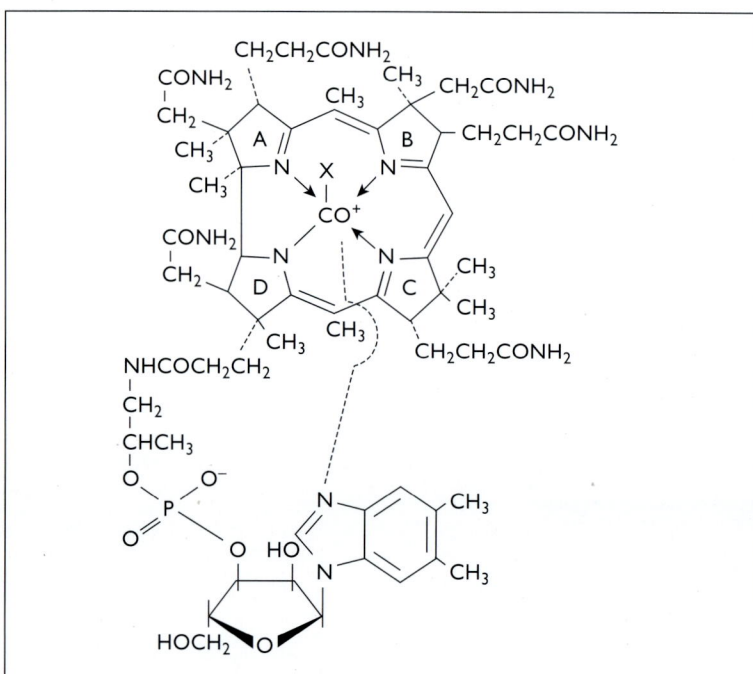

FIGURE 11-13. Structure of vitamin B_{12} (cobalamin). Vitamin B_{12} consists of a porphyrinlike ring structure (with cobalt in its central core) that is linked to two groups that provide specific functions. Vitamin B_{12} as methylcobalamin is the cofactor for methionine synthase. Vitamin B_{12} as adenosylcobalamin is a cofactor for methylmalonyl–coenzyme A (CoA) mutase, which is essential in myelin metabolism. Vitamin B_{12} deficiency is characterized by elevations in both plasma homocysteine (the precursor of methionine synthase) and methylmalonic acid (the precursor of methylmalonyl-CoA mutase). (*Adapted from* Chang et al. [3].)

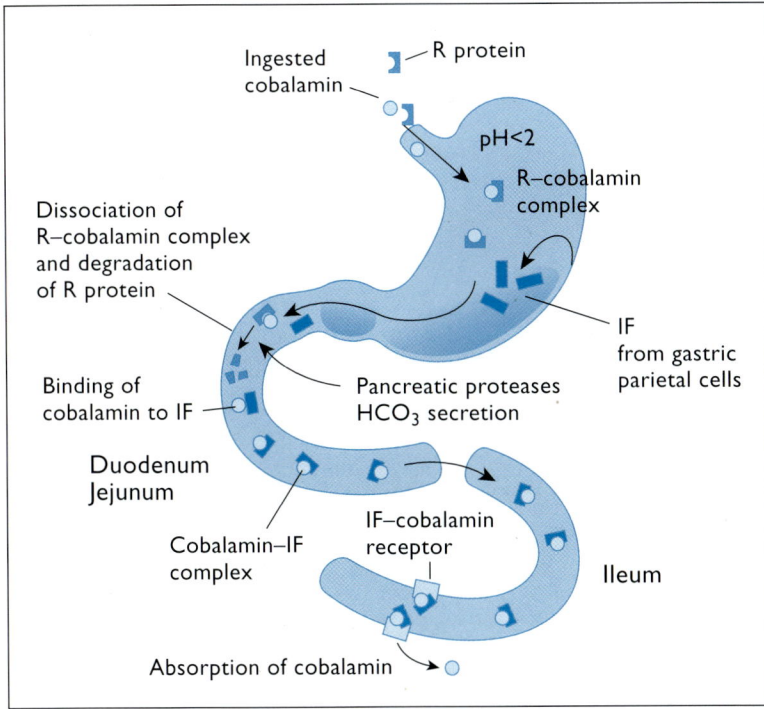

FIGURE 11-14. Overview of vitamin B$_{12}$ (cobalamin) absorption. The intestinal absorption of cobalamin is a complex progression of steps in the stomach and small intestine. In the stomach, cobalamin is released by gastric acid (pH < 2) from dietary protein and is then bound to salivary and gastric R protein before passage to the duodenum. The stomach also secretes a separate protein called *intrinsic factor* (IF). Within the duodenum, the higher pH releases cobalamin from its R complex, following which cobalamin is tightly bound to IF. The cobalamin–IF complex passes through the intestine to the terminal ileum where, at neutral pH and in the presence of calcium ions, it is bound to the brush border and then absorbed through the enterocyte. (*Adapted from* Chang et al. [3].)

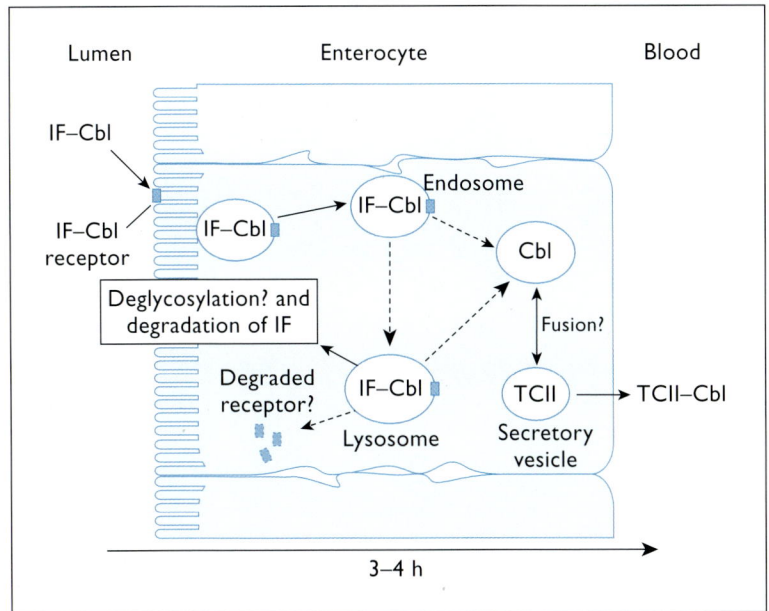

FIGURE 11-15. Uptake and transfer of vitamin B$_{12}$ (cobalamin [Cbl]) through the ileal enterocyte. After binding and internalization of the intrinsic factor (IF)–cobalamin complex within the ileal enterocyte, cobalamin is released and then bound to transcobalamin (TCII). This new complex is then secreted into the portal blood system for transport into the liver and other tissues. (*Adapted from* Chang et al. [2].)

Folate

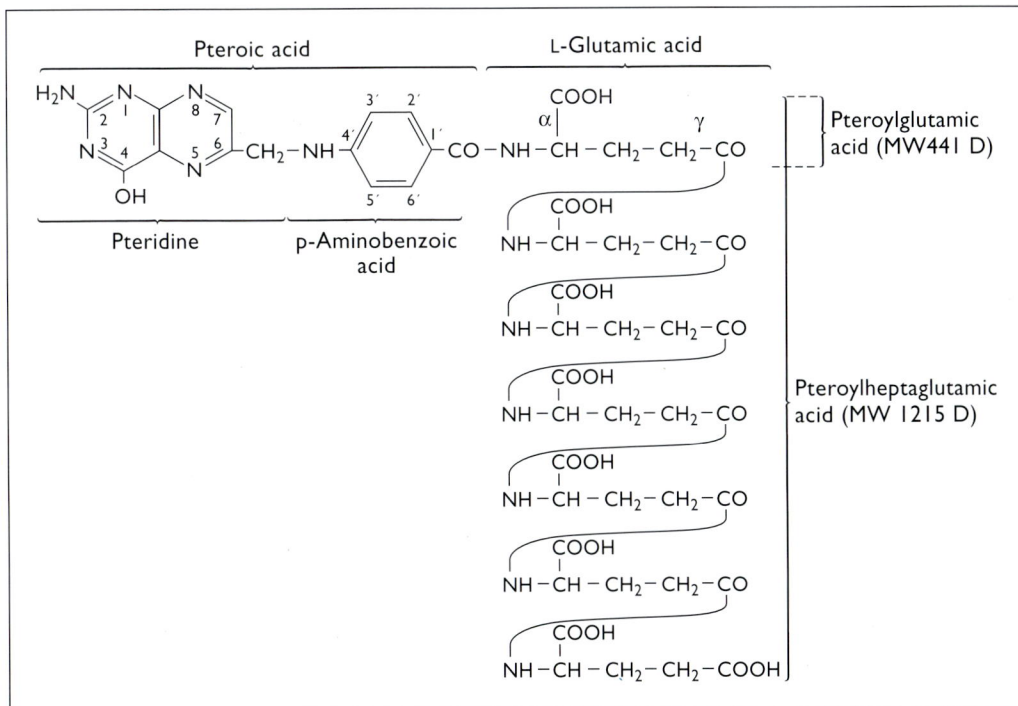

FIGURE 11-16. Structure of folate. The term *folate* refers to conjugated, reduced, and substituted forms of folic acid (pteroylglutamic acid). The structure of fully conjugated folate consists of pteroylglutamic acid, which is linked by γ-peptide bonds to six additional glutamates to form pteroylheptaglutamate. Folates exist in the diet in the conjugated form, whereas folates circulate in the blood as methylated and reduced forms of folic acid. Folates serve as substrates or coenzymes for reactions that transfer methyl groups and other carbon units among amino acids and ultimately are involved in nucleic acid synthesis. MW—molecular weight. (*Adapted from* Johnson et al. [4].)

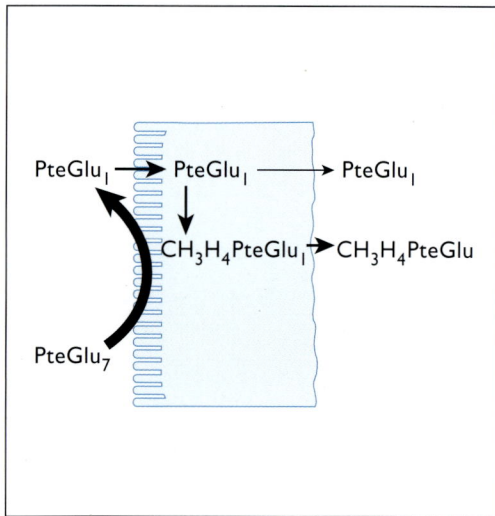

FIGURE 11-17. Intestinal absorption of folates. Dietary folates are absorbed in the duodenum and jejunum by a two-stage process. For example, pteroylheptaglutamate (PteGlu₇) is first hydrolyzed at the enterocyte surface by intestinal brush-border folate hydrolase to pteroylglutamate (PteGlu or folic acid), which is transported by the reduced folate carrier into the enterocyte. Here it undergoes further methylation and reduction to CH₃H₄PteGlu. The same reduced folate carrier protein transports both oxidized and reduced forms across the basolateral membrane, presumably to the capillary blood. Folate absorption is affected by diseases of the small intestinal mucosa (eg, celiac disease) and is decreased in chronic alcoholism. (*Adapted from* Johnson *et al.* [4].)

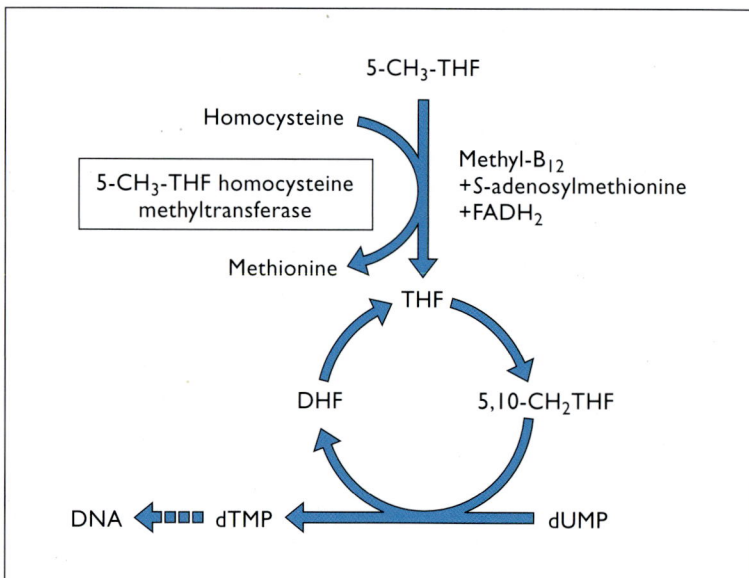

FIGURE 11-18. Metabolic interactions of folate and vitamin B_{12}. Folate and vitamin B_{12} interact in the methionine synthase reaction in which vitamin B_{12} serves as a cofactor and methyltetrahydrofolate (5-CH₃-THF) donates its methyl (CH₃) group to homocysteine. The resultant tetrahydrofolate (THF) is substrate for subsequent reactions involved in deoxynucleotide (dUMP, dTMP) metabolism and DNA synthesis. Methionine is substrate to S-adenosylmethionine, which is a principal methyl donor in many other cellular reactions (not shown). These reactions form the basis for measurement of serum homocysteine, which is elevated in both folate and vitamin B_{12} deficiency. DHF—dihydrofolate; FADH₂—flavin adenine dinucleotide (reduced) (*Adapted from* Chang *et al.* [3].)

Other Vitamins and Minerals

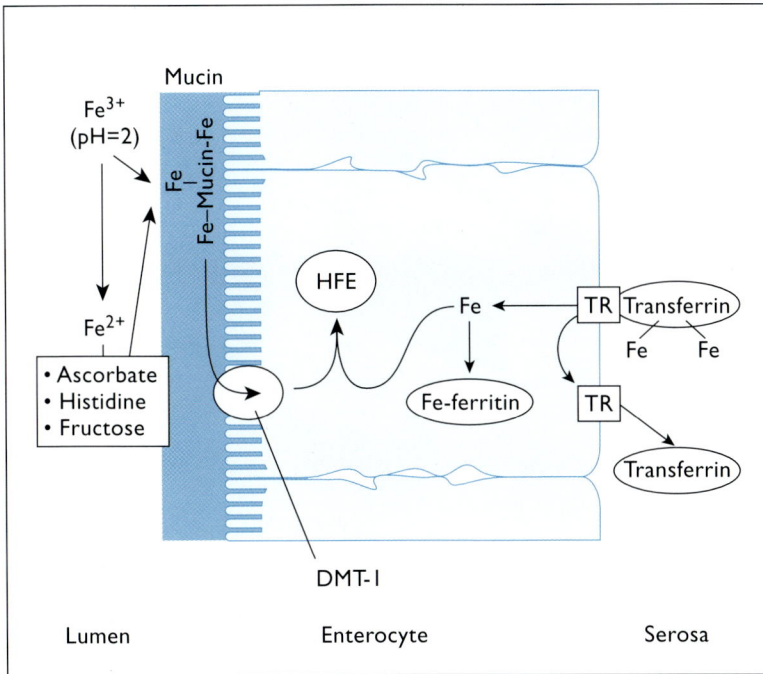

FIGURE 11-19. Intestinal absorption of iron. Dietary iron exists in two forms, as heme iron from animal sources in the reduced Fe^{2+} (ferrous) state, and as nonheme iron from plant sources in the Fe^{3+} (ferric) state. Ferric iron is soluble in gastric acid, but not at the neutral pH of the small intestine, and is solubilized, chelated, and reduced to ferrous iron by such dietary factors as amino acids, vitamin C, and fructose. Heme iron remains soluble in the intestinal environment. Reduced (Fe^{2+}) iron binds to mucins on the surface of the enterocyte and is then transported by divalent metal transporter–1 (DMT-1), a protein that also interacts with zinc, magnesium, and divalent aluminum. Iron also binds to the hemochromatosis gene protein (HFE) soon after transport through the brush border. HFE is internalized and may play a role with the transferrin receptor (TR) in the transfer of iron across the basolateral membrane. TR may also play a role in the reverse transport of circulating iron into the enterocyte. Body iron stores regulate the fate of enterocyte iron. When body iron stores are in excess, enterocyte iron is bound to intracellular ferritin and eventually sloughed with the cell into the intestinal lumen and out of the body. Heme iron enters the cell intact, where iron is released by heme oxygenase to enter the intracellular iron pool (not shown). Iron absorption is increased in patients with iron deficiency, chronic hypoxia, and chronic hemolytic diseases as well as the genetic disorder hemochromatosis. In health, the overall absorption of iron from all sources is efficient at only approximately 10%. (*Adapted from* Chang *et al.* [3].)

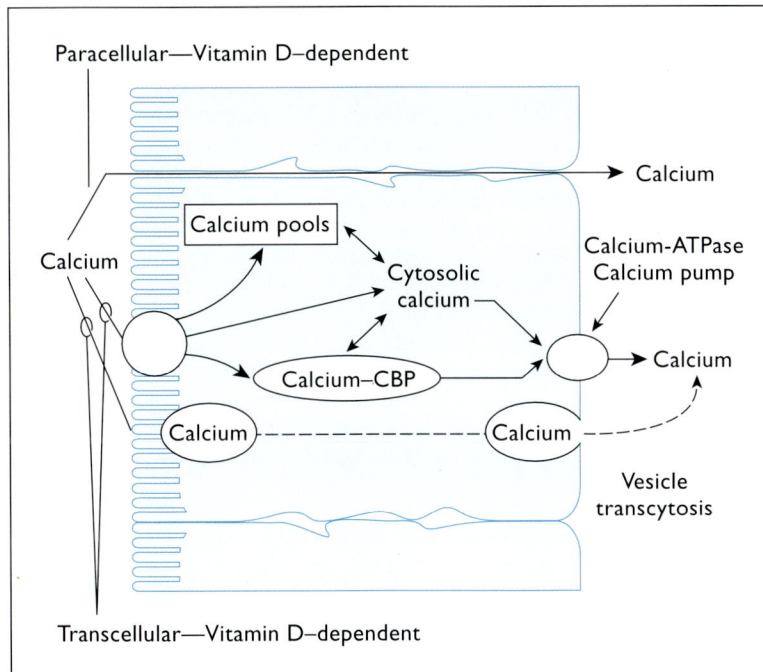

FIGURE 11-20. Calcium absorption. Through several regulatory steps, calcium (Ca^{2+}) is absorbed throughout the small intestine. Calcium crosses the brush-border membrane via a 10- to 100-fold electrochemical gradient. $1,25(OH)_2$ vitamin D, alkaline phosphatase, and calmodulin also regulate brush-border transport. Calcium binds to vitamin D–dependent calbindin-D or calcium-binding protein (CBP), which facilitates its movement across the cell. At the basolateral membrane, a vitamin D–stimulated pump known as calcium-transporting ATPase facilitates calcium extrusion. A concentration gradient is developed by the three-fold greater binding effect of calcium to the ATPase than to CBP. (*Adapted from* Chang *et al.* [3].)

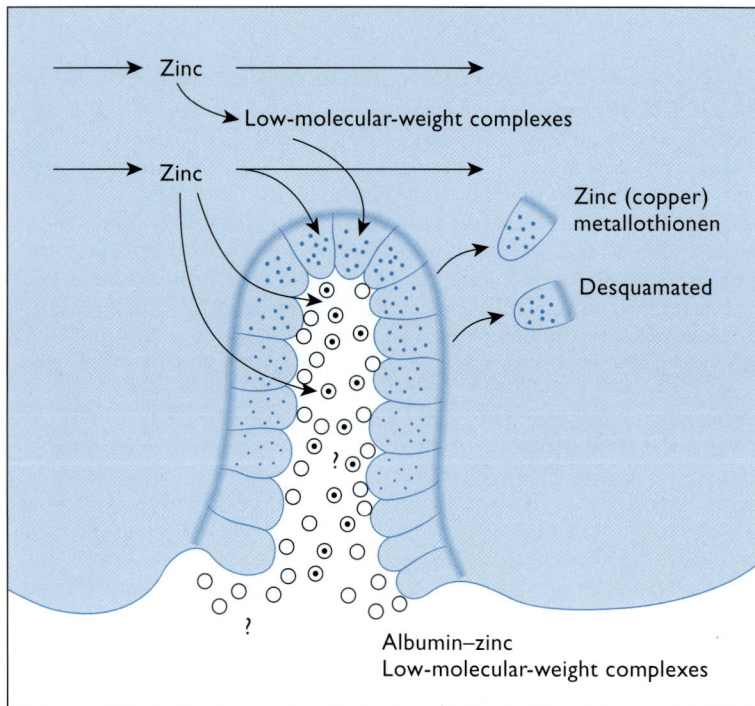

FIGURE 11-21. Zinc absorption. Dietary zinc is essential for appetite, wound healing, reproductive performance, and as a cofactor for many enzymes. The typical American diet provides 10 to 12 mg of zinc per day, of which about 25% is absorbed throughout the small intestine. Zinc transport across the brush border is mediated by divalent metal transporter–1 (not shown). Intracellular zinc associates first with cysteine-rich intestinal protein (CRIP, not shown) as the main transporter across the cell. When the intracellular binding protein metallothionen (MT) is low, more zinc is transported by CRIP, whereas high MT levels (indicative of high body zinc stores) reduce CRIP transport. Zinc absorption is decreased in alcoholics as well as in patients with Crohn's disease, celiac disease, and diabetes. The gut is also the major source of zinc excretion, with approximately 90% leaving the body through pancreatic and intestinal bile secretions and sloughed mucosal cells. (*Adapted from* Johnson *et al.* [4].)

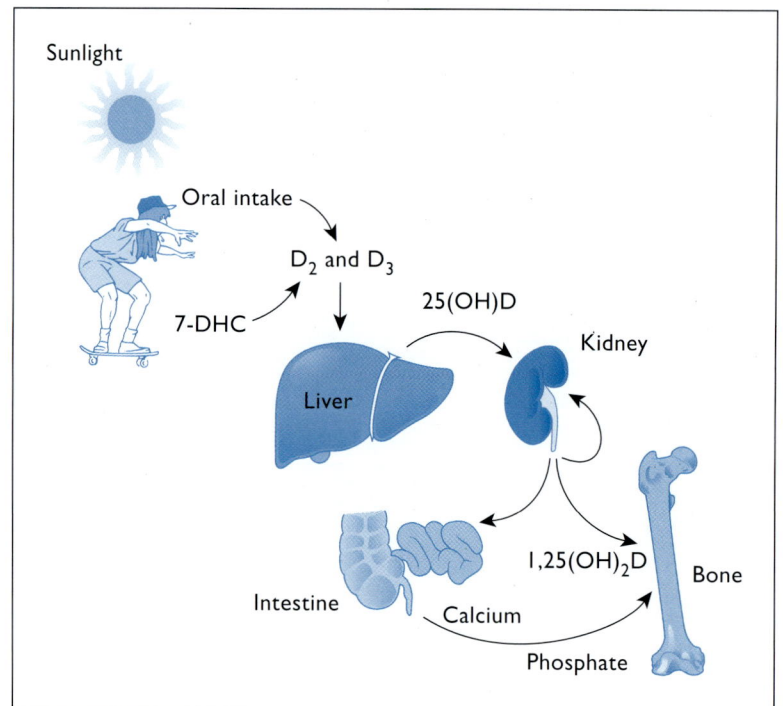

FIGURE 11-22. Vitamin D absorption. Vitamin D is ingested in the diet as vitamin D_2 (ergocalciferol) or D_3 (cholecalciferol). Vitamin D can also be synthesized from 7-dehydrocholesterol (7-DHC) in the skin after exposure to sunlight. For activation, vitamin D must undergo 25-hydroxylation in the liver followed by 1-hydroxylation in the kidneys. Once activated, vitamin D is free to act on bones, kidneys, and intestines to maintain calcium, phosphate, and bone homeostasis. Cholecalciferol and ergocalciferol found in the diet do not require intraluminal digestion. Bile salts are required to solubilize vitamin D_3 in the mixed-micellar phase and are subsequently incorporated into chylomicrons within the enterocyte. Studies in rats have shown that vitamin D absorption is greater in the proximal and mid-small intestine than in the distal small intestine. Vitamin D is absorbed into the lymphatics and enters the circulation bound to vitamin D–binding protein. Poor vitamin D absorption can be seen in patients with intraluminal bile salt deficiency or in those who have had intestinal resections causing malabsorption of bile salts.

The vitamin D metabolites $25(OH)D_3$ and $1,25(OH)_2D_3$ are not found in significant amounts in the diet but are used pharmacologically in the treatment of metabolic bone diseases and disorders of mineral metabolism. These forms are more readily absorbed than is vitamin D_3, especially in patients with intraluminal bile salt deficiency and steatorrhea. (*Adapted from* Reichel *et al.* [5].)

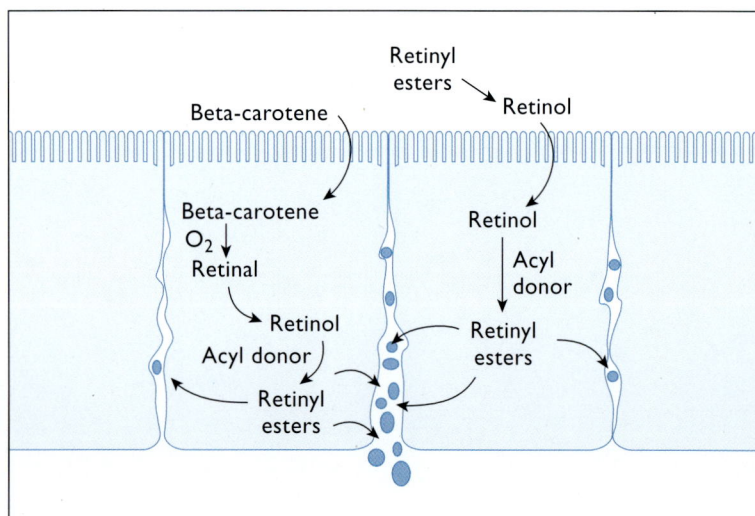

FIGURE 11-23. Absorption and metabolism of beta-carotene and retinyl esters. The term *vitamin A* refers to all-*trans*-retinol and a family of structurally related compounds. Other compounds such as retinol, retinoic acid, and retinaldehyde are termed *retinoids*. Dietary vitamin A is found in animal sources as long-chain fatty acyl retinol esters, and some animals fats are precursors of vitamin A. Fruits and vegetables contain some carotenoids that are precursors of vitamin A. There are over 500 carotenoids, of which only about 50 are precursors of retinol. Six micrograms of dietary beta-carotene or 12 µg of mixed carotenoids is equivalent to 1 µg of retinol due to factors including bioavailability, intestinal absorption, and limited conversion of carotenoids to vitamin A.

Dietary retinyl esters need to be hydrolyzed in order for intestinal absorption to occur. Pancreatic bile salt–activated lipase and intestinal brush-border membranes play a part in the hydrolysis. Retinol formed by the hydrolysis of retinyl esters and beta-carotene is contained in mixed micelles within the lumen. At low concentrations, retinol is taken up by enterocytes by carrier-mediated facilitated diffusion. At higher concentrations, uptake is through passive diffusion. Retinol uptake is greater in the jejunum than in the ileum. (*Adapted from* Ong [6].)

Intestinal Malabsorption Syndromes

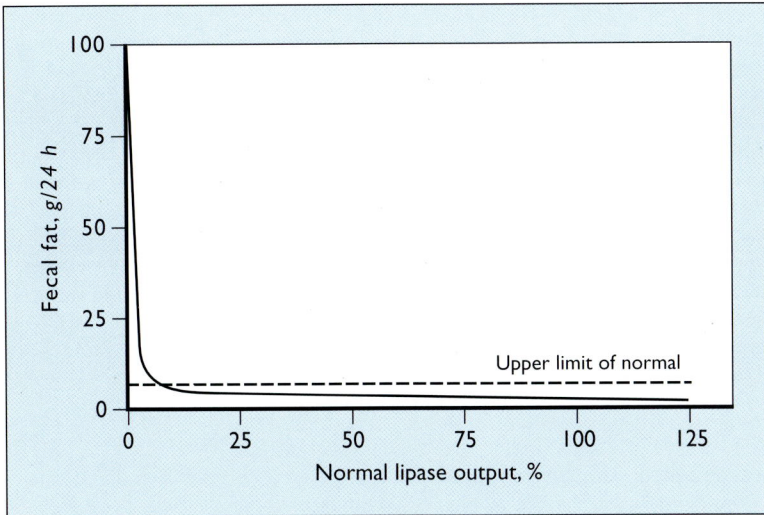

FIGURE 11-24. Relationship of steatorrhea (24-hour fecal fat over 7g when 100g of fat is ingested daily) to lipase output in chronic pancreatitis. Chronic pancreatitis is characterized by glandular damage resulting in various exocrine and endocrine dysfunctions and is accompanied by disabling pain. Chronic pancreatitis is caused by chronic alcoholism, heredity, cystic fibrosis, tropical (nutritional) trauma, and idiopathic etiologies. The medical treatment of chronic pancreatitis consists primarily of pain control, correction of maldigestion by oral enzyme replacement, and management of glucose intolerance. Diarrhea, steatorrhea, and azotorrhea occur when exocrine secretions of pancreatic enzymes are insufficient to maintain normal digestion. Typically, this occurs late in the course of chronic pancreatitis because malabsorption does not occur until enzyme secretion is reduced to less than 10% of normal. (*Adapted from DiMagno et al. [7].*)

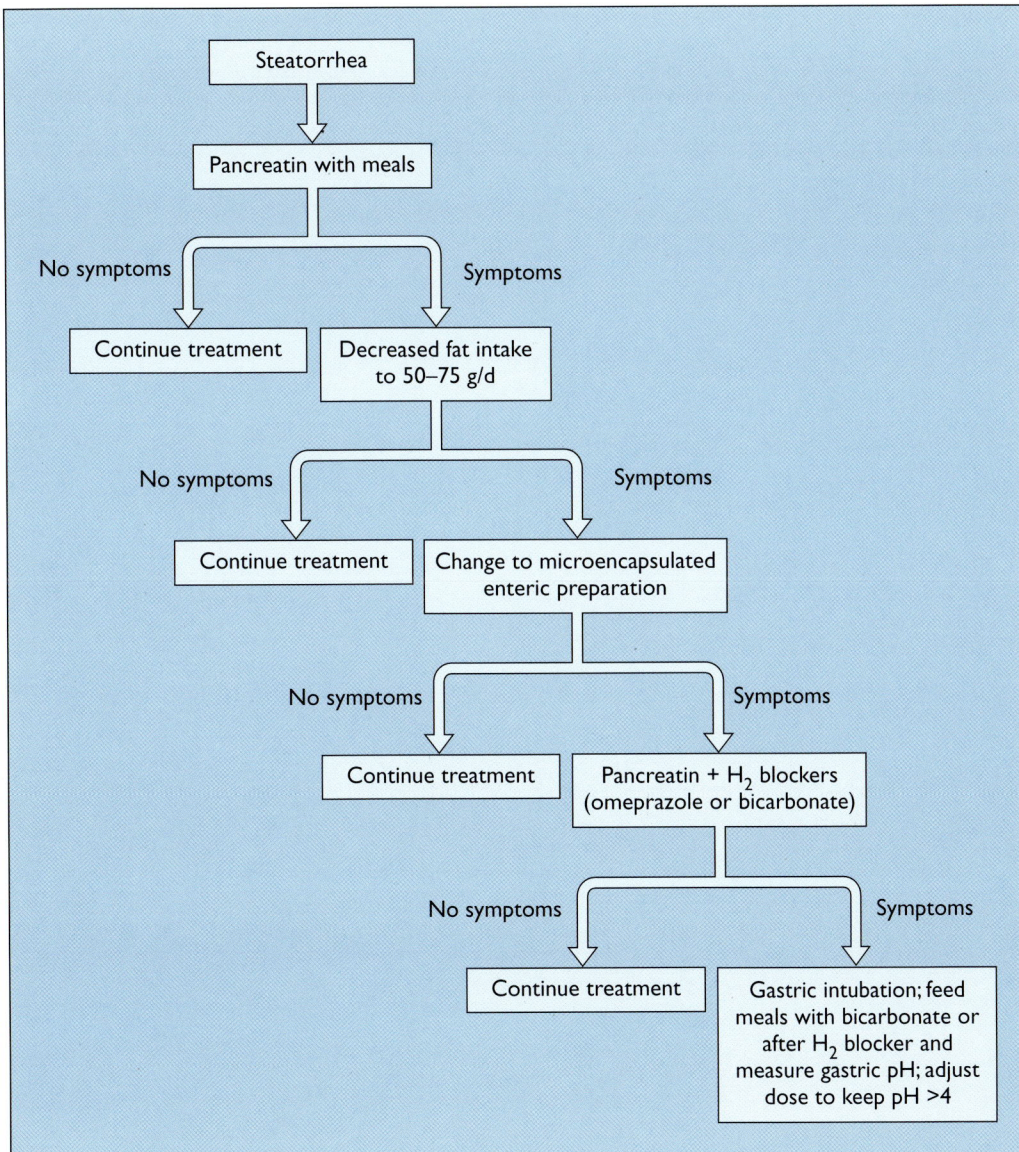

FIGURE 11-25. Treatment algorithm for malabsorption caused by pancreatic insufficiency. Many patients with exocrine pancreatic insufficiency are satisfactorily managed with standard pancreatin treatment consisting of eight tablets with each meal that contains 25 g of fat. In the remaining symptomatic patients, reducing dietary fat intake is usually effective in alleviating the symptoms. For those who may remain symptomatic, the addition of an H_2 blocker of gastric acid secretion (eg, omeprazole, bicarbonate) may eliminate steatorrhea. Difficult cases may require intraluminal studies of gastric pH levels to assess the correct dosage of medication.

High-potency lipase enteric-coated preparations with microspheres have recently become commercially available. These preparations can reduce the number of pancreatic enzyme tablets a patient needs to take per meal. Pancreatic enzyme therapy is also suggested for pain management in mild to moderate pancreatic insufficiency. However, various multicenter trial data yielded mixed results. Pancreatic enzyme therapy is used routinely for patients with cystic fibrosis associated with pancreatic insufficiency. (*Adapted from Go et al. [8].*)

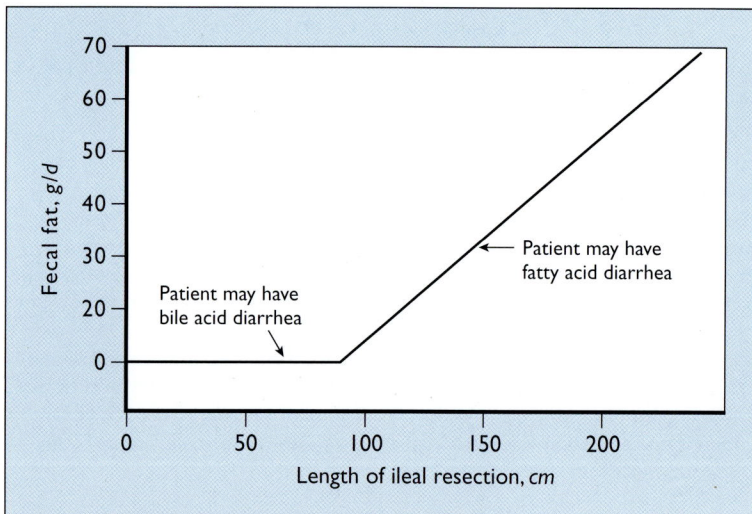

FIGURE 11-26. Etiology of short-bowel syndrome. Short-bowel syndrome is a condition in which a significant portion of the small intestine is severely diseased or surgically removed. The causes most commonly include inflammatory bowel disease (Crohn's disease), acute strangulation or infarction of the small bowel leading to emergent intestinal surgery, and previous elective jejunoileal bypass surgery in severely obese patients. As shown, under conditions of disease or surgical loss of the terminal ileum, conjugated bile salts are unabsorbed and, following deconjugation from taurine or glycine by colonic bacteria, stimulate water secretion in the colon with resultant diarrhea. When the length of ileal resection exceeds approximately 100 cm, the size of the circulating bile salt pool is contracted below the capacity of the liver for compensatory synthesis and secretion. As result, fewer bile salts are secreted by the liver, resulting in decreased micelle formation in the upper intestine and malabsorption of fat and fat-soluble vitamins. Unabsorbed fatty acids pass through the small intestine and result in steatorrhea (ie, a mixture of fat- and fatty acid–stimulated water secretion from the colon into the stool). (*Adapted from* the American Gastro-enterological Association Undergraduate Teaching Project [2].)

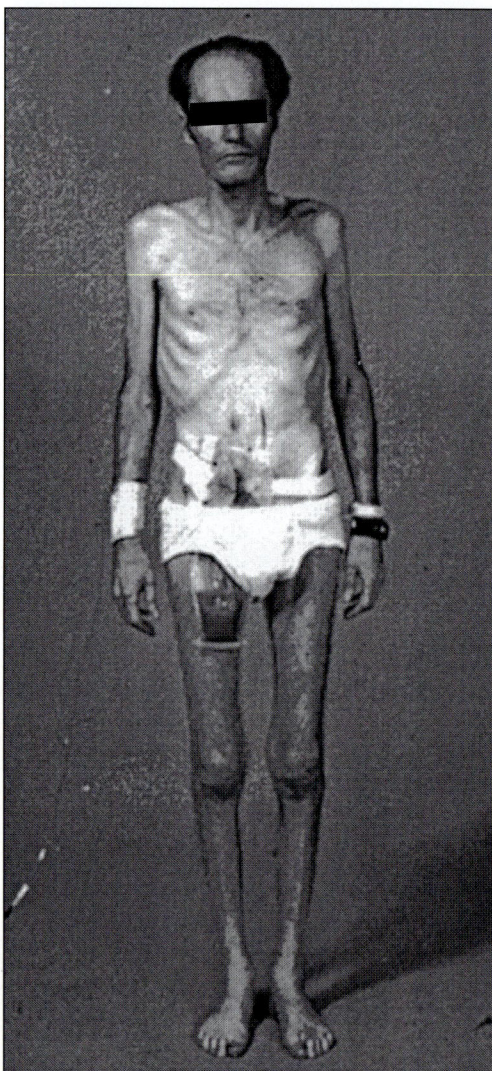

FIGURE 11-27. A malnourished patient with Crohn's disease, 12 months after surgical resection of the ileocecal valve and 100 cm of the distal ileum. The clinical picture is complicated further if the ileocecal valve is lost because colonic bacteria migrate upward to the small intestine and further impair bile acid effectiveness through deconjugation, thereby worsening fat losses in the stool. In addition, vitamin B_{12} absorption is impaired in both short-bowel syndrome and intestinal bacterial stasis syndrome through the loss of ileal receptors and by bacterial uptake or cleavage of the intrinsic factor complex. Consequently, the patient becomes progressively malnourished with a deficiency of body fat, fat-soluble vitamins, and vitamin B_{12}. Such patients typically suffer from extreme diarrhea and learn to restrict their food intake in order to reduce the frequency of their meal-stimulated stool evacuations, further compromising their nutritional state. This patient is severely malnourished, with loss of body fat and skeletal muscle mass; vitamin B_{12} deficiency was apparent by laboratory testing.

A. DISEASES OF THE INTESTINAL MUCOSA THAT CAUSE MALABSORPTION

Disease	Clinical Causes and Mechanisms
Celiac disease	Gluten sensitive enteropathy; loss of villus surface results in generalized malabsorption of macro and micronutrients
AIDS	Infection of mucosa with HIV, cryptosporidia, mycobacteria, microsporidia alters villus functions
Whipple's disease	Infection of mucosa with *Tropheryma whippelii* alters villus functions
Tropical sprue	Unknown, causes loss of villus surface with generalized malabsorption
Parasitism, especially *Giardia*	Causes loss of villus functions with generalized malabsorption
Intestinal lymphoma	Malignant infiltration of mucosa alters villus functions

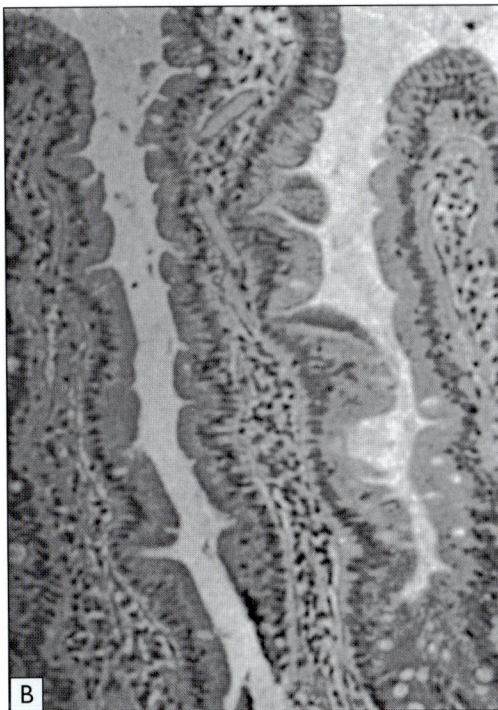

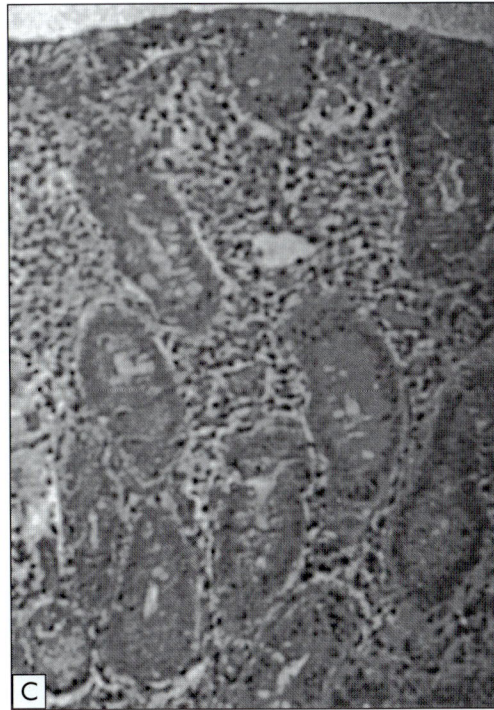

FIGURE 11-28. A, Diseases of the intestinal mucosa that cause malabsorption. Intestinal malabsorption syndromes occur when intestinal villus architecture and absorbing enterocytes are damaged or lost, resulting in severe compromise of the brush-border enzymes and transporters that regulate the absorption of carbohydrate, protein, fatty acids, and many vitamins and minerals. The patient experiences multinutrient deficiencies as well as chronic diarrhea owing to loss of electrolyte transporters.

In celiac disease, the small intestinal mucosa is characterized by a mucosal inflammatory response to gliadin, a protein present in the alcohol-soluble gluten fraction of many grains, including wheat, barley, and rye. Approximately one in 300 whites has one or more abnormalities in specific HLA complex genes (which regulate the immune recognition of dietary gliadin) and develops an intense inflammatory response in the mucosa of the duodenum and jejunum in response to ingestion of offending grains that include this protein.

B and **C**, Histopathology of the jejunal mucosa in health and in celiac disease. The normal intestinal mucosal architecture (*panel B*) shows orderly surface-absorbing enterocytes lining each villus. The jejunal mucosal features of untreated celiac disease (*panel C*) include complete loss of villus architecture, near-absence of absorbing enterocytes, intense inflammatory response to the lamina propria, and hypertrophy of the crypt regions.

Patients with celiac disease experience deficiencies of iron; folate; calcium; and vitamins D, E, and K. Such patients are characteristically generally malnourished as a result of malabsorption of fatty acids, peptides, and carbohydrates and experience chronic diarrhea owing to the osmotic effect of unabsorbed and fermented sugars. However, about half of affected individuals describe a less dramatic clinical experience and are underweight with moderate, chronic diarrhea and isolated abnormalities leading to iron deficiency and/or accelerated osteoporosis. Over 90% of patients with celiac disease are responsive to a strict dietary regimen of gluten exclusion from the diet.

Alcoholism and Alcoholic Liver Disease

RELATIVE RISK OF MORTALITY FROM MODERATE ALCOHOL CONSUMPTION

Drinks Per Day, n	Ethanol Per Day, g	Relative Risk
0	0	1.4
0–1	0–12	1.0
1–2	12–24	1.1
2–4	24–48	1.2
4–6	48–72	1.3
6–10	72–120	1.5
>10	>120	2.3

FIGURE 11-29. Relative risk of mortality from moderate alcohol consumption. As shown in data from Copenhagen, Denmark, when alcohol is quantified as drinks per day (one drink = 12 g of ethanol, such as in one can of beer, one glass of wine, or 1.25 oz of liquor), the overall mortality risk is least among those drinking one to two drinks daily [9]. Further, women have about twice the mortality risk from drinking as do men. Therefore, it is reasonable to advise women to have no more than one drink per day and men no more than two drinks per day. The protective effects of moderate alcohol intake relate to the reduced incidence of coronary heart disease and ischemic stroke that results from increased synthesis of high-density lipoproteins, reduced platelet adhesiveness, and flavonoids in wine that may protect low-density lipoproteins from oxidation.

Alcohol is a dietary substance with a caloric value of 7.1 kcal/g, providing 5% of the daily energy intake of Americans. Although 35% of the US population abstains, 60% are occasional to moderate drinkers, and 5% to 10% are addicted, heavy drinkers.

The Copenhagen study [9] has recently been updated to show that consumers of wine receive greater benefit than do drinkers of other alcoholic beverages because the diets of wine drinkers tend to include more fruits and vegetables and therefore increased levels of antioxidant flavonoids [10]. At higher drinking levels, mortality is increased through hypertension, many cancers, and a greater risk of cirrhosis among those consuming more than five drinks daily. (*Adapted from* Grønbæck, et al. [9].)

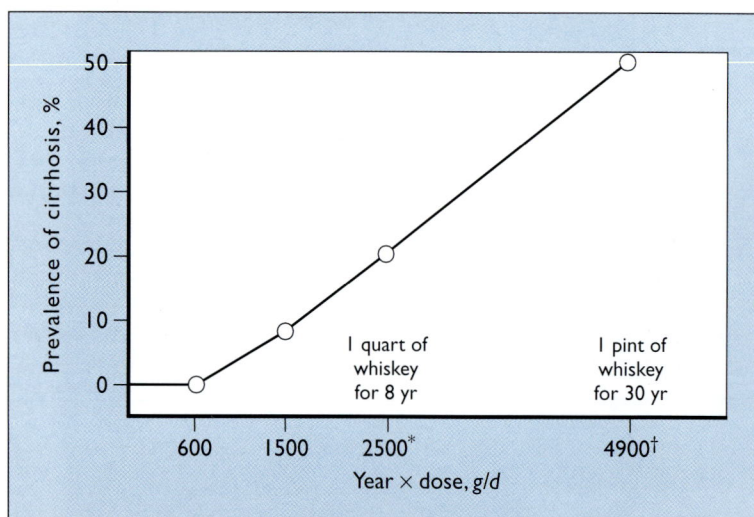

FIGURE 11-30. Risk of cirrhosis in relation to amount of alcohol consumed. The risk of alcoholic liver disease is related directly to the amount of alcohol consumed, regardless of the nutritional state of the drinker. In this study of over 300 well-nourished German executives, the prevalence of alcoholic cirrhosis was established by liver biopsy and related directly to historical consumption of alcoholic beverages. Thus an individual who consumed 150 g/d of alcohol (equivalent to 10 drinks) for 10 years would have a likelihood of cirrhosis of about 10%. Similarly, someone drinking 300 g or 20 drinks per day, roughly equivalent to one quart of whiskey, would have a 20% chance of being cirrhotic after 8 years [11]. (*Adapted from* the American Gastroenterological Association Undergraduate Teaching Project [12].)

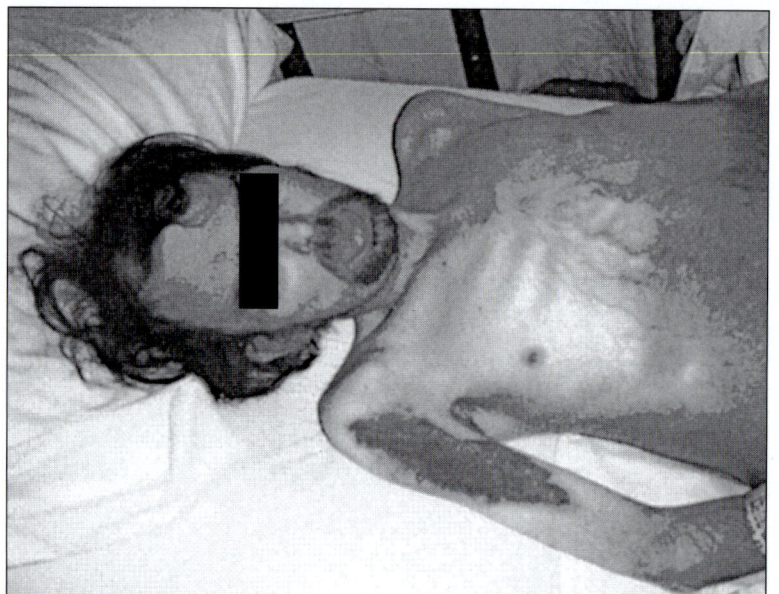

FIGURE 11-31. Severe protein malnutrition in a patient with end-stage liver disease. Although poor nutrition is not a recognized cause of alcoholic cirrhosis, the converse is true, that is, the presence of alcoholic liver disease increases the likelihood of malnutrition. The causes of malnutrition in alcoholic liver disease are diverse and include inadequate diet; intestinal malabsorption of many nutrients conditioned by chronic alcohol consumption; and abnormal metabolism of lipid, carbohydrate, and protein. Abstinence from alcohol may arrest the progression of cirrhosis within the liver, whereas the roles of diet and other modalities of nutritional support in reversing the progression of liver disease have not been conclusively shown.

References

1. American Gastroenterological Association Undergraduate Teaching Project: *Mucosal Digestive and Absorptive Function*, vol VI. Timonium, MD: Milner-Fenwick, Inc.; 1981.

2. American Gastroenterological Association Undergraduate Teaching Project: *Lipid Digestion and Absorption*, vol V. Timonium, MD: Milner-Fenwick, Inc.; 1974.

3. Chang EB, Sitrin MD, Black DD: *Gastrointestinal, Hepatobiliary, and Nutritional Physiology*. Philadelphia: Lippincott-Raven; 1996.

4. Johnson LR, Alpers DH, Jacobson ED, *et al.*, eds: *Physiology of the Gastrointestinal Tract*, edn 3. New York: Raven Press; 1994.

5. Reichel H, Koeffler HP, Norman AW: The role of the vitamin D endocrine system in health and disease. *N Engl J Med* 1989, 320:980.

6. Ong DE: Absorption of vitamin A. In *Vitamin A in Health and Disease*. Edited by Blomhoff R. New York: Marcel Dekker; 1994:37–72.

7. DiMagno EP, Go VLW, Summerskill WHJ: Relations between pancreatic enzyme outputs and malabsorption in severe pancreatic insufficiency. *N Engl J Med* 1973, 288:813.

8. Go VLW, DiMagno EP, Gardner JD, *et al.*, eds: *The Pancreas: Biology, Pathobiology and Disease*, edn 2. New York: Raven Press; 1993.

9. Grønbæck M, Deis A, Sørensen TIA, *et al.*: Mortality associated with moderate intakes of wine, beer, or spirits. *BMJ* 1995, 310:1165–1169.

10. Tjønneland A, Grønbæck M, Stripp C, Overvad K: Wine intake and diet in a random sample of 48,763 Danish men and women. *Am J Clin Nutr* 1999, 69:49–54.

11. Lelbach WK: Cirrhosis in the alcoholic and its relation to the volume of alcohol abuse. *Ann N Y Acad Sci* 1975, 252:85–105.

12. American Gastroenterological Association Undergraduate Teaching Project: *Alcohol*, vol XIV. Timonium, MD: Milner-Fenwick, Inc.; 1981.

12

NUTRITION FOR CANCER AND AGING

David Heber

A significant body of epidemiologic evidence associates certain dietary patterns with an increased risk for cancer. A diet rich in fat and meat and low in cereals, fiber, fruits, and vegetables is associated with an increased risk for colorectal, mammary, and other common forms of cancer. Limited diets in some countries that have evident micronutrient deficiencies are also associated with an increased risk for certain types of cancer. A genetic polymorphism of the *GSTM1* enzyme increases the risk for colon polyps, while the ingestion of cruciferous vegetables (broccoli, cauliflower, Brussels sprouts) cancels out the effects of the null genotype. Although the population studies from which these data were derived cannot establish a cause-and-effect relationship between nutrition and cancer, many studies in animals support the concept that cancer results from a gene–nutrient interaction.

The final common mechanism believed to mediate the effects of different diets on cancer and aging is the oxidation of the genome and other cellular and subcellular structures. Mutations induced by oxidative damage may then lead to increased cellular proliferation, reduced apoptosis, or both. Therefore, genes confer susceptibility to oxidative damage through absence or malfunction of the extensive antioxidant defense and DNA repair mechanisms, while the diet can affect whether and to what extent that oxidative damage occurs.

Oxidative damage is increased during the aging process, and aging is the predominant risk factor for cancer. The demonstration of the effects of nutrition on cancer requires using age-adjusted incidences. Furthermore, dietary restriction with vitamin and antioxidant supplementation can significantly extend maximum lifespan in rodents. In epidemiologic studies in humans, intake of 400 to 600 g of fruits and vegetables per day is associated with a reduced risk for gastric and other cancers. The most common cancers in developed societies are breast, prostate, and colon cancer. Obesity, high-fat diets, and reduced intake of fiber from cereals, grains, fruits, and vegetables make up a high-risk dietary pattern. For each of the most common cancers, extensive evidence suggests a variation in incidence as individuals move from low-risk to high-risk countries. The incidence of latent prostate cancer is the same in the United States and Japan, but clinical prostate cancer is five times more frequent in the United States. In animal experiments, nutrition affects the growth, progression, and metastasis of established tumors as well as the incidence of new tumors.

Limited information is available on nutrition intervention in humans, but a clear demonstration comes from a study of nonmelanoma skin cancer, the incidence of which is clearly affected by dietary fat. This human intervention study confirms data in animals that the risk for carcinogen-induced skin cancer is enhanced by high-fat diets. The antioxidant defenses are carried out by enzymes that are part of the drug-metabolizing enzyme family. These enzymes use dietary substances as co-factors and inactivate or activate carcinogens depending on their environment. Variations in nutritional intake can interact with these metabolic enzymes to provide a defense against carcinogenesis.

The Process of Carcinogenesis

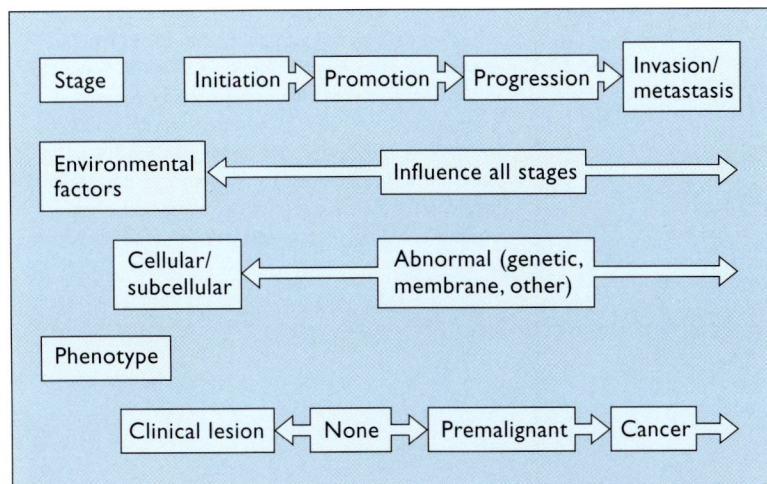

FIGURE 12-1. Factors that influence the stages of cancer. Cancer is due to accumulation of DNA mutations that confer a growth advantage and invasive properties on clones of cells. A variety of external factors, including the interaction between nutrients in the environment with genetic susceptibility, influence the accumulation of mutations in cells. Nutrition is important at every stage of carcinogenesis, from initiation to promotion to progression and metastasis.

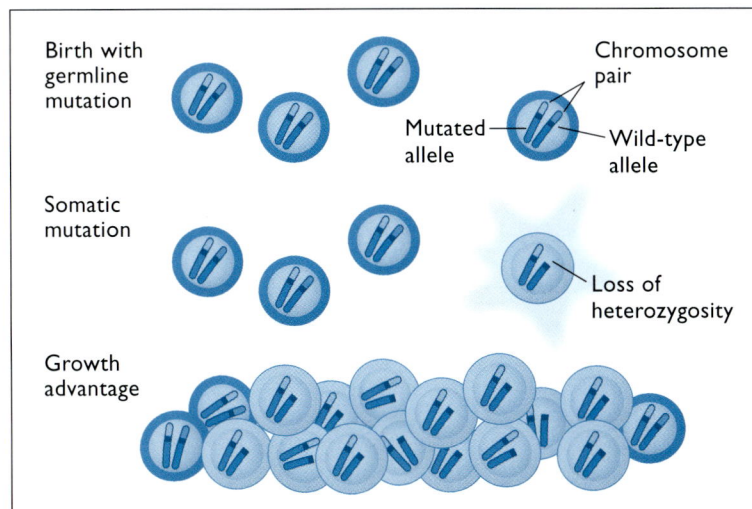

FIGURE 12-2. Cancer results from the growth of a clone of genetically susceptible cells that have been influenced by the environment, including nutrition to outgrow neighboring cells. A growth advantage is obtained by unregulated proliferation as the result of oncogene expression or by inhibited cell death (lack of apoptosis) due to mutated nonfunctional tumor suppressor genes.

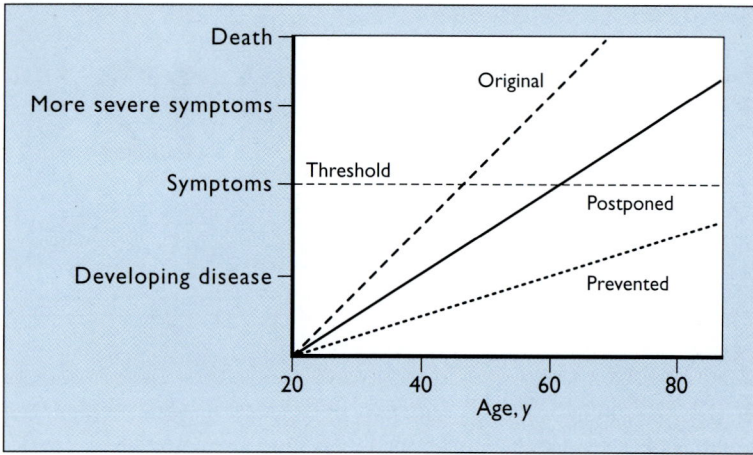

FIGURE 12-3. Compression of morbidity. The primary risk factor for cancer is aging. All data demonstrating nutritional influence use age-adjusted cancer incidence. Through primary prevention and nutritional effects on patients with early treated cancer, the hope is to reduce the duration of morbidity and lengthen survival. This has not yet been demonstrated in clinical trials but is the ultimate goal of research in nutrition and cancer.

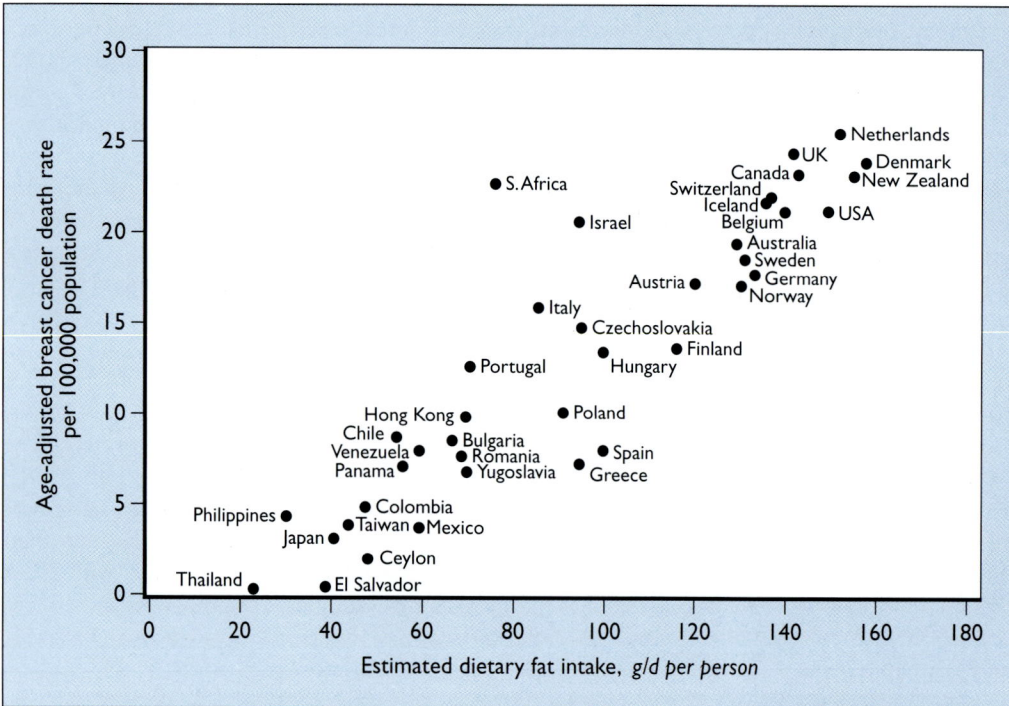

FIGURE 12-4. Dietary fat intake in relation to breast cancer–related mortality rate. International correlation data in the late 1960s demonstrated a relationship of age-adjusted breast cancer incidence to dietary fat intake. This correlation marked a dietary pattern rather than a specific effect of dietary fat. Later studies pinpointed a correlation with meat protein rather than vegetable protein intake. Migration data also indicate that individuals moving from a high-risk to a low-risk country (or vice-versa) take on the risk of the country to which they migrate within one generation.

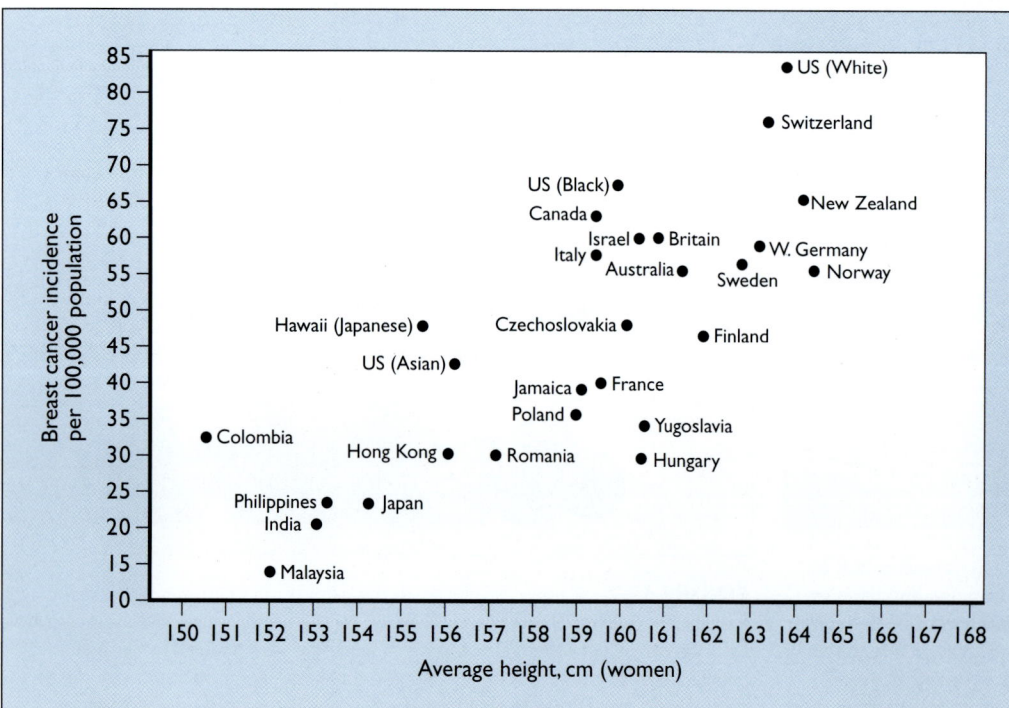

FIGURE 12-5. International correlation data showing a relationship of adult height to the age-adjusted rate of breast cancer. Adult height is a marker of prepubertal nutrition. With an increase in the incidence of childhood obesity, there is a concomitant increase in adult height. In Japan, the incidences of obesity and obesity-related cancer have increased in the past 20 years, as has adult height. Evidence suggests that childhood obesity confers a lifelong increased risk for common forms of cancer.

OBESITY AND CANCER

Mortality Ratios for Cancer Sites Relative to Percentage Over Average Weight

Cancer Type	Percentage Over Average Weight			
	10%–19%	20%–29%	30%–39%	≥ 40%
Men				
Colon, rectum	—	—	1.53	1.73
Prostate	—	1.37	1.33	1.29
Women				
Endometrium	1.36	1.85	2.30	5.42
Uterus (unspecified)	—	1.81	1.40	4.65
Cervix	—	1.51	1.42	2.39
Ovary	—	—	—	1.63
Gallbladder	1.59	1.74	1.80	3.58
Breast	—	—	—	1.53

Data from the 12-year prospective American Cancer Society study of 750,000 men and women were analyzed to determine the relationship between obesity and cancer site. Overweight men had a higher mortality rate from colorectal and prostate cancer than men of average weight. Overweight women had a higher mortality rate from cancer of the gallbladder and biliary passages, breast, cervix, endometrium, uterus (unspecified), and ovary than women of average weight.

FIGURE 12-6. Association between obesity and cancer. Obesity is a risk factor for common forms of cancer, including breast, prostate, colon, uterine, kidney, gallbladder, and pancreatic. Ad libitum intake of excess calories in animal models has also been associated with enhanced tumorigenesis for breast, colon, and skin cancer. Because laboratory animals tend to develop obesity with age, the preventive effects of calorie reduction in animals are likely to be analogous to the prevention and treatment of obesity in humans by reduction in caloric intake or an increase in physical activity. (*From* Garfinkel [1].)

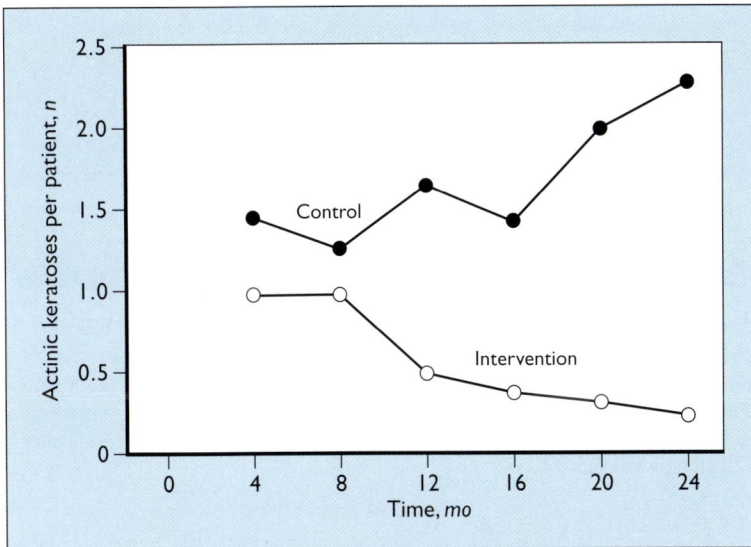

FIGURE 12-7. Data from an intervention study in humans with nonmelanoma skin cancer showing a striking effect of a high-fat (higher-calorie) diet on the development of new skin lesions. This study confirms findings from an early 1900s study in rodents, in which a carcinogen was painted on the skin and animals were fed either low-fat or high-fat diets. Similar proof is not yet available for breast and prostate cancer. (*From* Jaax et al. [2].)

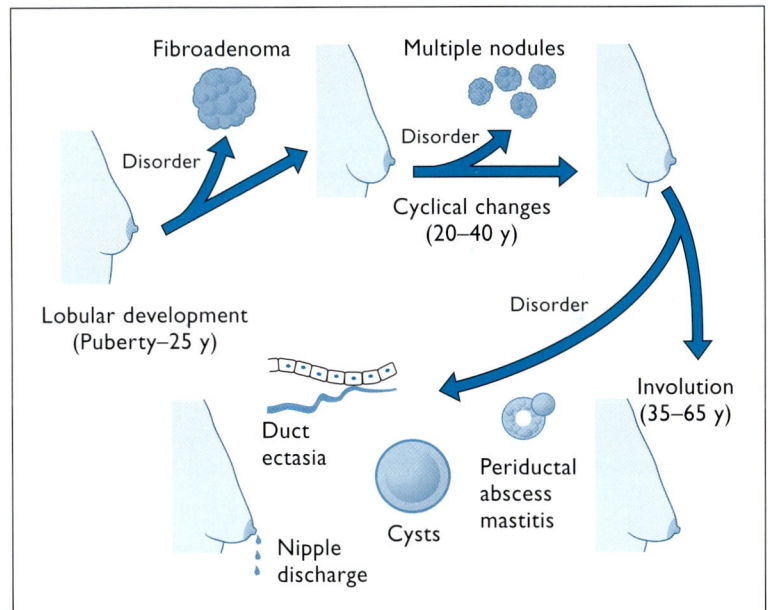

FIGURE 12-8. Changes that occur in breast tissue throughout the lifespan. Most breast cancer occurs after the menopause, but it is estimated that it requires 10 to 15 years for a breast cancer to develop from a single cell to a detectable tumor. Therefore, most cancers are developing during the period of breast involution between ages 35 and 55 when the fibrous stroma of the breast is differentiating into breast adipose tissue. In younger women, fibroadenomas and so-called fibrocystic conditions are frequently diagnosed. These are benign conditions and do not increase the risk for breast cancer (*Adapted from* Heber [3]).

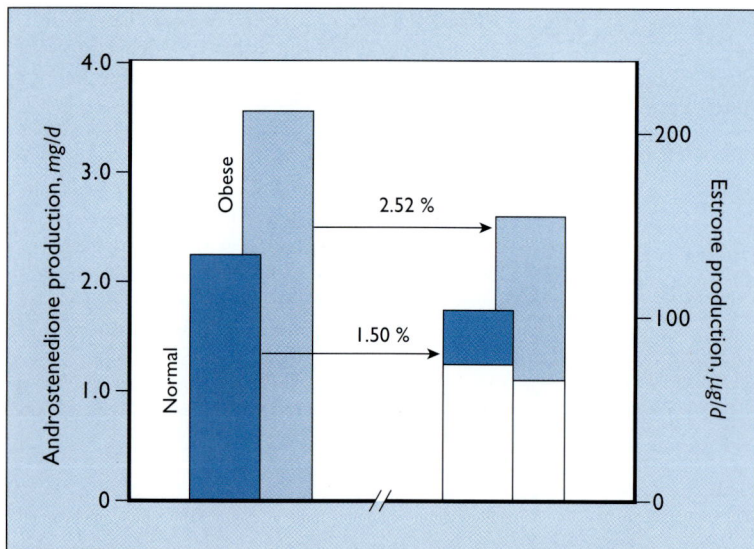

FIGURE 12-9. Androstenedione produced by the adrenal gland is converted into estrone by aromatase, a cytochrome P-450 enzyme, found in stromal tissues found in fat and muscle tissue stromal cells. The production of both androstenedione and estrone measured in 24-hour urine samples are makedly increased in obese compared with lean premenopausal women. The aromatase enzyme is positively regulated by insulin and glucocorticoids, both of which are increased in overnutrition and obesity. The conversion rates of androstenedione to estrone are also increased in obese compared to lean women (2.52% vs 1.50%), reflecting increased aromatase activity (Adapted from Heber [4]).

EFFECTS OF VLF (10%)/HFI (35–45 G/D) DIET ON ESTROGENS AND MENSTRUAL FUNCTION

	Control (30% AHA)	Month 1 VLF/Hfi	Month 2 VLF/Hfi
Menstrual cycle length, d	28.2 ± 3.4	28.2 ± 4.2	25.8 ± 5.2
Follicular phase, d	15.8 ± 4.2	16.2 ± 3.7	13.4 ± 4.1
Luteal phase, d	12.3 ± 3.0	12.0 ±1.7	12.4 ± 3.0
Estradiol (follicular), pg/mL	73.4 ± 16.7	60.2 ± 19.1	54.8 ± 29.9* [-26%]
Estradiol(luteal), pg/mL	193 ± 86	211 ± 84	151 ± 70* [-22%]
Estrone (follicular), pg/mL	73.4 ± 27	70.1 ± 40.5	59.4 ± 23.7* [-20%]
Estrone (luteal), pg/mL	86.7 ± 35	72.6 ± 27	71.4 ± 32.9* [-18%]

No significant effects on estrone sulfate and SHBG.
Significantly different from 30% AHA phase. P<0.05.

FIGURE 12-10. Effects of a low-fat diet fed ad libitum on estrogens and menstrual function. Many hormones are affected by such a diet; in this study the levels of the female hormones (estradiol and estrone) involved in breast tumorigenesis were reduced by about 25% in both the follicular and luteal phases of the cycle. This reduction is comparable to the difference in hormone levels seen between Chinese women living in Los Angeles and those living in Shanghai. Because the incidence of breast cancer is much higher in Chinese women living in the United States compared with those living in China, the effects of low-fat diet on breast cancer incidence may be mediated by effects of nutrition on reproductive hormone levels. AHA—American Heart Association; HFI—high fiber; SHBG—sex hormone–binding globulin; VLF—very low frequency. (From Bagga et al [5].)

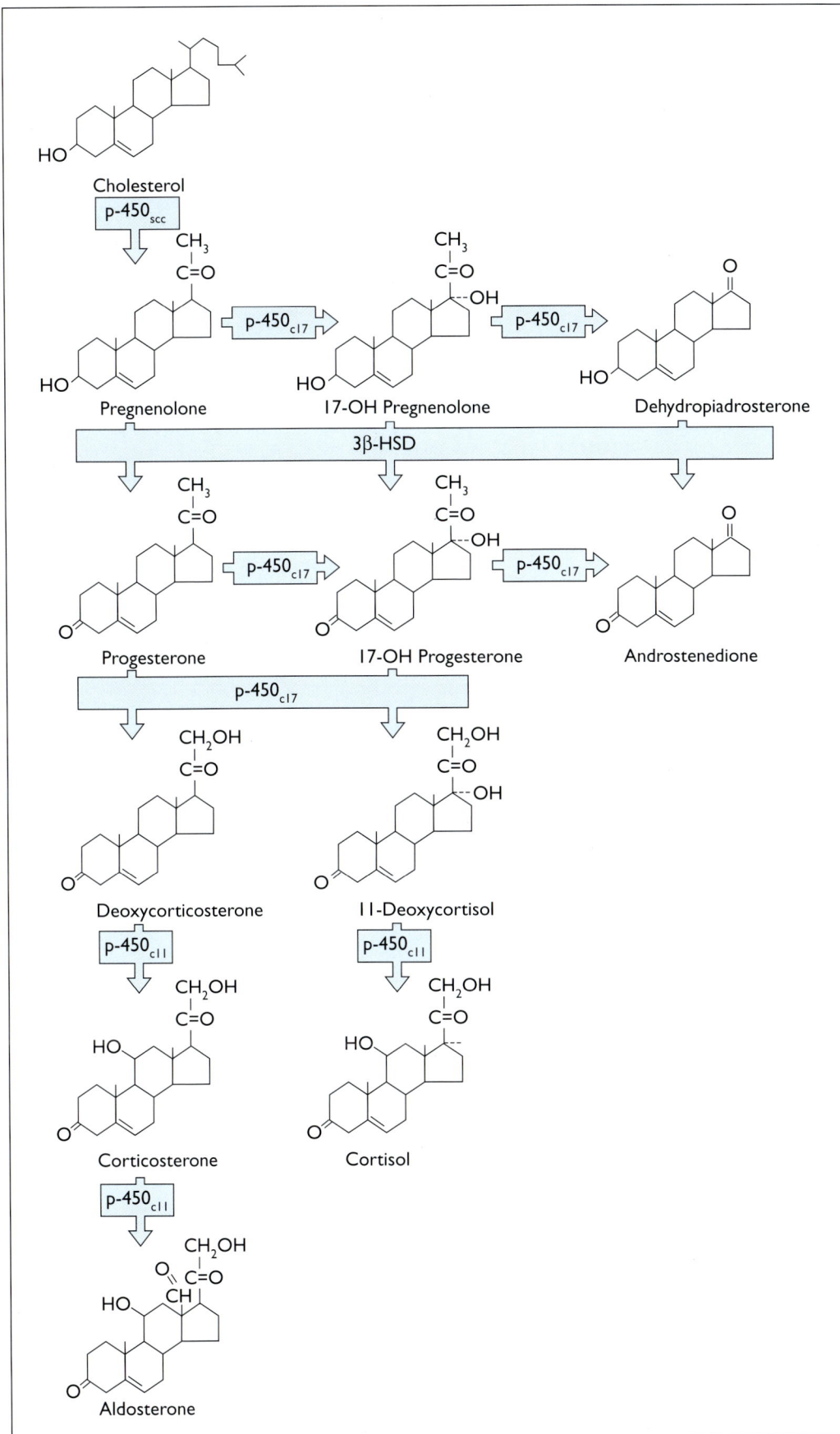

FIGURE 12-11. The interconversions of sex hormones, including estrogen and testosterone, that are involved in breast and prostate cancer are modulated by nutritional effects on substrates and products and by expression of enzymes such as aromatase. Some hormones, such as insulin and glucocorticoids, are modulated by nutrition and in turn affect the expression of various enzymes (eg, aromatase [cytochrome P-450 A19]). HSD—hydroxysteroid dehydrogenase. (*Adapted from* Orth et al [6].)

Evolution of Cancer: Genes and Environment

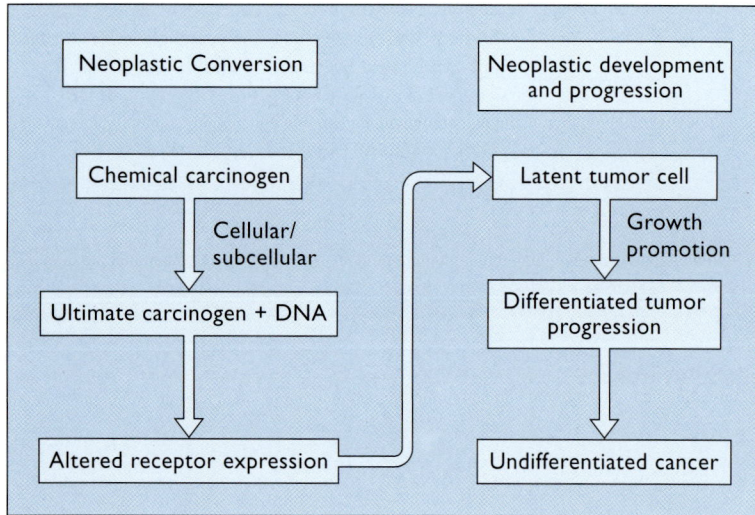

FIGURE 12-12. Components of the carcinogenesis process. This process is often divided into neoplastic conversion and neoplastic development and progression. For most human cancers, neoplastic conversion is estimated to occur 10 to 15 years before diagnosis. As diagnostic methods improve, diagnosis is made earlier. However, nutrition can influence both phases of carcinogenesis in experimental studies in animals.

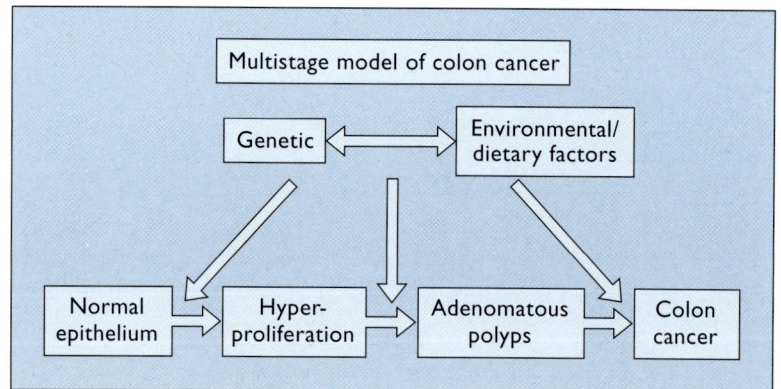

FIGURE 12-13. Multistage model of colon cancer. The multistage process of carcinogenesis has been defined best in colon cancer, where specific mutations have been related to each successive step in the development and progression of colon cancer. Nutrition can influence this process at every stage of carcinogenesis.

FIGURE 12-14. The metabolic activation of potential carcinogens. This activation results from the action of metabolizing enzymes, which, in turn, are affected by diet and the ingestion of a wide variety of phytochemicals. There are also genetic variations in the activity and distribution of these enzymes. (From World Cancer Fund [7].)

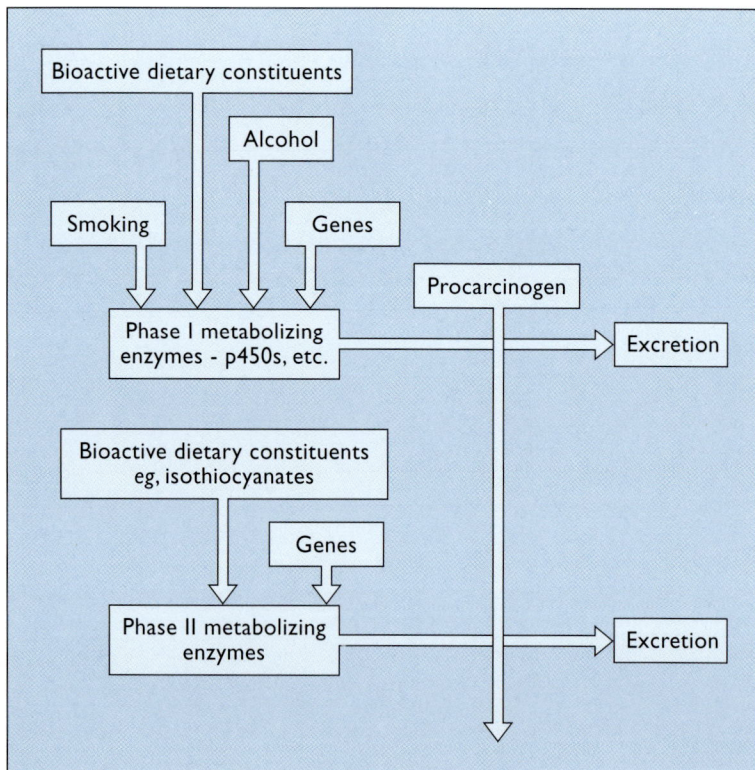

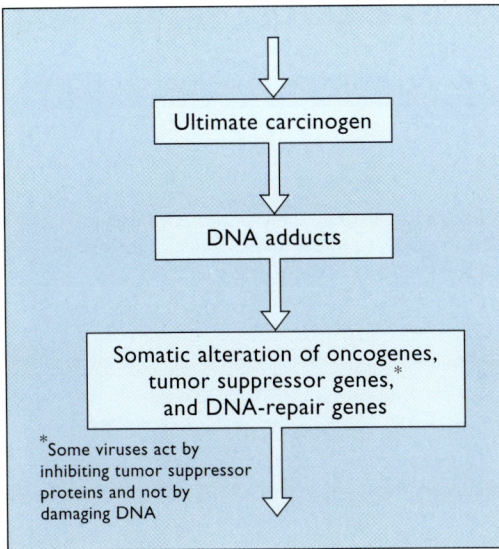

FIGURE 12-15. Pathway from ultimate carcinogen to gene alteration. Once the ultimate carcinogen is formed, it binds to DNA, forming an adduct that can then result in a mutation. The mutation, in turn, activates oncogenes, inactivates tumor suppressor genes, or modifies gene expression so as to promote carcinogenesis. (*From* World Cancer Fund [8].)

ODDS RATIOS FOR COLORECTAL ADENOMAS

	Broccoli Intake		
	Low	High	Overall
GSTM1 null	1.00	0.45*	0.94
GSTM1 Non-null	0.99	0.87	1.00

* P = 0.034

FIGURE 12-16. Odds ratios for colorectal adenomas. In studies of patients with colon polyps, the risk for developing cancer is increased twofold in patients with a null mutation at the GSTM1 enzyme locus. However, if these patients eat cruciferous vegetables such as broccoli, the effects of the GSTM1 mutation are obviated. (*From* Lin et al [9].)

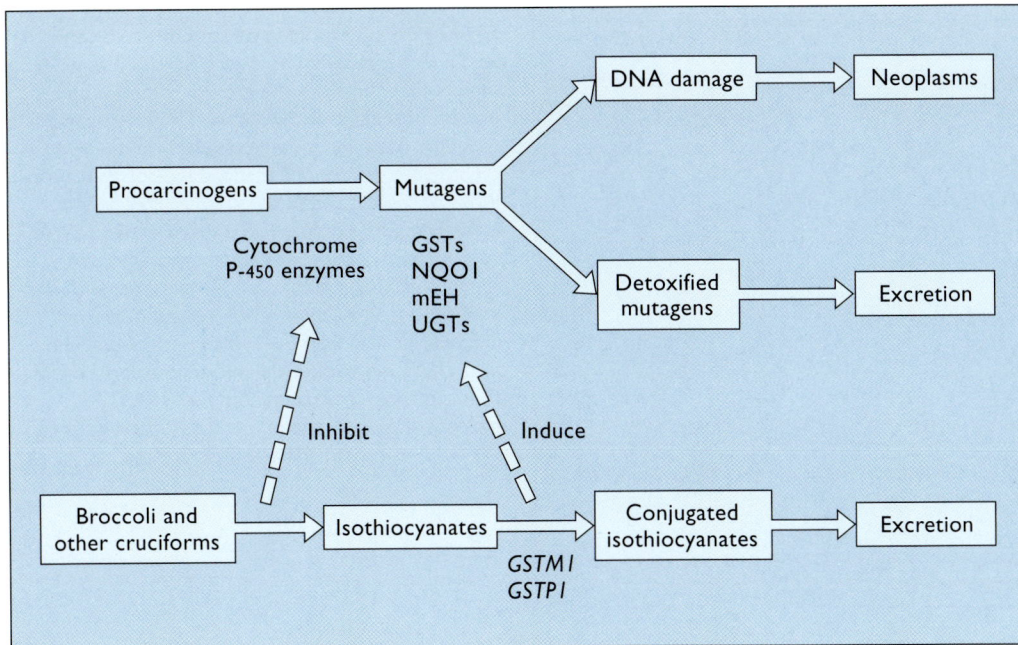

FIGURE 12-17. The observed gene–nutrient interaction for colon cancer. This interaction makes sense biochemically because broccoli constituents can inhibit the cytochrome P-450, which forms the carcinogens typically deactivated by GSTM1. The susceptibility to carcinogenesis may depend on such mutations in enzymes involved in carcinogen metabolism. The xenobiotic hypothesis of cancer posits that many such instances are to be discovered and that they will enhance our ability to prevent cancer. GST—glutathione S transferase; mEH—microsomal epoxide hydralase; NQO1—NAD(P)H: quinone oxidoreductase; UDP—glucuronosyl transferase. (*From* Lin et al [9].)

FOOD CONSTITUENTS WITH A SUSPECTED ROLE IN CANCER

Nutrient	Dietary sources	Action
Possibly carcinogenic agents in foods		
Fats	Meats, milk and milk products, vegetable oils	Excessive body fat is linked to increased synthesis of estrogen and other sex hormones, which in excess may themselves increase the risk for cancer
Alcohol	Beer, wine, liquor	Contribute to cancers of the throat, liver, and bladder, and possibly the breast. Increased cell turnover is the main mechanism
Nitrates, nitrites	Cured meats, especially ham, bacon, and sausages	Under very high temperatures will bind to amino acid derivatives to form nitrosamines, potent carcinogens
Multi-ringed compounds		
Aflatoxin	Formed when mold is present on peanuts and other grains	Multi-ringed compounds may alter DNA structure and inhibit its ability to properly respond to physiologic controls
Benzo-a-pyrene	Charcoal-broiled foods, especially meats	Aflatoxin is linked to liver cancer; benzo-a-pyrene is linked to stomach and other intestinal cancers

FIGURE 12-18. Food constituents with a suspected role in cancer. Known or suspected dietary carcinogens include aflatoxin (found in moldy foods), heterocyclic amines (found in meat cooked at high temperatures), N-nitroso compounds (found in spoiled foods, proteins, and endogenous sources), and polycyclic hydrocarbons (found in cooked foods and dark beer).

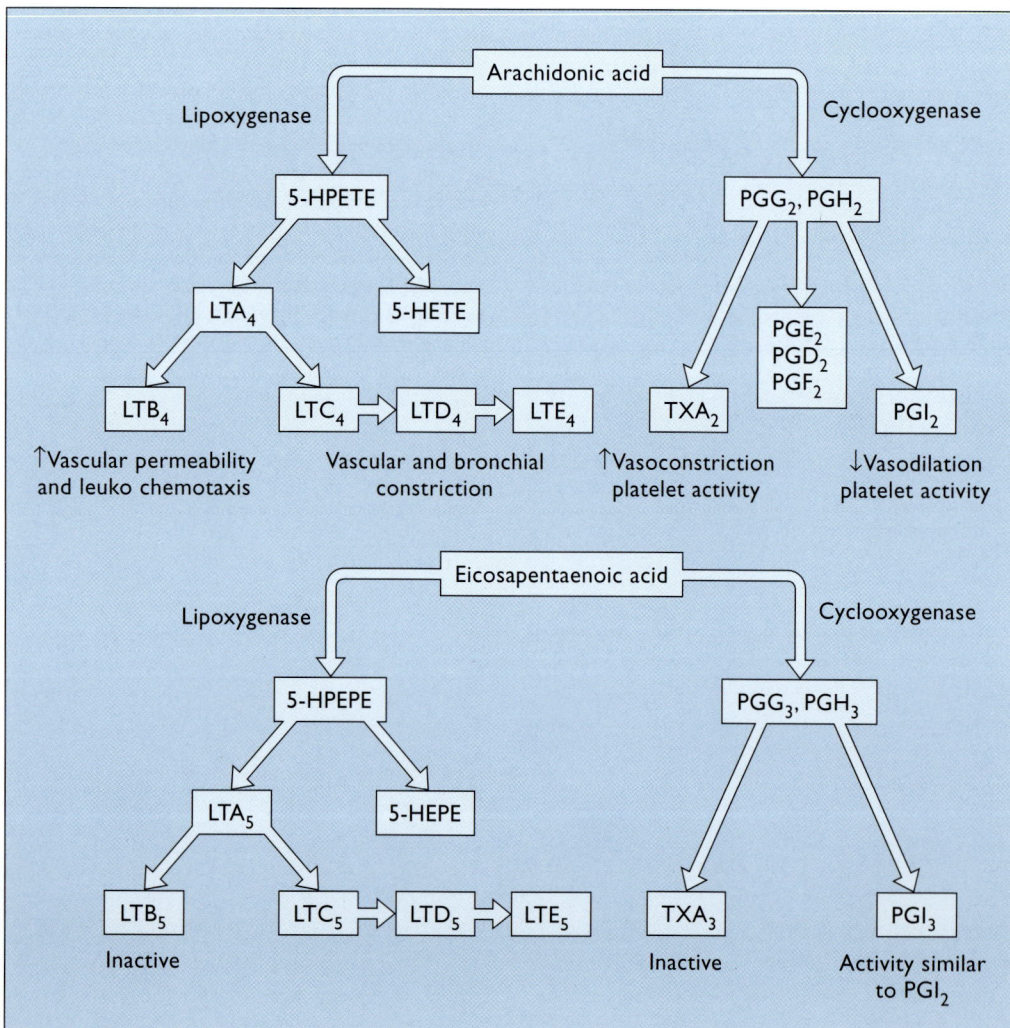

FIGURE 12-19. Chemical structure of arachidonic acid and eicosapentaenoic acid. Arachidonic acid metabolites promote the growth of breast and prostate cancer cells in culture. The PPAR-gamma receptor has been identified in both of these cell types and is believed to mediate the effects that high levels of linoleic acid in the western diet have on carcinogenesis. Linoleic acid is efficiently converted to arachidonic acid, but eicosapentaenoic acid, found in fish oil, competes and interferes with the metabolism and action of the eicosanoids from arachidonic acid. HEPE—hydroxyeicosapentaenoic acid; HETE—hydroxyeicosatetraenoic acid; HPEPE—hydroperoxyeicosapentaenoic acid; HPETE—hydroperoxyeicosatrienoic acid; LT—leukotriene; PG—prostaglandin; TXA—thromboxane.

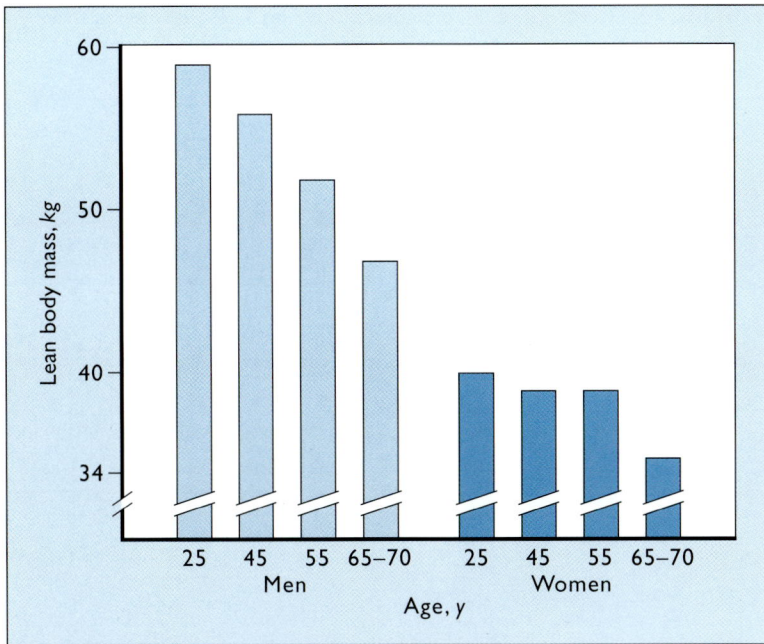

FIGURE 12-20. Lean body mass at selected ages in men and women. In both men and women, age is associated with a reduction in lean body mass. The decrease is associated with reduced calorie requirements and increased risk for developing common forms of cancer. The reduced muscle mass may be associated with increased insulin and reproductive hormone levels in some aging individuals.

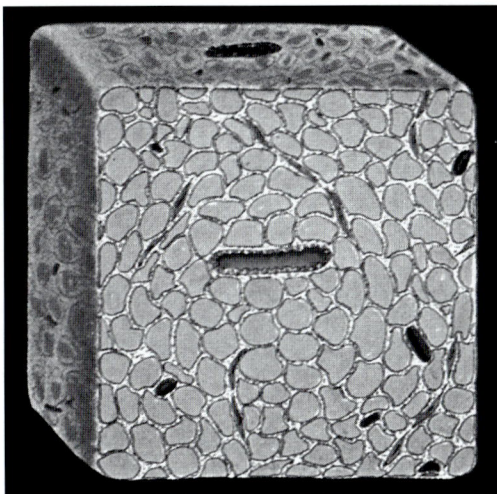

FIGURE 12-21. (see Color Plate) Adipocytes surround the breast duct and proliferate in aging breast tissue. Thus, the postmenopausal breast largely consists of adipocytes surrounding atrophic breast ducts. Because 75% of all breast cancers develop after menopause, it has been proposed that breast fat may have a local paracrine effect on the breast ductal cells that promote carcinogenesis. In support of this hypothesis, aromatase levels have been found to be increased in the stromal cells near a breast tumor compared with levels further away from the tumor. (*From* Lamarque [10].)

Phytochemicals and Cancer

ANTICANCER FOOD PHARMACY

Carotenoids	Lignans
Coumarins	Monoterpenes
Flavenoids	Phthalides
Phenolic acids	Phytates
Glucarates	Polyacetylenes
Indoles	Sulfides
Isothiocyanates	Triterpenes

FIGURE 12-22. The anticancer food pharmacy. This figure lists all the classes of substances found in plant-based foods that have an effect on cancer. These include the carotenoids found in yellow, green, and orange vegetables; isoflavones found in soy protein; isothiocyanates in broccoli; organosulfides in garlic and onion; and terpenoids found in the skin of citrus fruits.

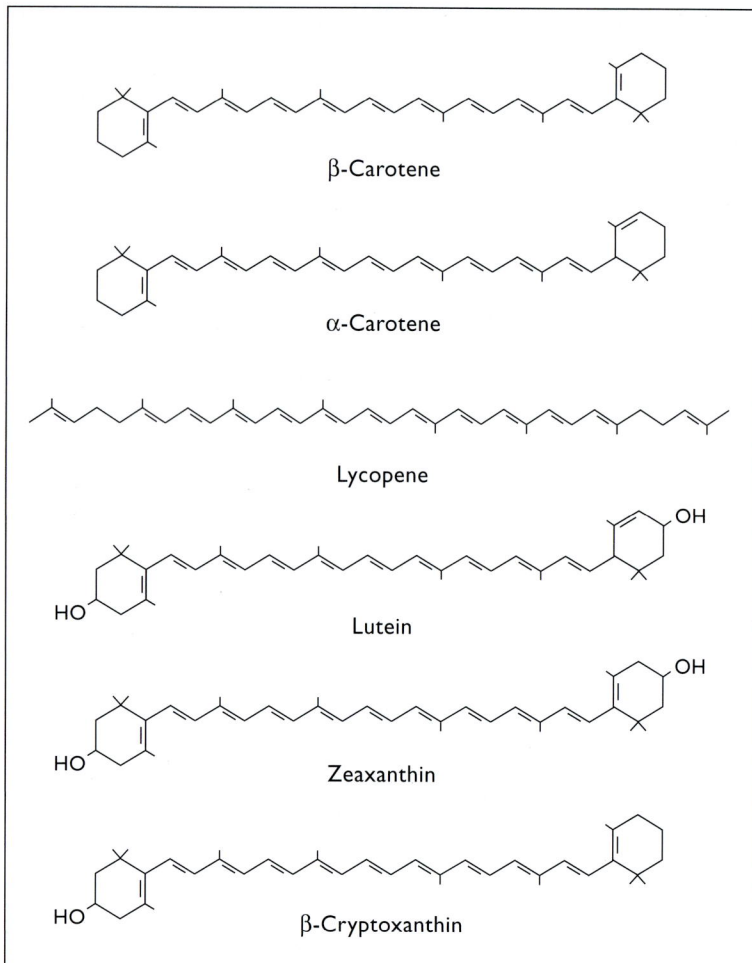

FIGURE 12-23. Structure of common carotenoids. These carotenoids share structural similarities and act as antioxidants. The metabolism of these carotenoids is complex, leading to more than 600 identified metabolites.

β-Carotene

α-Carotene

Lycopene

Lutein

Zeaxanthin

β-Cryptoxanthin

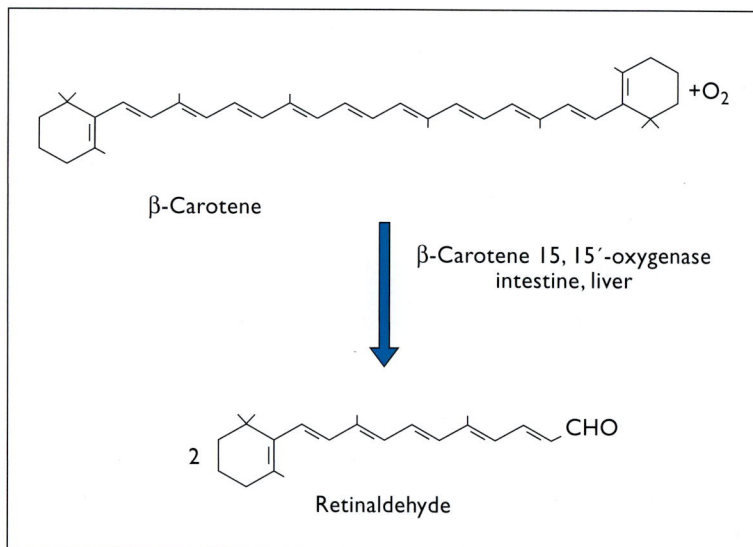

β-Carotene   +O₂

β-Carotene 15, 15′-oxygenase
intestine, liver

2   Retinaldehyde

FIGURE 12-24. Structure of beta-carotene. Beta-carotene, commonly found in carrots and many other vegetables, is the only carotenoid that can be converted to vitamin A.

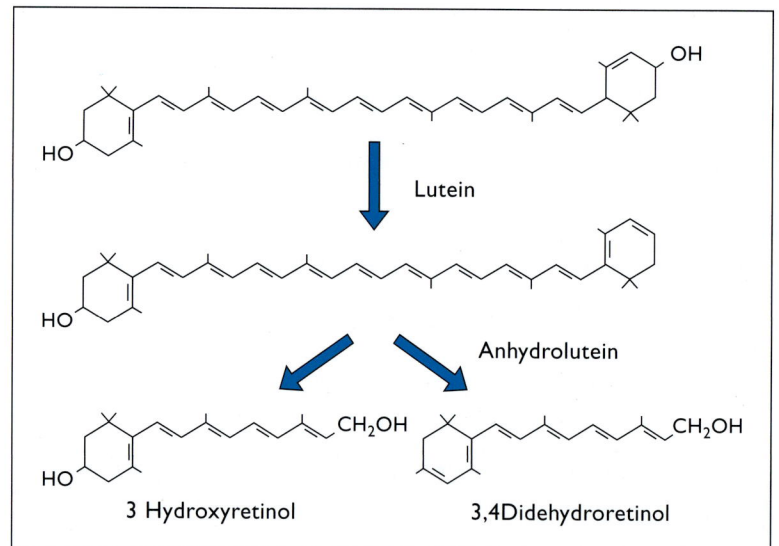

Lutein

Anhydrolutein

3 Hydroxyretinol

3,4Didehydroretinol

FIGURE 12-25. Structure and conversion of lutein. In a process that illustrates the complexity of carotenoid metabolism, lutein is converted into metabolites without vitamin A activity. However, lutein is extremely important in the retina, where it has been related to macular degeneration, a common cause of blindness in the elderly.

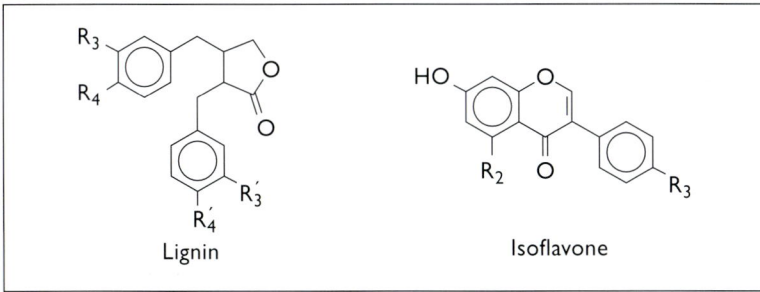

FIGURE 12-26. Structure of phytoestrogens. The phytoestrogens from soybean protein—genistein and daidzein—inhibit tyrosine kinase and act as selective estrogen response modifiers in cancer cells. The intake of soy protein is higher in countries with lower cancer incidence, and the effects of isoflavones suggest that soy may play an important role in inhibiting carcinogenesis in these populations.

Lignin

Isoflavone

Metabolic Effects of Tumors

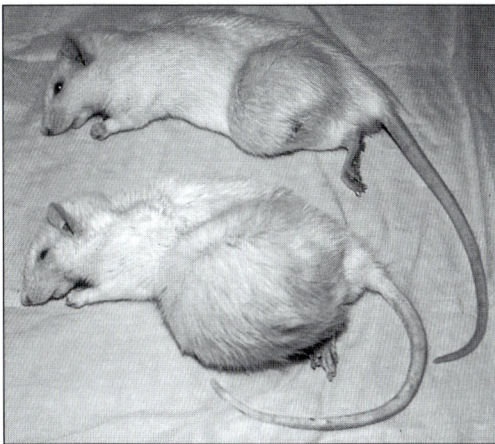

FIGURE 12-27. Tumor size in rats. In the early 1950s, it was believed that tumors stole protein from the host, causing starvation and death. As shown here, animal tumors grow to a significant fraction of total body weight and can trap host nutrients. In humans, however, tumors rarely increase beyond 1 to 2 kg, and most metabolic effects are mediated by humoral substances (including hormones and cytokines).

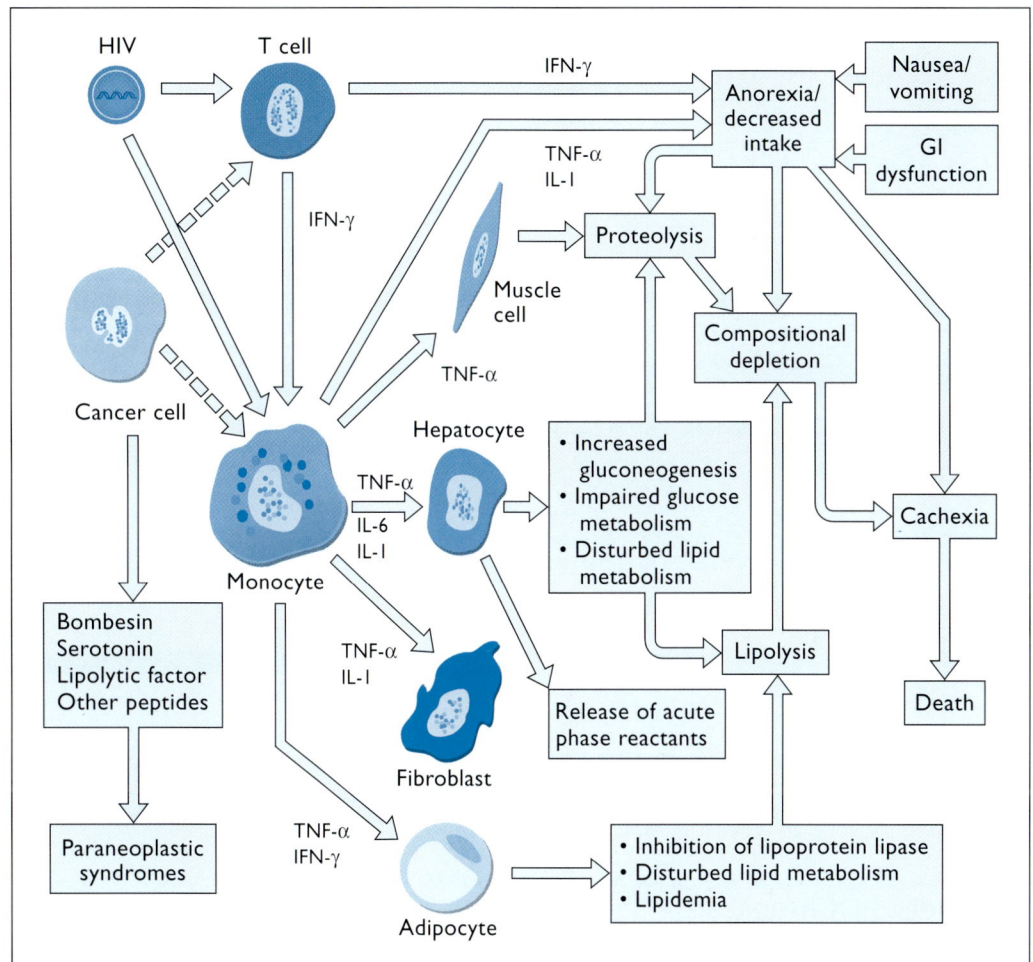

FIGURE 12-28. The multiple metabolic effects of tumors on host metabolism (including muscle catabolism, liver lipogenesis, fat cell lipolysis, anorexia, and reduced food intake), as mediated by a family of cytokines. Therapies for the anorexia and cachexia associated with cancer and AIDS are megestrol acetate, growth hormone, and anabolic hormones. GI—gastrointestinal; IFN-gamma—interferon-gamma; IL—interleukin; TNF-alpha—tumor necrosis factor-alpha.

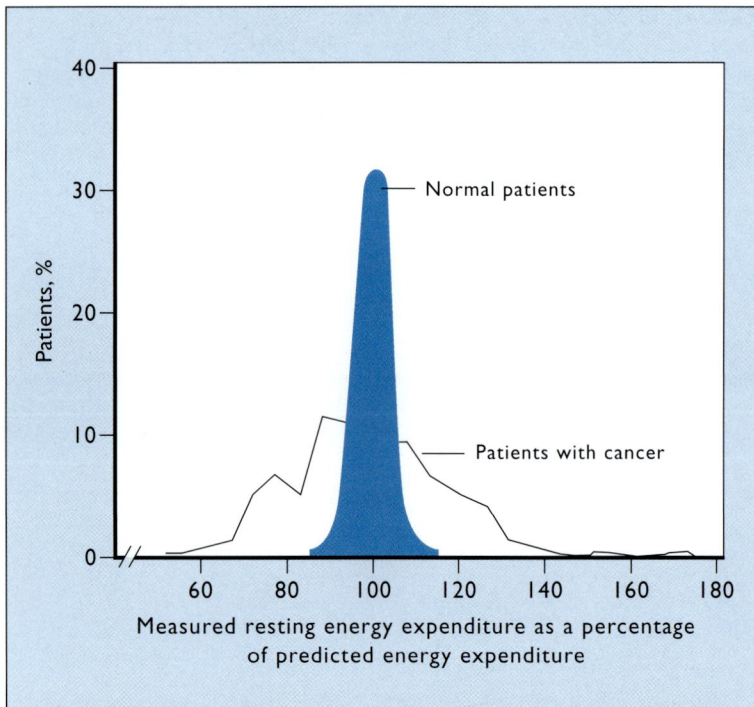

FIGURE 12-29. While lean body mass accurately predicts metabolic rate in normal persons (shown in *blue*), the measured metabolic rates in patients with cancer have a much wider distribution: one third are hypometabolic (presumably because of muscle wasting), and one third are hypermetabolic (presumably because of the effects of cytokines and the effects of the tumor on intermediary metabolism). It was once thought that all patients with cancer were hypermetabolic because of their failure to gain weight. This is clearly not the case.

AGE-RELATED CHANGES IN BODY COMPOSITION OF ADULT MEN

Age Group, y	Body Weight, *kg*	Body Fat, *kg*	Nonmuscle Mass, *kg*	Muscle Mass, *kg*
20–29	80	15	37	24
40–49	81	19	38	20
60–69	79	23	37	17
70–79	80	24	38	13

FIGURE 12-30. Age-related changes in body composition of men. As men age, lean body mass decreases because they tend to become less active. Age-related decreases may also occur in levels of hormones that mediate muscle growth and maintenance. These changes in body composition affect the levels of sex hormones, insulin, and growth factors, which may affect such chronic diseases as diabetes, cardiovascular disease, and common forms of cancer. Efforts aimed at diet and lifestyle change during aging to prevent chronic diseases (including cancer) must include interventions designed to maintain or increase lean body mass. (*From* Munro [11].)

References

1. Garfinkel L: Overweight and cancer. *Ann Intern Med* 1985, 103(6 [pt 2]):1034–1036.

2. Jaax S, Scott LW, Wolf JE, Jr, *et al.*: General guidelines for a low-fat diet effective in the management and prevention of nonmelanoma skin cancer. *Nutr Cancer* 1997, 27:150–156.

3. Heber D: Breast disease. In: *Current Practice of Medicine.* Volume 1. Edited by Roger C. Bone. Philadelphia: Current Medicine; 1996:IV:17.3.

4. Sherwin SA, Twardzik DR, Bohn WH, *et al.*: High-molecular-weight transforming growth factor activity in the urine of patients with disseminated cancer. *Cancer Res* 1983, 43:403–407.

5. Bagga D, Ashley JM, Geffrey S, *et al.*: Effects of a very low fat high fiber diet on serum hormones and menstrual function: implications for breast cancer prevention. *Cancer* 1995, 76:2491–2496.

6. Orth DN, Kovacs WJ, DeBold CR: The adrenal cortex. In: *Williams Textbook of Endocrinology*, edn 8. Edited by Wilson, Foster. Philadelphia: WB Saunders; 1992.

7. World Cancer Research Fund in Association with American Institute for Cancer Research: *Food, Nutrition, and the Prevention of Cancer: A Global Perspective.* Washington, DC: American Institute for Cancer Research; 1997:60.

8. World Cancer Research Fund in Association with American Institute for Cancer Research: *Food, Nutrition, and the Prevention of Cancer: A Global Perspective.* Washington, DC: American Institute for Cancer Research; 1997: 61.

9. Lin HJ, *et al.*: Glutathione transferase null genotype, broccoli, and lower prevalence of colorectal adenomas. *Cancer Epidemiol Biomark Prev* 1998, 7:647–652.

10. Lamarque JL: *An Atlas of the Breast.* Dobbs Ferry, NY: Sheridan Medical Books; 1985:69.

11. Munro H: Aging. In: *Nutrition and Metabolism in Patient Care.* Edited by Kinney, Jeejeebhoy, Hill, Owen. Philadelphia: WB Saunders; 1988.

13

DIETARY ASSESSMENT, DIETARY GUIDELINES, AND DIETS

Jennifer R. Eliasi and Johanna T. Dwyer

The major factors affecting nutritional status are anthropometric and biochemical measurements, clinical signs and symptoms of specific nutrient deficiencies, and dietary assessments of usual intakes. Comorbidities (especially those of the gastrointestinal tract and of metabolism) and compromised functional status (activities of daily living) are also useful parameters because they are often associated with secondary malnutrition.

Common height and weight standards for children and adults in the United States, updated to reflect current sizes, are presented in this chapter. Height and weight are useful for estimating lean body mass (the major contributor of resting energy expenditure). In addition, this chapter includes formulas to calculate estimates of resting energy expenditure based on height and weight. Measures of subcutaneous fat, such as the triceps skinfold test, permit more direct assessment of body fat. Midarm and calf circumferences provide a very rough estimate of the total contribution of bone, muscle, and fat. One commonly used method of assessing frame size is wrist breadth, and standards for this measurement are also included. Frame size, fat, and muscle vary between individuals of different somatotypes (ie, ectomorphs, endomorphs, mesomorphs).

Biochemical assessment measures of nutritional status are helpful in assessing both nutrient status (such as hemoglobin and other hematologic indices to measure anemia) and indicators of risk factors for such diet-related diseases as coronary artery disease or non–insulin-dependent diabetes mellitus. Blood pressure is another useful index.

Clinical signs and symptoms of nutrient deficiencies are not highly specific and may be mimicked by other environmental factors and disease. Nevertheless, they are useful to consider in the overall assessment of nutritional status.

Dietary assessment is another critical aspect of nutritional status. The DETERMINE checklist [1] of the Nutrition Screening Initiative helps to identify both social and medical factors that may be associated with undernutrition and malnutrition. This checklist provides a crude but useful indicator of risk factors for poor intake. More detailed dietary and nutritional histories may be needed in patients who are judged to be at risk of malnutrition. Eating disorders are increasingly common psychiatric problems with serious nutritional implications. Diagnostic criteria for two eating disorders, anorexia nervosa and bulimia, are provided.

The dietary reference intakes of the Food and Nutrition Board of the National Academy of Sciences and Health in Canada are undergoing review and updating. The latest standards and values, not yet updated, are provided. Dietary quality depends on the appropriate type, amounts, and balance of nutrients. A simple measure, the diet quality index, is discussed.

Various dietary guidelines and other food guidance systems for consumers are summarized. The Basic Four and Basic Five guides focus more specifically on getting enough nutrients. The latest US Department of Agriculture Food Guide Pyramid provides guidance on consuming adequate portions from the various food groups while emphasizing balance and moderation. The dietary guidelines and the Food Guide Pyramid are two useful tools for consumers in which serving sizes and number of portions per day are recommended. Other popular food-based dietary guidance systems developed for specific purposes are also provided.

The last section in the chapter addresses different types of diets. Guidelines for healthful weight loss and sample reducing diets are followed by several therapeutic regimens that involve modifications of sodium, protein, and other minerals. The types of fats and suggested amounts of intake are included.

Anthropometric, Biochemical, Clinical, and Other Tools to Assess Nutritional Status

REFERENCE HEIGHTS AND WEIGHTS FOR CHILDREN AND ADULTS IN THE UNITED STATES

Gender	Age	Median BMI	Reference Height, cm (in)	Reference Weight, kg (lb)
Male or female	2–6 mo	—	64(25)	7(16)
	7–12 mo	—	72(28)	9(20)
	1–3 yr	—	91(36)	13(29)
	4–8 yr	15.8	118(46)	22(48)
Male	9–13 yr	18.5	147(58)	40(88)
	14–16 yr	21.3	174(68)	64(142)
	19–30 yr	24.4	176(69)	76(166)
Female	9–13 yr	18.3	148(58)	40(88)
	14–16 yr	21.3	163(64)	57(125)
	19–30 yr	22.8	163(64)	61(133)

FIGURE 13-1. Reference heights and weights for children and adults in the United States. The values provided are based on data from the Third National Health and Nutrition Examination Survey, 1988–1994 [1]. BMI—body mass index. (*Adapted from* Yates *et al.* [2]; with permission.)

DAILY ENERGY REQUIREMENTS

Daily energy requirement = Resting metabolic rate x Activity factor
  Male: 10 x Weight (kg) + 900
  Female: 7 x Weight (kg) + 800
Activity level factors
  Sedentary = 1.2
  Moderate = 1.5
  Heavy = 1.7
Harris-Benedict Equation
  Male: 66.5 + [13.5 x Weight (kg)] + [5.0 x Height (cm)] - [6.75 x Age (yr)]
  Female: 65.5 + [9.56 x Weight (kg)] + [1.85 x Height (cm)] - [4.68 x Age (yr)]
FAO/WHO/UNU
  Male: 11.6 x Weight (kg) + 879
  Female: 8.7 + Weight (kg) + 829

FIGURE 13-2. Daily energy requirements. Caloric needs can be determined using a variety of formulas, based on the available information and the needs of the individual. When determining the energy requirements of an individual, it is necessary to account for activity; illness; and the need for weight gain, maintenance, or loss. The resting energy expenditure is derived by a formula and multiplied by an activity factor to assess total needs per day. The Harris-Benedict equation uses height, weight, and age to determine resting metabolic rate. The outcome is multiplied by an activity factor to determine total daily needs. For use in an obese individual, an adjusted body weight is substituted in calculation.

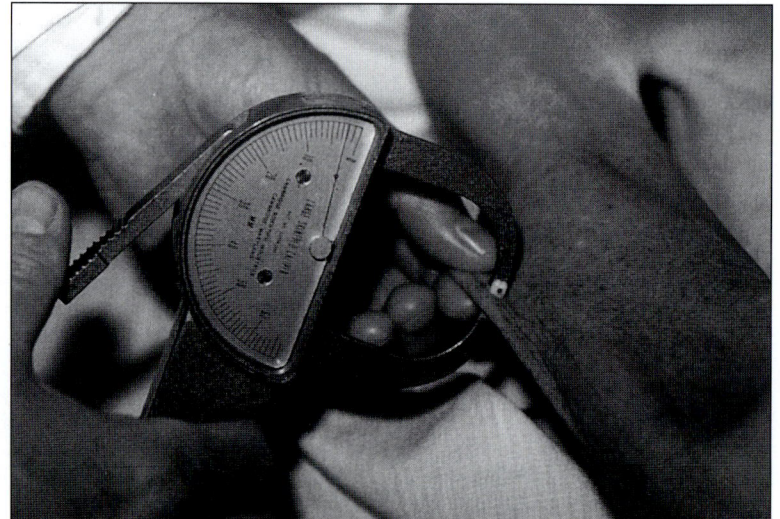

FIGURE 13-3. (*see* Color Plate) Measurement of the triceps skinfold with calipers. The triceps skinfold test is a simple, noninvasive method of estimating general fatness and determining the distribution of subcutaneous adipose tissue because all fat deposits are not equal in contribution to disease risks associated with obesity. Measurement of a skinfold of the triceps is taken at the midline of the arm, over the triceps muscle, with the arm hanging loosely at the subject's side. (*From* Weinsier and Morgan [3]; with permission.)

TRICEPS SKINFOLD THICKNESS IN ADULTS

Percent of Standard	Men, mm	Women, mm	Calorie Reserves
100	12.5	16.5	Adequate
90	11.0	15.0	Adequate
80	10.0	13.0	Adequate
70	9.0	11.5	Adequate
60	7.5	10.0	Adequate
50	6.0	8.0	Borderline
40	5.0	6.5	Borderline
30	4.0	5.0	Borderline
20	2.5	3.0	Severely depleted

FIGURE 13-4. Triceps skinfold thickness in adults [2]. Commonly measured because of arm accessibility, triceps skinfold thickness is closely correlated with total body fat and percentage of body fat. Borderline or depleted calorie reserve may indicates illness, wasting, or malnutrition, suggesting the need for aggressive nutrition intervention. (Adapted from Weinsier and Morgan [3].)

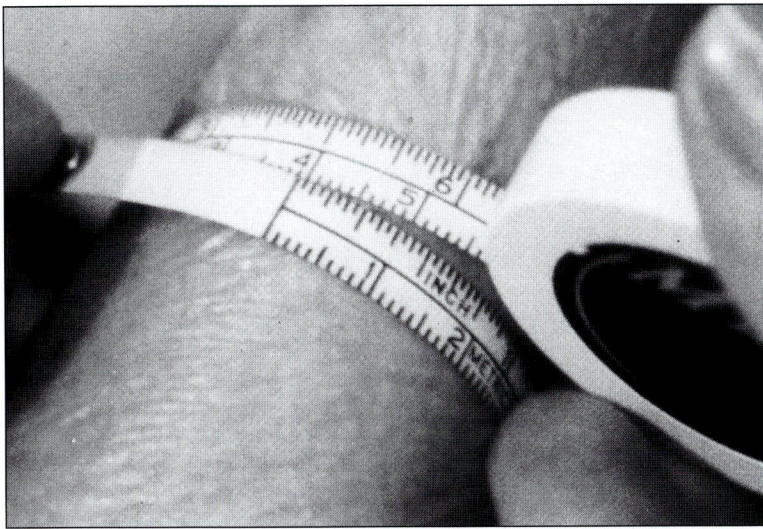

FIGURE 13-5. (*see* Color Plate) Measurement of midarm circumference. A measurement is taken to locate the midpoint between the lateral tip of the acromion to the elbow while the subject's elbow is flexed at a right angle. A small mark is indicated at the midpoint, and at this point the circumference of the arm is measured. (*From* Weinsier and Morgan [3].)

MIDARM MUSCLE CIRCUMFERENCE IN ADULTS

Percent of Standard	Men, cm	Women, cm	Muscle Mass
100	25.5	23.0	Adequate
90	23.0	21.0	Adequate
80	20.0	18.5	Borderline
70	18.0	16.0	Borderline
60	15.0	14.0	Severely depleted
50	12.5	11.5	Severely depleted
40	10.0	9.0	Severely depleted

FIGURE 13-6. Midarm muscle circumference in adults [2]. Midarm circumference values are used as an index of protein mass and body energy stores. A low value is interpreted as a cause to investigate protein–energy malnutrition. A high value indicates sufficient muscle mass. This value can distinguish an athletic person from an obese person, so both may have identical body weight and height. (Adapted from Weinsier and Morgan [3].)

DETERMINATION OF FRAME SIZE

Height, *in*	Wrist Size, *in*		
	Small Frame	Medium Frame	Large Frame
56	<5.5	5.5–5.75	>5.75
57	<5.5	5.5–5.75	>5.75
58	<5.5	5.5–5.75	>5.75
59	<5.5	5.5–5.75	>5.75
60	<5.5	5.5–5.75	>5.75
61	<5.5	5.5–5.75	>5.75
62	<5.5	5.5–5.75	>6.25
63	<6.0	6–6.25	>6.25
64	<6.0	6–6.25	>6.25
65	<6.0	6–6.25	>6.25
66	<6.25	6.25–6.5	>6.5
67	<6.25	6.25–6.5	>6.5
68	<6.25	6.25–6.5	>6.5
69	<6.25	6.25–6.5	>6.5
70	<6.25	6.25–6.5	>6.5
71	<6.25	6.25–6.5	>6.5
72	<6.25	6.25–6.5	>6.5

FIGURE 13-7. Determination of frame size [3]. Frame type provides a more accurate determination of weight range for a patient because the wrist is relatively clear of adipose tissue and muscle. To determine the correct frame size for an individual, the wrist is measured in front of the styloid process of the ulna and radius at the smallest portion with a measuring tape. To determine frame type, the height of the subject without shoes is compared with the wrist size. (Adapted from Day [4].)

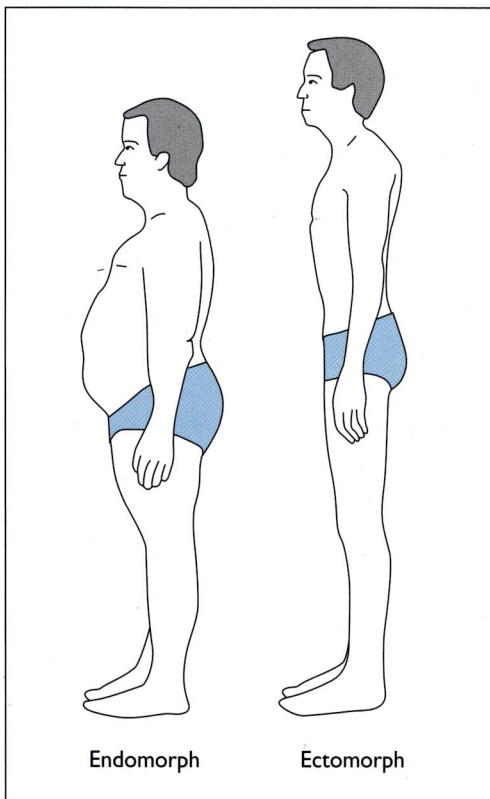

FIGURE 13-8. Somatotypes. Endomorphs have a tendency toward obesity, whereas ectomorphs tend to be thin [5].

LABORATORY VALUES FOR NORMAL NUTRITIONAL STATUS

Test	Normal Range
Hemoglobin, *g/dL*	
Men	14–17
Women	12–15
Hematocrit, %	
Men	39–57
Women	36–45
Leukocyte count	4000–11,000 mm^3
Serum iron	42–135 µg/dL
Ferritin	10–300 ng/mL
Total protein	6–8.4 g/dL
Albumin	3.3–5.0 g/dL
Calcium	8.5–10.5 mg/dL
Magnesium	1.4–2.3 mEq/L
Sodium	136–145 mEq/L
Potassium	3.5–5.0 mg/dL
Chloride	100–106 mEq/L
Blood urea nitrogen	4–22 mg/dL
Creatinine	0.7–1.5 mg/dL
Triglycerides	40–150 mg/dL

FIGURE 13-9. Laboratory values for normal nutritional status.

BLOOD CHOLESTEROL LEVELS AND CUTOFF POINTS

Level	Total Cholesterol	LDL	HDL
Desirable	< 200 mg/dL	< 130 mg/dL	> 35 mg/dL
Borderline-high	200–239 mg/dL	130–159 mg/dL	
High	> 240 mg/dL	> 160 mg/dL	

FIGURE 13-10. Blood cholesterol levels and cutoff points [5]. It is optimal to keep patients' cholesterol levels within the desirable range. A step I or step II diet (see Fig. 13-33) should be initiated for those with borderline-high or high cholesterol levels. Although diet does play a role in determining blood cholesterol levels, exercise and medication may be necessary to bring them to a sound level. Once optimal cholesterol levels are achieved, appropriate maintenance of diet and weight is necessary to prevent an increase. HDL—high-density lipoprotein; LDL—low-density lipoprotein. (From American Heart Association, National Institute of Health [6].)

BLOOD PRESSURE LEVELS AND CUT-OFF LEVELS

	Systolic, *mm Hg*	Diastolic, *mm Hg*
Optimal	< 120	< 80
Normal	< 130	< 85
High normal	130–139	85–89
Hypertension		
Stage 1	140–159	90–99
Stage 2	160–179	100–109
Stage 3	> 180	> 110

FIGURE 13-11. Blood pressure levels and cutoff points. Blood pressure can be lowered to optimal levels through weight loss; a low-sodium, high-potassium diet; decreased fat consumption; and smoking cessation. Similar to hypercholesterolemia, blood pressure may also be improved with exercise and medicine.

BLOOD GLUCOSE VALUES

Biochemical Index	Normal	Diagnosis of Diabetes
Fasting/preprandial glucose	< 115 mg/dL	> 140 mg/dL
Postprandial glucose	60–140 mg/dL	> 200 mg/dL
Hemoglobin A1C	< 6%	

FIGURE 13-12. Blood glucose values. Testing of blood sugar concentration before and after meals can help to evaluate the release of insulin and determine whether a person is diabetic. A fasting blood glucose value of more than 126 mg/dL indicates the need for additional testing. A second fasting plasma glucose test should then be administered to determine the diagnosis of diabetes.

NUTRITIONAL HISTORY: DETECTION OF DEFICIENCY

Mechanism of Deficiency	If There Has Been a History of:	Then Suspect Deficiency of:
Inadequate intake	Alcoholism	Calories, protein, thiamin, niacin, folate, pyridoxine, riboflavin
	Avoidance of meat, dairy, and eggs	Protein, vitamin B_{12}
	Avoidance of fruit, vegetables, and grains	Vitamin C, thiamin, niacin, folate
	Constipation, hemorrhoids, diverticulosis	Dietary fiber
Inadequate absorption	Malabsorption (diarrhea, steatorrhea, weight loss)	Vitamins A, D, K; calories, protein; calcium; magnesium; zinc; vitamin B_{12}
	Pernicious Anemia	
Increased requirements	Fever	Calories
	Surgery, trauma, infection, burns	Calories, protein, vitamin C, zinc
	Cigarette smoking	Vitamin C, folic acid
	Hyperthyroidism	Calories
	Physiologic demands (infancy, adolescence, pregnancy, lactation)	Various nutrients
Increased losses	Blood loss	Iron
	Alcohol abuse	Zinc, magnesium
	Uncontrolled diabetes	Calories
	Diarrhea	Protein, zinc, electrolytes
	Wounds, draining abscesses	Protein, zinc
	Peritoneal or hemodialysis	Protein, water-soluble vitamins, zinc

FIGURE 13-13. Nutritional history: detection of deficiency [3]. The nutritional history portion of the client interview may be used to lead the practitioner in the right direction for detection of deficiency. In such instances, suspected deficiencies should be further investigated with laboratory workups and anthrpometric measurements.

A. THE NUTRITION CHECKLIST

Use the word *determine* to remind you of the warning signs.

Disease

Any disease, illness, or chronic condition that causes you to change the way you eat, or makes it difficult for you to eat, puts your nutritional health at risk. Four of five adults have chronic diseases that are affected by diet. Confusion or memory loss that keeps getting worse is estimated to affect one of five (or more) older adults. This can make it difficult to remember what, when, or whether you have eaten. Feeling sad or depressed, which happens to about one in eight older adults, can cause big changes in appetite, digestion, energy level, weight, and well-being.

Eating poorly

Eating both too little and too much can lead to poor health. Eating the same foods day after day or not eating fruit, vegetables, and milk products daily will also result in poor nutritional health. One in five adults skips meals daily. Only 13% of adults eat the minimum amount of fruits and vegetables needed. One in four older adults drinks too much alcohol. Many health problems worsen in individuals who drink more than one or two alcoholic beverages per day.

Tooth loss/Mouth pain

A healthy mouth, teeth, and gums are needed to eat. Missing, loose, or rotten teeth or dentures that do not fit well or cause mouth sores make it difficult to eat.

Economic hardship

As many as 40% of older Americans have incomes of less than $6000 per year. Having less—or choosing to spend less—than $25 to $30 per week for food makes it very difficult to get the foods you need to stay healthy.

Reduced social contact

One third of all older people live alone. Spending time with people every day has a positive effect on morale, well-being, and eating.

Multiple medicines

Many older Americans must take medicines because of health problems. Almost half of all older Americans take multiple medications daily. Growing old may change the way we respond to drugs. The more medicines you take, the greater the chance for side effects such as increased or decreased appetite, change in taste, constipation, weakness, drowsiness, diarrhea, nausea, and others. Vitamins or minerals, when take in large doses, act like drugs and can cause harm. Alert your doctor to every medication you take.

Involuntary weight loss/gain

Losing or gaining a lot of weight when you are not trying to is an important warning sign that must not be ignored. Being overweight or underweight also increases the risk of poor health.

Needs assistance in self-care

Although most older people are able to eat, one of every five has trouble walking, shopping, buying, and cooking food, especially as they get older.

Elder years above 80

Most older people lead full and productive lives. As age increases, however, risk of frailty and health problems increase. Regularly checking your nutritional health makes good sense.

FIGURE 13-14. The Nutrition Checklist. The warning signs of poor nutritional health are often overlooked.

(*Continued on next page*)

B. DETERMINE YOUR NUTRITIONAL HEALTH

The warning signs of poor nutritional health are often overlooked. Use this checklist to find out whether you or someone you know is at nutritional risk.

Read the statements below. Circle the number in the "yes" column for statements that apply to you or someone you know. For each yes answer, score the number in the box. Total your nutritional score.

Warning signs	Yes
I have an illness or condition that made me change the kind and/or amount of food I eat.	2
I eat fewer than two meals per day.	3
I eat few fruits or vegetables or milk products.	2
I have three or more drinks of beer, liquor, or wine almost every day.	2
I have tooth or mouth problems that make it hard for me to eat.	2
I don't always have enough money to buy the food I need.	4
I eat alone most of the time.	1
I take three or more different prescription or over-the-counter drugs every day.	1
Without wanting to, I have lost or gained 10 pounds in the last 6 months.	2
I am not always physically able to shop, cook, or feed myself.	2
Total	

Total your nutritional score. If it's

0–2:   Good! Recheck your nutritional score in 6 months.

3–5:   You are at moderate nutritional risk. See what can be done to improve your eating habits and lifestyle. Your office on aging, senior nutrition program, senior citizens center, or health department can help. Recheck your nutritional score in 3 months.

6 or more: You are at high nutritional risk. Bring this checklist the next time you see your doctor, dietitian, or other qualified health or social service professional. Talk with them about any problems you may have. Ask for help to improve your nutritional health.

Remember that warning signs suggest risk but do not represent diagnosis of any condition.

FIGURE 13-14. (*Continued*) **A** and **B**, The Nutrition Checklist is based on common warning signs and can be used to determine nutritional risk. (*Adapted from* Nutrition Screening Initiative [1].)

ISSUES TO CONSIDER WHEN TAKING A NUTRITIONAL HISTORY

Usual meal pattern
Snack consumption
Appetite
Satiety
Changes in weight
Any discomfort after eating
Chewing/swallowing ability
Likes/dislikes
Taste changes/aversions
Allergies
Nausea/vomiting

Bowel habits
Living conditions
Ability to purchase and prepare food
Access to and ability to pay for health care
Alcohol/drug use
Previous diet restrictions
Surgery/chronic disease
Vitamin/mineral use
Cultural religious beliefs
Comprehension

FIGURE 13-15. Issues to consider when taking a nutritional history. A comprehensive approach is needed in the evaluation of a patient's nutritional history. The interviewer must address eating habits, recent weight changes, and the patient's current state of health. Previous diets, affordability of foods, and religious and cultural beliefs are also important. A complete picture is needed to best counsel the patient.

DIETARY REFERENCE INTAKES: RECOMMENDED LEVELS FOR INDIVIDUAL INTAKE

Life-stage group	Calcium, mg/d	Phosphorus, mg/d	Magnesium, mg/d	Vitamin D†‡, mg/d	Fluoride, mg/d	Thiamin, mg/d	Riboflavin, mg/d	Niacin§, mg/d	Vitamin B6, mg/d	Folate¶, µg/d	Vitamin B12, µg/d	Pantothenic acid, mg/d	Biotin, µg/d	Choline**, mg/d
Infants, mo														
0–6	210*	100*	30*	5*	0.01*	0.2*	0.3*	2*	0.1*	65*	0.4*	1.7*	5*	125*
7–12	270*	275*	75*	5*	0.5*	0.3*	0.4*	4*	0.3*	80*	0.5*	1.8*	6*	150*
Children, yr														
1–3	500*	460	80	5*	0.7*	0.5	0.5	6	0.5	150	0.9	2*	8*	200*
4–8	800*	500	130	5*	1*	0.6	0.6	8	0.6	200	1.2	3*	12*	250*
Males, yr														
9–13	1300*	1250	240	5*	2*	0.9	0.9	12	1.0	300	1.8	4*	20*	375*
14–18	1300*	1250	410	5*	3*	1.2	1.3	16	1.3	400	2.4	5*	25*	550*
19–30	1000*	700	400	5*	4*	1.2	1.3	16	1.3	400	2.4	5*	30*	550*
31–50	1000*	700	420	5*	4*	1.2	1.3	16	1.3	400	2.4	5*	30*	550*
51–70	1200*	700	420	10*	4*	1.2	1.3	16	1.7	400	2.4‡	5*	30*	550*
>70	1200*	700	420	15*	4*	1.2	1.3	16	1.7	400	2.4‡	5*	30*	550*
Females, yr														
9–13	1300*	1250	240	5*	2*	0.9	0.9	12	1.0	300	1.8	4*	20*	375*
14–18	1300*	1250	360	5*	3*	1.0	1.0	14	1.2	400‡	2.4	5*	25*	400*
19–30	1000*	700	310	5*	3*	1.1	1.1	14	1.3	400‡	2.4	5*	30*	425*
31–50	1000*	700	320	5*	3*	1.1	1.1	14	1.3	400‡	2.4	5*	30*	425*
51–70	1200*	700	320	10*	3*	1.1	1.1	14	1.5	400	2.4‡	5*	30*	425*
>70	1200*	700	320	15*	3*	1.1	1.1	14	1.5	400	2.4‡	5*	30*	425*
Pregnancy, yr														
≤18	1300*	1250	400	5*	3*	1.4	1.4	18	1.9	600§	2.6	6*	30*	450*
19–30	1000*	700	350	5*	3*	1.4	1.4	18	1.9	600§	2.6	6*	30*	450*
31–50	1000*	700	360	5*	3*	1.4	1.4	18	1.9	600§	2.6	6*	30*	450*
Lactation														
≤18	1300*	1250	360	5*	3*	1.5	1.6	17	2.0	500	2.8	7*	35*	550*
19–30	1000*	700	310	5*	3*	1.5	1.6	17	2.0	500	2.8	7*	35*	550*
31–50	1000*	700	320	5*	3*	1.5	1.6	17	2.0	500	2.8	7*	35*	550*

*Adequate intake values

†As cholecalciferol {1 µg cholecalciferol = 40 IU vitamin D).

‡In the absence of adequate exposure to sunlight.

§As niacin equivalents (NE); 1 mg of niacin = 60 mg of tryptophan; 0–6 mo = preformed niacin [not NE].

¶As dietary folate equivalents (DFE); 1 mg of niacin = 60 mg of tryptophan; 0–6 mo = preformed niacin [not NE]. 1 DFE = 1 µg food folate = 0.6 µg of folic acid [from fortified food or supplement] consumed with food = 0.5 µg of synthetic [supplemental] folic acid taken on an empty stomach.

**Although AIs have been set for choline, there are few data to assess whether a dietary supply of choline is needed at all stages of the life cycle, and it may be that the choline requirement can be met by endogenous synthesis at some of these stages.

††Because 10% to 30% of older people may malabsorb foodbound vitamin B12, it is advisable for those older than 50 years of age to meet their RDA mainly by consuming foods fortified with B12 or by taking a supplement containing B12.

‡‡In view of evidence linking folate intake with neural tube defects in the fetus, it is recommended that all women capable of becoming pregnant consume 400 µg of synthetic folic acid from fortified foods and/or supplements in addition to intake of food folate from a varied diet.

§§It is assumed that women will continue consuming 400 µg of folic acid until their pregnancy is confirmed and they enter prenatal care, which ordinarily occurs after the end of the periconceptional period—the critical time for formation of the neural tube.

FIGURE 13-16. Dietary reference intakes: recommended levels for individual intake [7]. This table presents the recommended dietary allowances (RDAs) in bold type and adequate intakes (AIs) in regular type followed by an asterisk. RDA and AI may both be used as goals for individual intake. For healthy breastfed infants, the AI is the mean intake. The AI for other life-stage and gender groups is believed to cover the needs of all individuals in the group, but lack of data or uncertainty in the data prevent being able to specify with confidence the percentage of individuals covered by this intake. (Adapted from the Food and Nutrition Board of the National Research Council [7].)

RDAs are set to meet the needs of almost all (97% to 98%) individuals in a group.

DIETARY REFERENCE INTAKES

Recommended Dietary Allowance (RDA)

  The average daily dietary intake level that is sufficient to meet the nutrient requirement of nearly all healthy individuals in a group.

Adequate Intake (AI)

  A recommended daily intake level based on observed or experimentally determined approximations of nutrient intake by a group of healthy people. It is used when a RDA cannot be determined

Tolerable Upper Intake Level (UI)

  The highest level of daily nutrient intake that is likely to pose no risks of adverse health effects to almost all individuals in the general population. As intake increases above the UL, the risk of adverse effects increases.

Estimated Average Requirement (EAR)

  A nutrient intake value that is estimated to meet the requirements of half the healthy individuals in a group. It is used to assess adequacy of intakes of population groups and, along with knowledge of the distribution of requirements, to develop RDAs.

FIGURE 13-17. Dietary reference intakes (*Adapted from* Yates, *et al.* [2].)

DIET QUALITY INDEX SCORING GUIDELINE

Recommendation	Intake	Score
Reduce total fat intake to 30% or less of energy	< 30%	0
	31%–40%	1
	> 40%	2
Reduce saturated fatty acid intake to less than 10% of energy	< 10%	0
	10%–13%	1
	13%	2
Reduce cholesterol to less than 300 mg daily	< 300 mg/d	0
	300–400 mg/d	1
	400 mg/d	2
Eat five or more servings daily of a combination of vegetables and fruits	5+ servings	0
	3–4 servings	1
	0–2 servings	2
Increase intake of starches and other complex carbohydrates by eating six or more servings daily of breads, cereals, and legumes	6+ servings	0
	4–5 servings	1
	0–3 servings	2
Maintain protein intake at a moderate level	< 100% RDA	0
	101%–150%	1
	> 150% RDA	2
Limit total daily intake of salt to 6 grams	< 2400 mg sodium	0
	2401–3400 mg sodium	1
	> 3400 mg sodium	2
Maintain adequate calcium intake	> 100% RDA	0
	67%–99% RDA	1
	< 67% RDA	2

FIGURE 13-18. Diet quality index (DQI) scoring guidelines [8]. One method of assessing dietary intake, the DQI, classifies people by final score. The higher the score (the maximum is 16), the more work the diet needs. A lower score reflects a better-balanced diet. RDA—recommended dietary allowance. (*Adapted from* Lee and Nieman [8].)

Dietary Guidelines and Food Guidance Systems

DIAGNOSTIC CRITERIA FOR EATING DISORDERS

Bulimia

Recurrent episodes of binge eating (rapid consumption of a large amount of food in a discrete period of time)

A feeling of lack of control over eating behavior during eating binges

Regularly engaging in self-induced vomiting, use of laxatives or diuretics, strict dieting or fasting, or vigorous exercise in order to prevent weight gain

A minimum average of two binge-eating episodes a week for at least 3 months

Persistent overconcern with body shape and weight

Anorexia nervosa

Refusal to maintain body weight over a minimal normal weight for age and height

Intense fear of gaining weight or becoming fat, even though underweight

Disturbance in the way in which one's body weight is experienced; the person may claim to feel fat even when emaciated or believe that one body part is too fat even when underweight

In girls and women, the absence of at least three consecutive menstrual cycles when otherwise expected to occur

FIGURE 13-19. Diagnostic criteria for eating disorders: bulimia and anorexia nervosa [3]. These criteria are by no means all-inclusive as there are patients who exhibit symptoms of both illnesses or who may have a type of eating disorder not documented in this chapter. Eating disorders in men are not uncommon, and "eating disorder" is not limited to anorexia and bulimia. (*Adapted from* Weinsier and Morgan [3].)

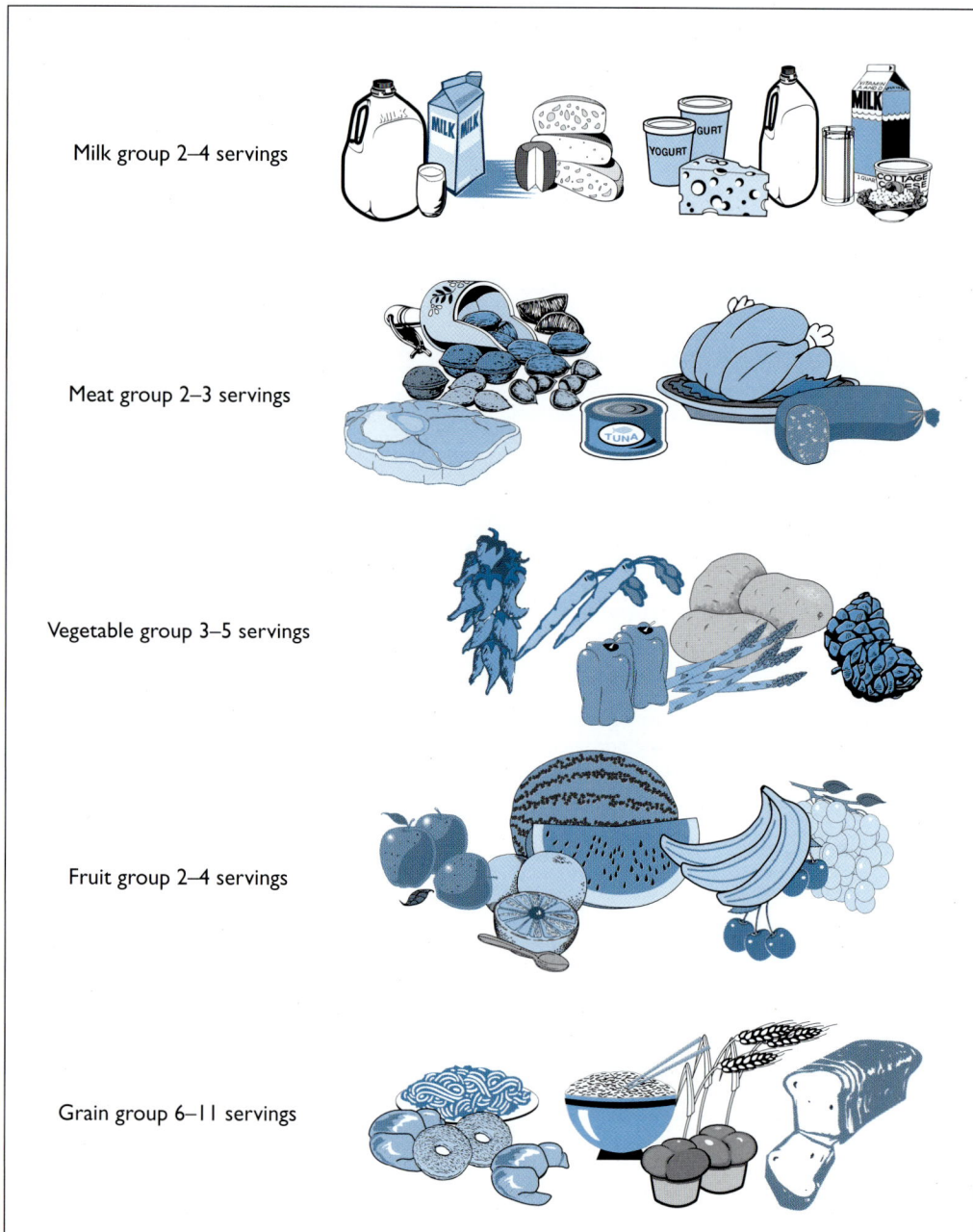

Milk group 2–4 servings

Meat group 2–3 servings

Vegetable group 3–5 servings

Fruit group 2–4 servings

Grain group 6–11 servings

FIGURE 13-20. The National Dairy Council's Guide to Good Eating [9]. Before the advent of the US Department of Agriculture (USDA) Food Guide Pyramid [10] (see Fig. 13-21), foods were classified into one of four food groups: milk, meat, vegetables and fruits, and breads and cereals. The 1964 Guide to Good Eating differentiated dairy needs by age but made no mention of fat or condiments. The 1989 version initiated low-fat eating and the consumption of a "wide variety of foods in moderation." The most recent Guide to Good Eating (1994) continues to stress low-fat eating and moderation. Fruits and vegetables are grouped separately to stress their individual importance. (*Adapted from* the National Dairy Council [9]; with permission.)

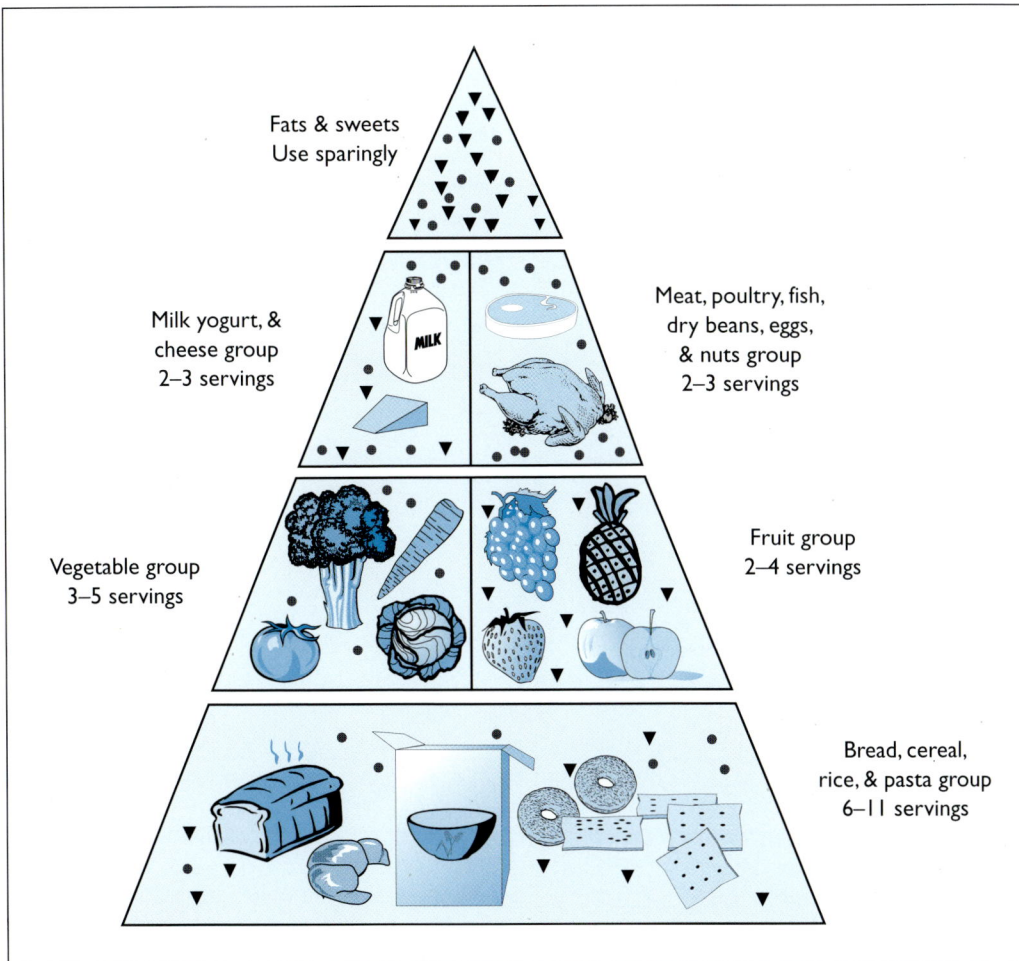

FIGURE 13-21. The USDA Food Guide Pyramid [10]. The Food Guide Pyramid was devised to offer a pattern for food choices from the various food groups. The groups closer to the base of the pyramid should be eaten more often than those closer to the top. The pyramid may be used to help patients visualize the greater need for grains and decreased need for fats and sweets. Because sodium, alcohol, and weight are not addressed in the Food Guide Pyramid, however, it should only be used as a supplement to other educational methods and materials. (*Adapted from* the National Livestock and Meat Board [10].)

Pyramid labels:
- Fats & sweets Use sparingly
- Milk yogurt, & cheese group 2–3 servings
- Meat, poultry, fish, dry beans, eggs, & nuts group 2–3 servings
- Vegetable group 3–5 servings
- Fruit group 2–4 servings
- Bread, cereal, rice, & pasta group 6–11 servings

WHAT COUNTS AS A SERVING?

Food Group	Serving
Bread, cereal, rice, and pasta	1 slice of bread
	1 oz of ready-to-eat cereal
	½ cup of cooked cereal, rice, or pasta
Vegetable	1 cup of raw, leafy vegetables
	½ cup of other vegetables, cooked or chopped raw
	¾ cup of vegetable juice
Fruit	1 medium apple, banana, or orange
	½ cup of chopped, cooked, or canned fruit
	¾ cup of fruit juice
Milk, yogurt, and cheese	1 cup of milk or yogurt
	1–1½ oz. of natural cheese
	2 oz of processed cheese
Meat, poultry, fish, dry beans, eggs, and nuts	2–3 oz of cooked, lean meat, poultry, or fish
	½ cup of cooked dry beans, 1 egg, or 2 tbsp of peanut butter count as 1 oz of lean meat

FIGURE 13-22. Serving size guidelines [11]. These serving sizes are used as a supplement to the various dietary guidelines to indicate the quantity of food that is equivalent to one serving. Serving sizes are meant to be used as a general guide. A smaller portion would count as a partial serving; a larger amount, multiple portions. For example, half a medium apple would count as half a fruit serving, whereas a large bowl of pasta could actually be 2 cups of pasta (four servings of grains). (*Adapted from* the USDA, USDHHS [11].)

More consistent serving sizes, in both household and metric units, replace those that used to be set by manufacturers.

Nutrients required on nutrition panel important to today's consumers, most of whom need to reduce intake of certain items (eg, fat, cholesterol) and increase intake of other items (eg, dietary fiber).

These vitamins and minerals of current concern are still mandatory.

Conversion guide helps consumers learn of the energy-yielding nutrients.

Nutrition Facts

Serving Size 1 cup (228g)
Servings Per Container 2

Amount Per Serving

Calories 260   Calories from fat 120

	% Daily Value*
Total Fat 13g	20%
Saturated Fat 5g	25%
Cholesterol 30mg	10%
Sodium 660mg	28%
Total Carbohydrate 31g	10%
Dietary Fiber 0g	0%
Sugars 5g	
Protein 5g	

Vitamin A 4%	•	Vitamin C 2%	
Calcium 15%	•	Iron 4%	

• Percent Daily Values are based on a 2,000 calorie diet. Your daily values may be higher or lower depending on your calorie needs:

	Calories	2,000	2,500
Total Fat	Less than	65g	80g
Sat Fat	Less than	20g	25g
Cholesterol	Less than	300mg	300mg
Sodium	Less than	2,400mg	2,400mg
Total Carbohydrate		300g	375g
Dietary Fiber		25g	30g

Calories per gram:
Fat 9 • Carbohydrate 4 • Protein 4

This mandatory component helps consumers meet dietary guidelines recommending that no more than 30% of energy come from fat.

Percent of daily value for mandatory dietary components shows how the food fits into the overall diet. If a food is fortified or enriched with any of the optional dietary components, or if a claim is made about any of them, the pertinent nutrition information then becomes mandatory.

Daily reference values help consumers learn good diet basics. They can be adjusted, depending on a person's energy needs.

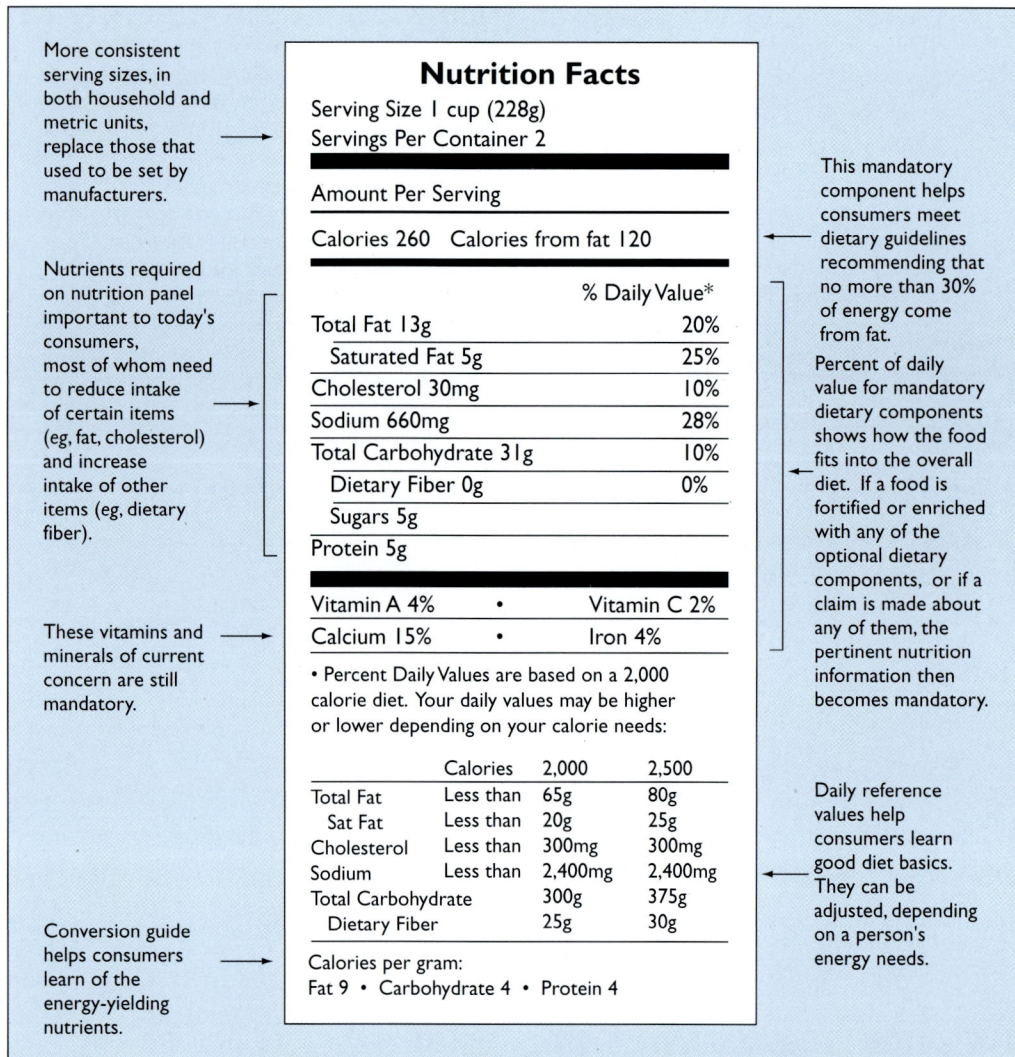

FIGURE 13-23. Key aspects of the Food and Drug Administration (FDA) nutrition label. In 1994, Congress made it mandatory that all foods carry this food label format. Serving sizes on the label are standardized based on amounts commonly consumed. The percentage of daily values is based on a 2000-calorie diet, which may be more or less than an individual needs. (*Adapted from* the USDA [12].)

NUTRIENT CONTENT CLAIMS CURRENTLY ALLOWED BY THE FDA: LABELING TERMS

High	> 20% of desired daily value per serving
Light	Half the fat or one third the calories of the regular product
Healthy	Low total and saturated fat, cholesterol, and sodium; > 10% daily value of vitamin A, C, calcium, iron, protein, or fiber
Free	Insignificant amount (< 1 g fat or < 0.5 g sugar per serving, or none)
Low-fat	≤ 3.5 g per serving
Low saturated fat	≤ 1 g per serving, <15% of calories
Low-calorie	< 40 calories per serving

FIGURE 13-24. Nutrient content claims currently allowed by the FDA: labeling terms [13]. These terms have been approved for use on food labels. For a label to carry one of these claims, the food must meet specific definitions set by the government. Although these terms can serve as an aid for consumers who have a hard time with decision making, they may also serve as a trap. For example, a box of cookies labeled as "fat-free" will likely have a deceptively high calorie count because of the high sugar content. (*Adapted from* Mahan and Escott-Stump [13].)

NUTRIENTS AND DISEASE PREVENTION: RELATIONSHIPS PERMITTED BY THE FDA

Soluble fiber and cholesterol

Calcium and osteoporosis

Lipids and cardiovascular disease

Dietary lipids and cancer

Sodium and hypertension

Folate and birth defects

Fiber and cancer

Fiber and cardiovascular disease

Fruits and vegetables and cancer

Psyllium and coronary heart disease

Dental caries and "sugarless" sugar alcohols

FIGURE 13-25. Permissible health claims. Eleven health claims and relationships between nutrients and disease have been approved by the FDA for product labeling. These 11 claims were approved to call attention to the relationship between diet and disease. Listed here are the 11 nutrients that have been linked to the prevention of disease. Health claims may not be used in foods that provide more than 20% of the daily value for fat, saturated fat, sodium, or cholesterol and may not be used to imply that consumption of the food can single-handedly prevent or cure disease.

DIET AND HEALTH: IMPLICATIONS FOR REDUCING CHRONIC DISEASE RISK

Reduce total fat intake to ≤ 30% of calories. Reduce saturated fatty acid intake to < 10% of calories and cholesterol intake to <300 mg/d. Fat and cholesterol intake can be reduced by substituting fish, poultry without skin, lean meats, and low-fat or nonfat dairy products for fatty meats and whole-milk dairy products; by choosing more vegetables, fruits, cereals, and legumes; and by limiting oils, fats, egg yolks, and fried and other fatty foods.

Eat ≥5 servings every day of a combination of vegetables and fruits, especially green and yellow vegetables and citrus fruits. Also, increase intake of starches and other complex carbohydrates by eating ≥ 6 daily servings of a combination of breads, cereals, and legumes.

Maintain protein intake at moderate levels.

Balance food intake and physical activity to maintain appropriate body weight.

The committee does not recommend alcohol consumption. The committee recommends limiting alcohol consumption to the equivalent of <1 oz of pure alcohol in a single day. Pregnant women should avoid all alcoholic beverages.

Limit total daily intake of salt to ≤ 6 g. Limit the use of salt in cooking and avoid adding salt to food at the table. Salty, highly processed salty, salt-preserved, and salt-pickled foods should be consumed sparingly.

Maintain adequate calcium intake.

Avoid taking dietary supplements in excess of the recommended dietary allowance in any one day.

Maintain an optimal intake of fluoride, particularly during the years of primary and secondary tooth formation and growth.

FIGURE 13-26. Diet and health: implications for reducing chronic disease risk [14]. (*Adapted from* the National Research Council [14].)

DIABETIC EXCHANGE LIST: MACRONUTRIENTS PROVIDED

Food groups	Carbohydrate, g	Protein, g	Fat, g	Calories
Carbohydrate				
Starch	15	3	≤1	80
Fruit	15	—	—	60
Milk				
Skim	12	8	0–3	90
Reduced-fat	12	8	5	120
Whole	12	8	8	150
Other carbohydrates	15	Varies	Varies	Varies
Vegetables	5	2	—	25
Meat and meat-substitute				
Very lean	—	7	0–1	35
Lean	—	7	3	55
Medium-fat	—	7	5	75
High-fat	—	7	8	100
Fat	—	—	5	45

FIGURE 13-27. Diabetic exchange list. Formulated by the American Diabetes Association and the American Dietetic Association [15], this table can be used as a tool to count calories and determined various macronutrient components of the diet. Each food falls into a category (carbohydrate, milk, fruit, vegetable, meat, or fat). The serving size determines caloric value. The exchange list is used for people with diabetes to measure carbohydrate intake. It may also be used for protein-restricted diets. (*Adapted from* the American Diabetes Association [15].)

RECOMMENDED AMOUNTS OF TOTAL AND SATURATED FAT

Dietary Fat, g	Daily Calorie Intake						
	1200	1500	1800	2000	2200	2500	3000
Total	≤40	≤50	≤60	≤67	≤73	≤83	≤100
Saturated	11–13	13–17	16–20	18–22	20–24	22–28	27–33

FIGURE 13-28. Recommended amounts of total and saturated fat. This table is based on a diet in which 30% of calories are derived from fat, 10% of which are provided by saturated fats.

DIETARY GUIDELINES FOR HEALTHY AMERICANS

Total fat intake should not exceed 30% of total calories.

Saturated fat intake should not exceed 8% to 10% of total calories.

Polyunsaturated fat intake should not exceed 10% of total calories.

Monounsaturated fat intake should not exceed 15% of total calories.

Cholesterol intake should not exceed 300 mg/d.

Sodium intake should not exceed 2400 mg/d, which is about 1 1/4 teaspoons of salt.

Carbohydrate intake should make up 55% to 60% of calories, with emphasis on increased sources of complex carbohydrates.

Total calories should be adjusted to achieve and maintain a healthy body weight.

FIGURE 13-29. Dietary guidelines for healthy Americans. In formulating guidelines for dietary practices for reducing the risk of cardiovascular disease in the general population, the American Heart Association Nutrition Committee limited their recommendations to those for which the scientific evidence provided satisfactory support [16]. Although these guidelines were developed specifically for prevention of heart and blood vessel disease, they are also applicable to the prevention of other diseases, including osteoporosis, renal disease, and some forms of cancer. These chronic diseases, in which nutrition plays a role, account for the majority of the morbidity and mortality in the population, highlighting the importance of providing the public with scientifically based dietary and lifestyle guidelines. (*Adapted from* the American Heart Association [16].)

Foods are indicated with
amount equal to one serving.

Fats, oils, and sweets
Use sparingly

Jelly
Candy
Soda
Margarine
Mayonnaise
Salad dressing

Dairy products
Eat 2-3 servings daily

Milk: 1 cup	Eggs: 1 cup
Yogurt: 1 cup	Hot dog: 1 cup
Frozen yogurt\	Fish sticks: 2 oz
Ice cream: 1/2 cup	Chicken: 2 oz
Pudding: 1/2 cup	Hamburger: 2 oz
Milkshake: 1 cup	Peanut butter: 2 tbsp
Cheese spread: 2 oz	Baked beans: 1/2 cup
American chese: 2 oz	

Meat, poultry, fish,
and dry beans
Eat 2-3 servings daily

Vegetables
Eat 3-5 servings
daily

Carrots: 1	Apple: 1
Corn: 1/2 cup	Banana: 1
Lettuce: 1 cup	Grapes: 1/2 cup
Broccoli: 1/2 cup	Fruit juice: 3/4 cup
Green beans: 1/2 cup	Watermelon: 1/2 cup
Tomato sauce: 1/2 cup	Fruit cocktail: 1/2 cup
Mashed potatoes: 1/2 cup	Strawberries: 1/2 cup

Fruits
Eat 2-4
servings
daily

Grains
eat 6-11
servings
daily

Bagel: 1/2	Tortilla: 1
Spaghetti: 1/2 cup	Rice: 1/2 cup
Macaroni: 1/2 cup	Bread: 1 slice
Hamburger: 1/2	Pretzels: 1 oz
Graham crackers: 3-4	Muffin: 1
Ready-to-eat cereal: 1/2 cup to 3/4 cup	

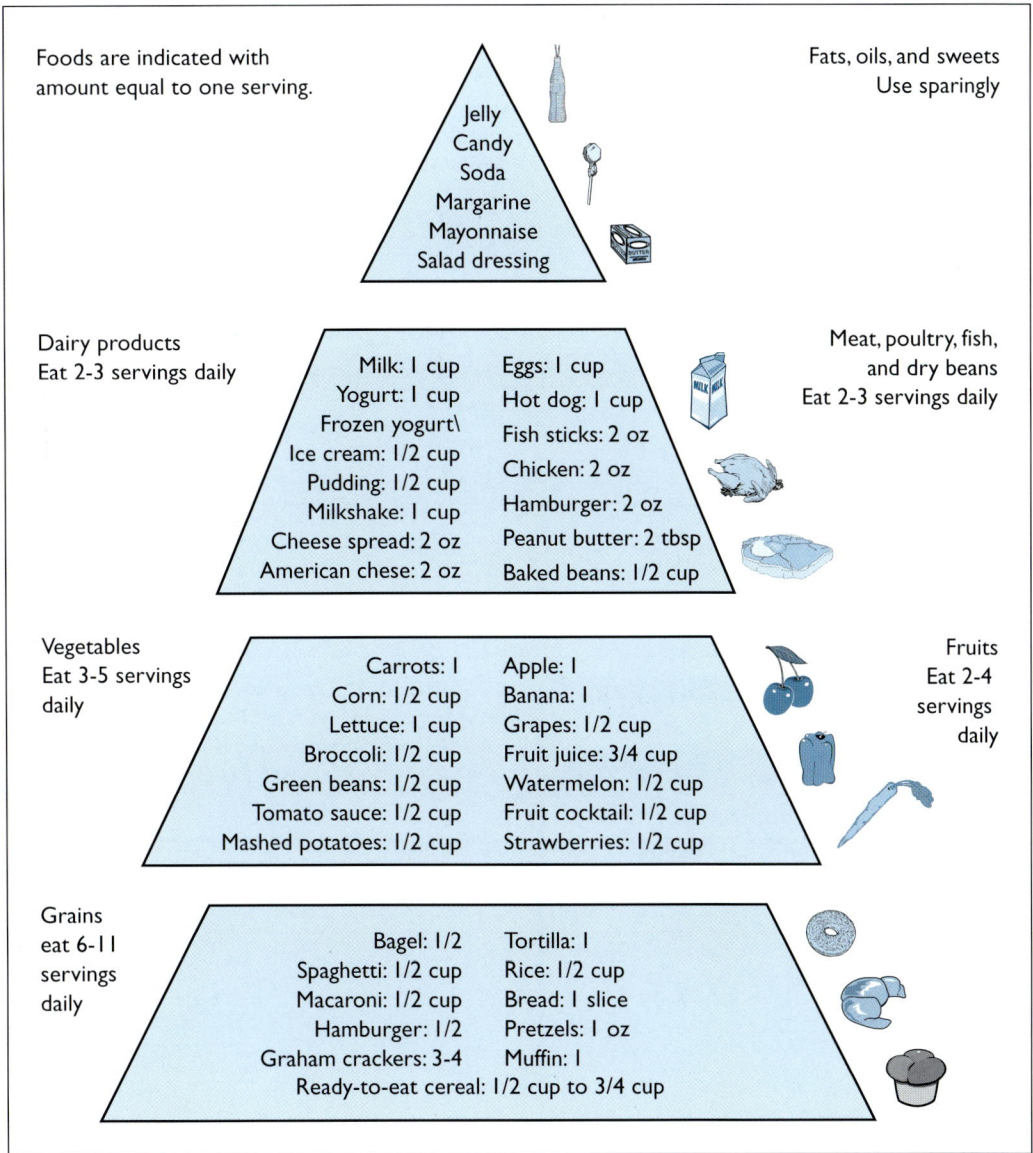

FIGURE 13-30. Food Guide Pyramid for Children [17]. Easier to read, the Food Guide Pyramid for Children was developed as a teaching tool for school-age youth. This pyramid indicates the food amounts that are equal to one serving.

Taking into consideration that different people eat different foods based on practices and culture, a variety of culturally sensitive food guidance systems have been developed. Beuna alimentación, the Spanish Food Guide Pyramid, is a vivid snapshot of the foods eaten in Latino culture and serves as a tool for Spanish-speaking patients and consumers. The Mediterranean Food Guide Pyramid, developed by the Harvard School of Public Health, is based on the eating habits of the inhabitants of Southern Italy, Crete, and Greece, who have low levels of disease and higher longevity. Olive oil, wine, fish, and physical activity are highlighted in this pyramid. The Asian Food Guide Pyramid takes into account the different eating habits of Asian populations and incorporates the need for fluids. Salt is included in the pyramid in the same category as sugar and fats. The Soul Food Guide Pyramid follows the same guidelines as the USDA pyramid but boasts more of the foods that are used to prepare soul food. "More grains and vegetable, less fats and sweets" is the key to the Israel Food Guide Pyramid, in which protein-rich foods are sandwiched between fruits and vegetables. The Vegetarian Food Guide Pyramid is tailored for the needs of vegetarians; the meat group is replaced with a legume, nut, seed, and meat-alternative group. (*Adapted from* the American Diabetes Association [17].)

Diets

THE SEVEN Cs OF HEALTHFUL WEIGHT LOSS

Calories allotted

Composition of the diet

Cost associated with following the diet

Consumer friendliness

Coping with coexisting conditions

Components of sound weight management

Continuation provisions for long-term
  maintenance

FIGURE 13-31. The seven C's of healthful weight loss [18]. In order for a weight loss program to be successful, it must be both healthful and follow the seven C's. Adequate calories must be allotted in the diet plan to prevent starvation. The diet must be affordable for the patient using it. It must also be easy to follow so patients will continue with it for maintenance. The diet must be sound and address comorbid conditions where appropriate. (*Adapted from* the US Department of Agriculture and US Department of Health and Human Services [18].)

DIETS FOR VARYING ENERGY LEVELS

Food Group	Number of Servings Needed Each Day to Provide		
	1600 calories+	2200 calories‡	2800§
Bread	6	9	11
Vegetable	3	4	5
Fruit	2	3	4
Milk*	2–3	2–3	2–3
Meat, oz	5	6	7
Total fat, g	53	73	93

*Women who are pregnant or breastfeeding, teenagers, and young adults to 24 years of age need three servings.
+Women and some older adults.
‡Children, teenage girls, active women, most men.
§Teenage boys and active men.

FIGURE 13-32. Diets for varying energy levels. Based on the USDA Food Guide Pyramid, the calorie levels presented in this table are based on low-fat, lean food choices from the food groups.

DAILY FOOD GUIDE

Food Group	Servings, n	Serving Size
Lean meat, poultry, fish, and shellfish	≤ 6 oz/d on step 1 diet ≤ 5 oz/d on step 2 diet (leanest cuts only)	
Skim/low-fat dairy foods	2–3	1 cup skim or 1% milk 1 cup nonfat or low-fat yogurt 1 oz low-fat or fat-free cheese that has ≤ 3 g of fat per serving
Eggs	≤ 4 yolks/wk on step 1 diet* ≤ 2 yolks/wk on step 1 diet*	
Fats and oils	≤ 6–8*	1 teaspoon soft margarine or vegetable oil 1 tbsp salad dressing 1 oz nuts
Fruits	2–4	1 piece fruit 1/2 cup diced fruit 3/4 cup fruit juice
Vegetables	3–5	1 cup leafy or raw 1/2 cup cooked 3/4 cup juice
Breads, cereals, pasta, rice, dry peas and beans, grains, and potatoes	6–11	1 slice bread 1/2 bun, bagel, muffin 1 oz dry cereal 1/2 cup cooked cereal, dry peas or beans, potatoes, or rice or other grains 1/2 cup tofu
Sweets and snacks	Occasionally	

*Includes food preparation; for fats and oils also includes salad dressings and nuts.

FIGURE 13-33. Daily food guide for step I and step II diets. The step diets, developed by the National Cholesterol Education Program, are designed to lower cholesterol levels through decreased intake of fat, saturated fat, cholesterol, and in some cases, calories [5]. A step I diet is usually the first choice; for those who do not experience desired results with the step I diet or are at higher risk for cormorbidities, however, a step 2 is implemented. The step 2 diet calls for fewer egg yolks per week and smaller servings of leaner cuts of meat than in the step I diet. (*Adapted from* the American Heart Association, National Institutes of Health [6].)

LIFESTYLE MODIFICATION FOR HYPERTENSION CONTROL OR OVERALL CARDIOVASCULAR RISK

Lose weight, if overweight.

Limit alcohol intake to no more than 1 oz/d.

Exercise regularly.

Reduce sodium intake to <100 mmol/d (<2.3 g of sodium or <6 g of salt).

Maintain adequate dietary potassium, calcium, and magnesium intake.

Stop smoking and reduce dietary saturated fat and cholesterol for overall cardiovascular health.

Reducing fat intake also helps reduce caloric intake, which is important for weight control and type 2 diabetes.

FIGURE 13-34. Lifestyle modifications for hypertension control or overall cardiovascular risk [19]. (*Adapted from* the National Institute of Health [19].)

References

1. Nutrition Screening Manual for Professionals Caring for Older Americans. Washington, DC: Greer, Margolis, Mitchell, Grunwald, and Associates; 1991.

2. Yates, Schlicker S, Suitor C: Dietary reference intakes: the new basis for recommendations for calcium and related nutrients, B vitamins, and choline. *J Am Diet Assoc* 1998, 98:699–706.

3. Weinsier M, Morgan S, eds: *Fundamentals of Clinical Nutrition*. New York: Mosby–Year Book; 1993.

4. Day B: *High Energy Eating: Sports Nutrition Workbook for Active People*. Louisville, KY: An Apple A Day; 1995.

5. Guthrie HA, Picciano MF: *Human Nutrition*. St. Louis: Mosby–Year Book; 1995.

6. American Heart Association, National Institutes of Health: *Step by Step: Eating to Lower Your High Blood Cholesterol*. 1994.

7. Food and Nutrition Board of the National Research Council: *Dietary Reference Intakes*. Washington, DC: National Academy of Sciences; 1998.

8. Lee R, Neiman D: *Second Edition Nutritional Assessment*. New York: Mosby–Year Book; 1996.

9. National Dairy Council: *Guide to Good Eating*. Rosemont, IL: 1994.

10. The Human Nutrition Information Services and the USDA: *USDA Food Guide Pyramid*. The Home and Garden Bulletin, no. 249, Washington DC: US Government Printing Office; 1992.

11. USDA, USDHHS: *United States Department of Agriculture Dietary Guidelines for Americans*, edn. 3. The Home and Garden Bulletin, no. 332. Hyattesville, MD; 1990.

12. USDA: *Nutrition Facts*.

13. Thomas PR: Guidelines for Dietary Planning. In *Krause's Food, Nutrition, and Diet Therapy*, edn 9. Edited by Maham L, Escott-Stump S: Philadelphia, WB Saunders; 1996.

14. National Research Council Food and Nutrition Board: *Diet and Health: Implications for Reducing Chronic Disease Risk*. Washington, DC: National Academy Press; 1989.

15. American Diabetes Association: *Food Exchange List [System]*: 1995.

16. American Heart Association: *The American Heart Association's Eating Plan for Healthy Americans*; 1996.

17 The American Diabetes Association: *Food Guide Pyramid for Children*. 1996.

18. USDA, USDHHS: *Nutrition and Your Health: Dietary Guidelines for Americans*, edn 4; 1995.

19. National Institutes of Health: *National High Blood Pressure Education Program*. NIH Publication #93-1088. January 1993.

PARENTERAL AND ENTERAL NUTRITION

Lalita Khaodhiar, Manoj K Maloo, and George L. Blackburn

The use of parenteral nutrition dates back to the 1930s [1], when amino acid infusions were first made possible with the development of protein hydrolysates. However, the institution of a hypertonic infusion that met goal caloric needs was only possible after Aubaniacs' description [2] of subclavian vein cannulation in 1952. With the landmark demonstration by Dudrick *et al* [3–5]. of growth and development in patients receiving parenteral nutrition as the sole source of nutrition, hyperalimentation came to be adapted into common clinical practice. Hyperalimentation has evolved into a route of nutrition delivery for those who cannot eat, should not eat, or cannot eat enough. Like the discoveries of insulin and antibiotics and the development of heart–lung bypass and transplantation, hyperalimentation is considered one of the top five discoveries of modern medicine.

The decision to initiate nutrition support in hospitalized patients is based on the presence of clinically significant malnutrition and the patient's inability to take adequate food by mouth. Enteral feeding refers to the provision of nutrient solutions into the gastrointestinal tract through a tube [6]. This route of nutrition support is typically used in patients who cannot ingest or digest sufficient food but have an intact absorptive capacity. Parenteral nutrition provides nutrients, energy, and metabolic requirements directly through the venous system for patients who are unable to tolerate or absorb adequate nutrients by the enteral route. Enteral nutrition is preferred in patients with a functional gastrointestinal tract because it is more physiologic, associated with fewer complications, and less expensive than is the parenteral route. In patients with severe metabolic derangement, however, total parenteral nutrition may play a role in the correction of severe electrolyte and acid–base disturbances.

In order to provide effective nutrition support, patients must be individually assessed and nutrition therapy should be directed by taking into account the patient's underlying diseases; baseline nutritional status; protein and energy requirements; and the presence of fluid, electrolyte, and acid–base abnormalities. The goal of nutrition support is to provide sufficient nutrients and metabolic support and to prevent further loss of lean body mass.

Malnutrition

PROTEIN AND PROTEIN–CALORIE MALNUTRITION

Parameter	Protein Malnutrition (Kwashiorkor)	Protein–calorie Malnutrition (Marasumus)
Causes	Diarrhea, gastrointestinal fistula, kidney/liver failure, infection, severe trauma, major burns, critical illness	Low intake (ie, anorexia, cancerous cachexia, short-gut syndrome, chronic pain, chronic obstructive pulmonary disease)
Results	Low serum albumin, sequelae of anemia, edema, muscle wasting, decline in cardiac function, delayed wound healing (decreased chemotaxis, phagocytosis, and serum complement)	Weight loss, decreased basal metabolic rate, loss of tissue turgor, bradycardia, hypothermia
Development time	Rapidly over a few weeks	Months to years
Features	May appear well (secondary to edema), low protein levels	Appears emaciated, protein levels usually normal
Mortality	High (visceral protein depletion)	Low

FIGURE 14-1. Protein and protein–calorie malnutrition. Protein–calorie malnutrition, which is common in hospitalized patients, can lead to significant increases in morbidity and mortality. Identification and treatment of malnutrition can improve patient outcome and should be a standard part of patient care [7–9].

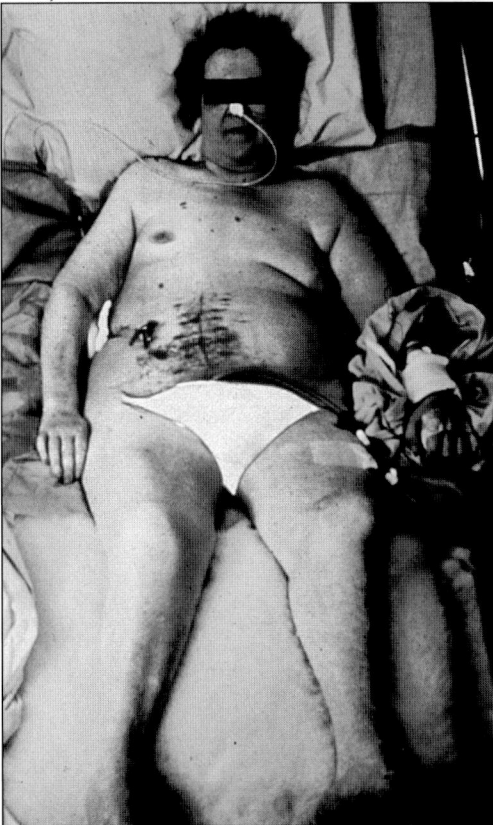

FIGURE 14-2. Kwashiorkor. Protein malnutrition, also known as kwashiorkor or hypoalbuminemic malnutrition, is common in hospitalized patients. Usually caused by low food intake, kwashiorkor is accompanied by the stress response to infection or injury. Common causes include infection, trauma, burns, kidney failure, liver failure, and critical illness [7]. Patients usually have marked hypoalbuminemia, anemia, edema, and impaired wound healing. Weight loss may not occur because of edema. This condition is associated with a significant increase in morbidity and mortality [8].

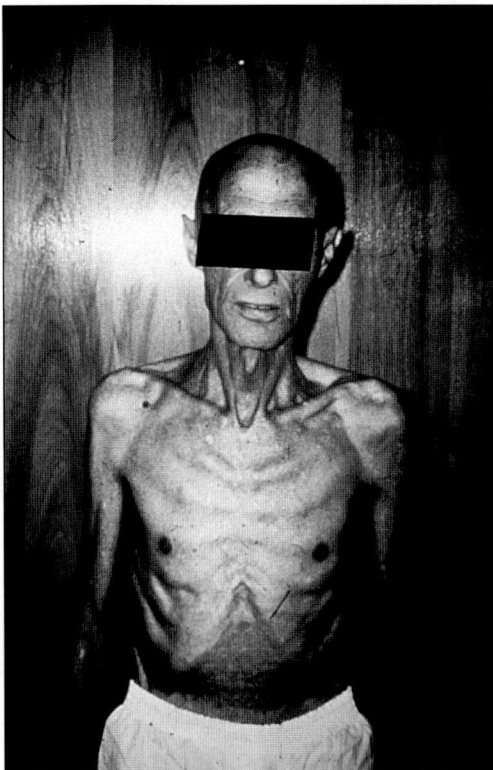

FIGURE 14-3. Marasmus. Protein–calorie malnutrition, or marasmus, is typically seen in patients with prolonged starvation (eg, anorexia nervosa, cancer cachexia, drug addiction, alcoholism)[7,8]. Patients usually have significant weight loss, a decreased basal metabolic rate, bradycardia, and depleted subcutaneous fat and lean body tissue. The serum albumin level is usually normal. The mortality rate is low, but significant morbidity can be seen after refeeding these patients (see Fig. 14-22).

Nutrition Assessment

GOALS OF NUTRITION ASSESSMENT

Identify patients who require nutrition support during their hospital stay.

Determine the degree and causes of malnutrition.

Determine the risk of complications or death from malnutrition.

Assess the patient's response to therapy.

FIGURE 14-4. Goals of nutrition assessment [9].

NUTRITION ASSESSMENT PARAMETERS

History and physical examination
  Subjective global assessment
  Body weight
Anthropometrics
  Triceps skinfold thickness
  Midarm muscle circumference
Biochemical parameters
  Albumin
  Prealbumin
  Transferrin
  Retinal binding protein
  Insulinlike growth factor–1
Immunologic determinants
  Lymphocyte counts (<3000)
  Anergy
  Cutaneous hypersensitivity
Nutritional indices
  Prognostic nutritional index
  Catabolic index
  Diagnosis of cancer (limited accuracy)
Body composition studies
  Distribution of fat, protein, and water
    K scanning
    Water space measurements
    Total body protein (neutron activation)
  Muscle mass
    Creatinine/height index
Bioelectrical impedence analysis
Muscle function
  Electrical stimulation of adductor pollicis

FIGURE 14-5. Nutrition assessment parameters. The diagnosis of malnutrition is usually made clinically in conjunction with some of the most commonly used parameters (eg, serum protein, upper-arm anthropometry) [9–13]. Other parameters have also been used, some of which are more helpful than others. For normal values and details on individual parameters, readers should refer to standard nutrition textbooks.

EVALUATION OF WEIGHT CHANGE

Time	Significant Weight Loss, %	Severe Weight Loss, %
1 wk	1–2	>2
1 mo	5	>5
3 mo	7.5	>7.5
6 mo	10	>10

Percent weight change = [(Usual weight - Actual weight)/(Usual weight) x 100]

FIGURE 14-6. Evaluation of weight change [8]. Nutrition assessment should begin with a careful history and physical examination. Weight loss is usually one of the first clues to underlying malnutrition [12]. Recent unintentional weight loss should prompt physicians to complete a nutrition assessment. (*Adapted from* Blackburn et al. [8].)

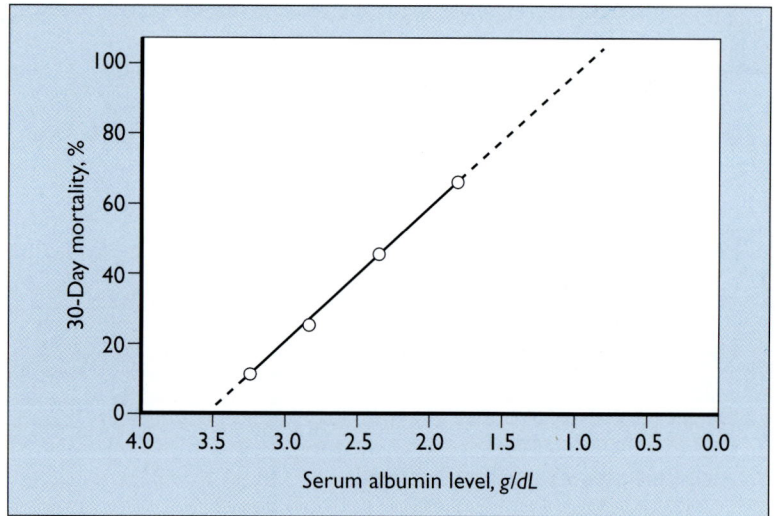

FIGURE 14-7. Correlation of serum albumin levels and 30-day mortality rate. The 30-day mortality rate increased with increasing levels of malnutrition in hospitalized men who did not receive TPN (*n* = 494) [14]. In this study, the index of malnutrition was serum albumin. (*Adapted from* Reinhardt et al. [14].)

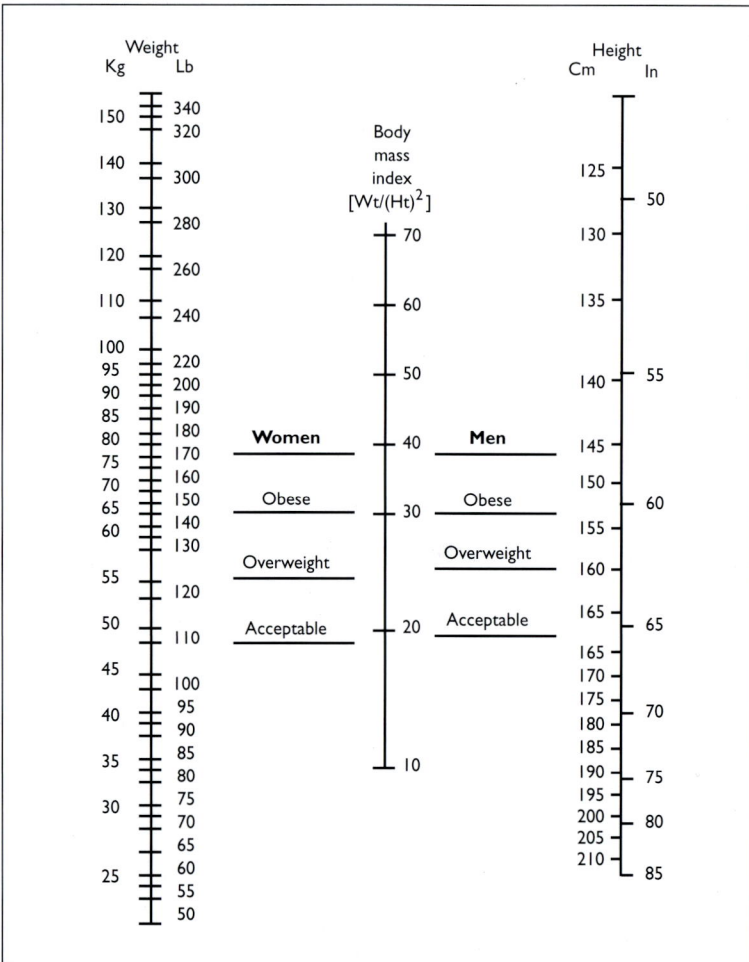

FIGURE 14-8. Nomogram for determining body mass index (BMI). To use this nomogram, connect the weight and height values with a ruler. The BMI is the value at which the ruler crosses the middle line. Normal BMI is 18.5 to 25 kg/m^2. A BMI of 18.5 kg/m^2 or less indicates malnutrition, whereas a BMI of greater than 30 kg/m^2 defines obesity. (*Adapted from* Bray [15].)

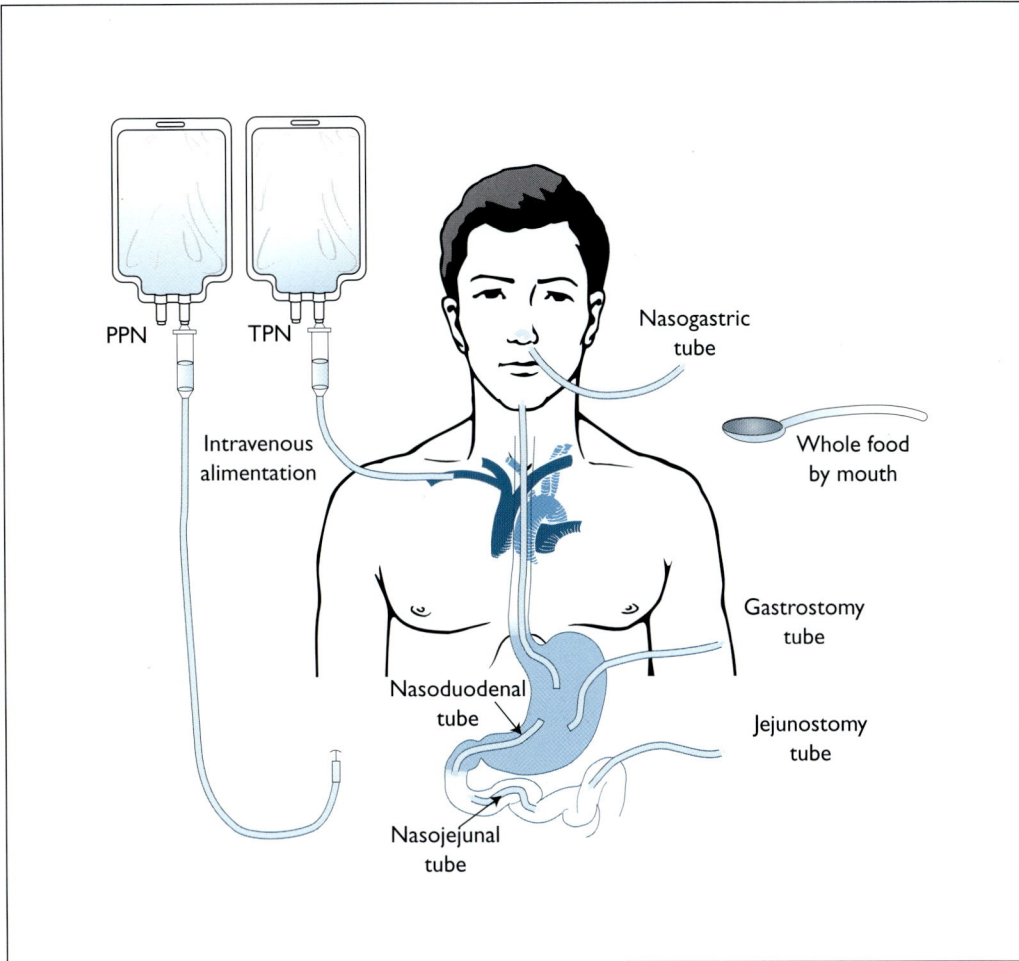

FIGURE 14-9. Routes of nutrition support. Nutrition support can be provided orally, enterally, or parenterally. Nasogastric, nasoduodenal, or nosojejunal tube feeding is used for short-term enteral nutrition, while a gastrostomy or jejunostomy tube is used for long-term enteral nutrition. Parenteral nutrition can be given via peripheral (peripheral parenteral nutrition; PPN) or central (total parenteral nutrition; TPN) venous access. (*Adapted from* Hardy [16].)

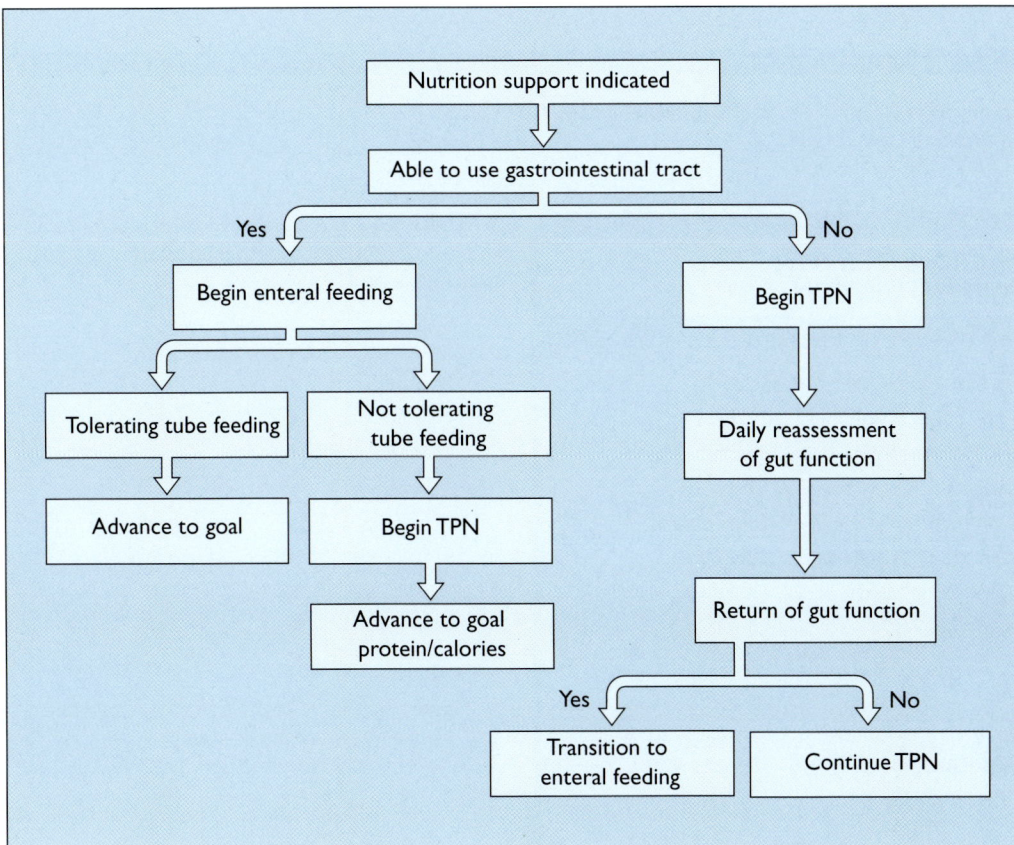

FIGURE 14-10. Nutritional support algorithm. A flow diagram is used to determine the route of feeding [17]. TPN—total parenteral nutrition.

Parenteral Nutrition

INDICATIONS FOR STANDARD TPN IN ADULTS

General indications

Long-term (>10 d) supplemental nutrition in patients who are unable to receive all of their daily energy protein and other nutrient requirements through oral or enteral feedings

Total nutrition because of severe gut dysfunction or an inability to tolerate enteral feedings

Specific indications

Inability to eat or absorb nutrients through the gastrointestinal tract because of massive small bowel resection, diseases of the small bowel, radiation enteritis, severe diarrhea, or intractable vomiting

Malnourishment in patients undergoing high-dose chemotherapy or radiation therapy or recent bone marrow transplantation

Severe necrotizing pancreatitis when enteral feeding is not possible or tolerated

Severe malnutrition and a nonfunctional gut

Malnourishment in patients with AIDS or AIDS-related complex who have intractable diarrhea and no other HIV-related infection or other pathology, particularly when they are undergoing definitive chemotherapy for diarrhea and enteral feeding is unsuccessful

Severe catabolism (ie, closed head injury, major trauma, or severe burn), with or without malnutrition, in patients whose guts cannot be used within 5–7 d

When enteral feeding cannot be established

After major surgery (in severely malnourished patients preoperative TPN should be continued for 5–7 postoperative days; TPN should begin 5 days after surgery in moderately malnourished patients)

Moderate stress 7–10 d after the injury

Enterocutaneous fistula (both high and low)

Inflammatory bowel disease

Hyperemesis gravidarum

Moderate malnourishment in patients who require intensive medical or surgical intervention within 3–5 d of treatment

When adequate enteral nutrition cannot be established within 1 wk of hospitalization

Small bowel obstruction secondary to inflammatory adhesions

Moderate to severe malnourishment in patients undergoing chemotherapy

FIGURE 14-11. Indications for standard total parenteral nutrition (TPN) in adults [18]. (*Adapted from* the American Society for Parenteral and Enteral Nutrition Board of Directors [18].)

GUIDELINES FOR TPN MACRONUTRIENTS: CALORIE AND FLUID ADMINISTRATION

Fluid	25–35 mL/kg/d unless patient has volume overload or deficit
Calories	25–30 kcal/kg/d for medical and surgical nonobese patients
	25–35 kcal/kg/d for patients following trauma (including major burns)
	20–25 kcal/kg/d for obese patients
	30–35 kcal/kg/d for patients on hemodialysis or peritoneal dialysis
Glucose	Provide most of the calories in the TPN admixtures (50%–75%)
	Caloric value = 3.4 kcal/g
	Rate of infusion = 2.5–4 mg/kg/min
Protein	Caloric value = 4 kcal/g
	Protein requirement
	Healthy adults: 0.8–1 g/kg/d
	Chronically ill and surgical patients: 1.2–1.5 g/kg/d
	Patients on hemodialysis: 1.2–1.5 g/kg/d
	Patients with nephropathies: 0.8 g/kg/d
Lipid	Caloric value = 9 kcal/g
	<30% of total calories or 1–1.5 g/kg/d

FIGURE 14-12. Guidelines for total parenteral nutrition (TPN) macronutrients: calories and fluid administration [12,19–21].

GUIDELINES FOR MICRONUTRIENT ADMINISTRATION

Micronutrient	Daily RDA For Adults	Recommended Daily Intravenous Formulation
Vitamin*		
A	4000–5000 IU	3000 IU
D	400 IU	200 IU
E	12–15 IU	10 IU
C (ascorbic acid)	45 mg	100 mg
Folic acid	200µg	400 µg
Niacin	12–20 mg	40 mg
B_1 (thiamine)	1.0–1.5 mg	3.0 mg
B_2 (riboflavin)	1.1–1.8 mg	3.6 mg
B_6 (pyridoxine)	1.6–2.0 mg	4.0 mg
B_{12} (cobalamine)	3µg	5 µg
Pantothenic acid	5–10 mg	15 mg
Biotin	150–300 µg	60 µg
Trace element		
Zinc	2.5–4.0 mg	2.5–4.0 mg[†]
Copper	0.5–1.5 mg	0.5–1.5 mg
Manganese	150–800 µg	150–800 µg
Chromium	10–15 µg	10–15 µg

*Vitamin K is administered separately once a week by intramuscular or subcutaneous injection.
[†]Adults in acute catabolic states should receive an additional 2.0 mg of zinc.

FIGURE 14-13. Guidelines for micronutrient administration [22]. RDA—recommended dietary allowance. (*Adapted from* the American Medical Association Department of Foods and Nutrition [22].)

FIGURE 14-14. How to start total parenteral nutrition (TPN).

HOW TO START TPN*

Day 1

Start with: 70–80 g amino acids

100–150 g dextrose   7%–8% amino acid and 10%–14%
1-L volume   dextrose in 1–1.5 L volume

Day 2 and subsequently:

Increase volume

Increase protein content to goal amount

Increase dextrose as tolerated, and add insulin as needed to keep
  blood sugar <220 mg/dL

Add fat

*This protocol is used for the majority of patients requiring TPN at Beth Israel Deaconess Medical Center.

VENOUS ACCESS FOR TPN

Catheter type	Advantages	Disadvantages
Peripherally inserted central	Low cost, can be inserted at bedside, good for patients with neck wounds	Skin site irritation, tendency of catheter to break at hub, patients require assistance with weekly dressing change
Centrally inserted externalized catheters	Relatively low cost, can be inserted at bedside, can be changed over a guidewire if clinically indicated	10% incidence of mechanical complication with insertion, multilumen catheters increase incidence of sepsis
Tunneled central catheter (Broviac or Hickman) or subcutaneous implanted port	Stable for long-term use, patients can swim or shower	More expensive, requires operating room insertion or subcutaneous implanted port

FIGURE 14-15. Venous access for total parenteral nutrition (TPN) [23]. Several types of catheters can be used for TPN. Single- or multilumen, nontunneled catheters are often used in hospitalized patients; tunneled catheters or subcutaneous implanted ports are used primarily in patients requiring home TPN [24,28]. Peripherally inserted central catheters can be used for several weeks or months for patients both at home and in the hospital. (*Adapted from* Howard [23].)

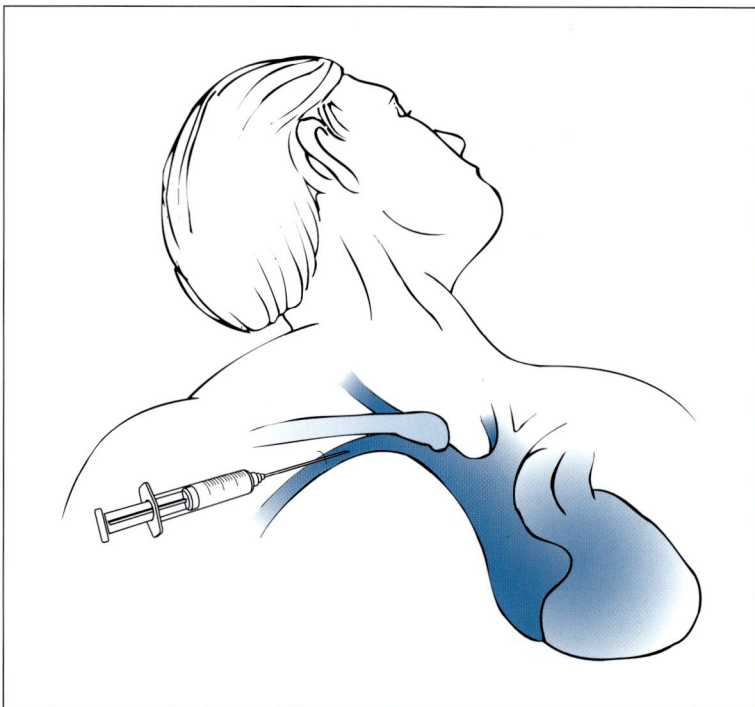

FIGURE 14-16. Correct positioning of the total parenteral nutrition (TPN) catheter. Safe and effective administration of hypertonic TPN solution requires access to the central venous system. The preferred site for TPN infusion is via a subclavian vein catheter, with the tip advanced to the superior vena cava. This can be done safely at bedside. (*Adapted from* Bistrian [25].)

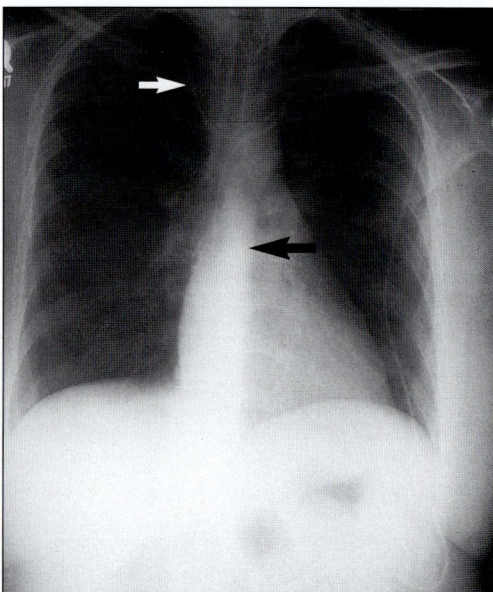

FIGURE 14-17. Chest radiograph demonstrating proper positioning of the tip of a central venous catheter in the superior vena cava (*large arrow*) and a misplaced central venous catheter in a vein in the neck (*small arrow*).

TYPICAL CONSIDERATIONS WHEN TPN BEGINS

Considerations	Possible Status at Initiation of TPN	Comments
Protein, carbohydrate, and energy needs	Dynamic, fluctuating	Must be established to initiate therapy, may be estimated or measured directly
Fluid balance	Fluid overloaded	Common finding in many critically ill patients, may be exacerbated by multiple intraveous medication, may preclude initial administration of optimal calculated protein and coloric needs, may increase morbidity and mortality if exacerbated by too vigorous TPN fluid administration
Glucose and electrolyte abnormalities	Present	Must be identified and corrected, must be quantified and all losses assessed (nasogastric, stool, urine)
Acid–base status	Abnormal	TPN alone is not associated with acidosis or alkalosis, possible to add specific substance (ie, sodium or potassium acetate, hydrochloric acid) to nutrition solution to manipulate serum pH
Concurrent illness	Present	May require specific modification or tailoring of TPN solution to match clinical requirements
Micronutrient deficiency	Present	Administer appropriate trace elements, cofactors, and vitamins
Venous access	Require sterile, dedicated site	Perform central venous cannulation (subclavian, internal jugular, external jugular vein)
Availability of functioning enteral access	Present, not delivering full enteral diet	Protocol for transitional (combination) feeding considered, pending full enteral diet

FIGURE 14-18. Typical considerations when total parenteral nutrition (TPN) begins [25]. (*Adapted from* Bistrian [25].)

MECHANICAL COMPLICATIONS OF TPN

Complications	Prevention or Treatment
Catheter misplacement	Perform chest radiography after central venous catheter placed
Pneumothorax	Perform end-expiratory chest radiography; observe whether pneumothorax is small (5%–10%), perform closed-tube thoracotomy if pneumothorax is large or tension
Bleeding	Evaluate and treat for bleeding disorders before line is placed
Arterial laceration	Repair surgically
Air embolism	Secure the integrity of the catheter system and fix all connections; position the patient in the Durant position (on left side, head down, feet elevated); and aspirate blood and air through the catheter
Pulmonary embolism	Perform ventilation–perfusion scan; administer anticoagulants
Cardiac arrhythmia	Withdraw catheter to superior vena cava; treat arrhythmia
Myocardial perforation	Perform chest radiography for catheter position
Venous thrombosis	Administer anticoagulants; remove catheter

FIGURE 14-19. Mechanical complications of total parenteral nutrition (TPN) [26,27,29]. Complications of TPN are generally divided into three categories: mechanical, infectious, and metabolic [30]. Mechanical complications are not specific to TPN but are those related to central venous catheter placement. The reported incidence of mechanical complications has ranged from 0.3% to 12% [31]. When skilled, experienced physicians perform the procedure, the complication rate is substantially reduced.

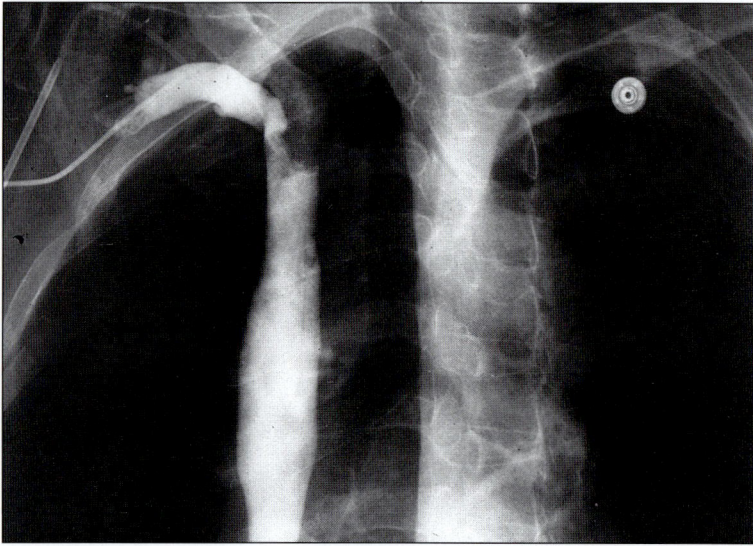

FIGURE 14-20. Venous thrombosis. Venous thrombosis is one of the most common complications of central venous catheterization. Although the incidence of catheter-related thrombosis diagnosed on the basis of clinical symptoms alone is only 0% to 4.8%, venography has detected mural thrombi in 28% to 54% in patients with central venous catheters [32]. Complications of catheter-related thrombosis include catheter-related infection, septic thrombophlebitis, superior vena cava syndrome, pulmonary embolism, and loss of venous access [33]. Patients may present with pain in the neck area, swelling of the face and arms, or dyspnea from a pulmonary embolism. The diagnosis is usually confirmed by venous contrast study. Treatment requires removal of the catheter with or without anticoagulation. The use of an anticoagulant (heparin and/or warfarin) [34] in a small dose [32] reduces the risk of thrombosis.

INFECTIOUS COMPLICATIONS OF TPN: CATHETER-RELATED SEPSIS

Culture Result				Treatment	
Catheter Tip	**Peripheral Blood Count**	**Aspirate Blood Culture**	**Interpretation**	**Temporary Catheter**	**Long-Term Catheter***
Negative	Negative	Negative	No infection	None	None
Negative	Positive	Positive	Sepsis, not related to catheter	Systemic antibiotic, catheter change over guidewire	Systemic antiobiotics
Negative	Positive	Negative			
Positive	Negative	Negative	Catheter colonization or infection[†]	Catheter change over guidewire	Culture-specific antibiotic through catheter, catheter removal or change over guidewire
Negative	Negative	Positive			
Positive	Negative	Positive			
Positive	Positive	Positive	Catheter sepsis	Catheter removal, culture-specific antibiotics, resite catheter	Catheter removal, culture-specific antibiotics, resite catheter, culture-specific antibiotics through catheter, and catheter change over guidewire (only patients with severe limitation of central venous access)
Positive	Positive	Negative			

*Tunneled catheter or implantable venous infusion port.
[†]Colonization or infection with virulent bacteria (eg, Staphylococcus aureus) or fungi warrants treatment as catheter sepsis.

FIGURE 14-21. Infectious complications of total parenteral nutrition (TPN): catheter-related sepsis [35]. Catheter-related bloodstream infections remain an important cause of nosocomial infection and produce significant morbidity and mortality [36]. Although fever is the only sign of catheter-related infection in most patients, hypothermia, tachycardia, tachypnea, hypotension, and a decrease in mental status may also be present. Leukocytosis with increasing band forms [37] is usually seen. When patients who are receiving TPN develop a new or changing fever pattern, a fever workup should be performed. Blood culture should be drawn through the catheter, from the catheter tip after exchanging over a guidewire for a temporary catheter, and from peripheral blood. Treatment is based on culture results. *Adapted from* Lowell and Bothe [35]; with permission.

METABOLIC COMPLICATIONS OF TPN

Complication	Cause(s)	Prevention/Treatment
Hyperglycemia	Abnormal glucose homeostasis in critically ill patients (increased stress hormone)	Monitor blood sugar; start with 100–150 g glucose on day 1, then increase by 50 g/d if glucose control is acceptable (100–220 mg/dL), particularly in critically ill or diabetic patients; do not provide excess glucose; add insulin as needed
Hypoglycemia	Abrupt withdrawal of TPN	Slowly taper TPN in 1–2 hr before discontinuing
Hypertriglyceridemia	Excessive fat administration	Do not give >1–1.5 g/kg/d
Refeeding syndrome	Glucose-induced hypophosphatemia leading ot cardiac dysfunction; fluid overloaded (usually seen in patients who lose >30% of their usual weight)	Start with small amount of dextrose and volume, then gradually increase over a few days; provide adequate amount and monitoring of electrolytes, particularly Na^+, K^+, PO_4
Fluid overloaded	Excess fluid administration	Monitor fluid intake/output and daily weight
Hypophosphatemia	Inadequate phosphorus administration	Monitor PO_4; provide as needed
Hypocalcemia, hypercalcemia, hypokalemia, hyperkalemia, hypomagnesemia, hypermagnesemia	Excess/inadequate TPN administration	Monitor serum levels; provide as needed
Cholestatic hepatitis	Decreased water content of bile; excess fat administration	Do not give excess fat
Abnormal liver function	Excess glycogen and fat deposition in liver from overfeeding or sepsis	Do not overfeed; monitor liver function test

FIGURE 14-22. Metabolic complications of total parenteral nutrition (TPN). With better knowledge of nutrition support among specialists who prescribe TPN and the development and use of nutrition support teams, many metabolic complications of TPN (eg, electrolyte abnormalities, vitamin and mineral deficiency) have become more manageable. However, hyperglycemia is still a common problem [38,39].

A PRACTICAL TECHNIQUE TO PROVIDE TPN TO PATIENTS WITH DIABETES MELLITUS

Estimated caloric requirement: 20–25 kcal/kg/d

Optimal rate of glucose infusion: 2–4 mg/kg/min

Glucose control goal: 100–200 mg/dL

In patients with diabetes mellitus or abnormal glucose tolerance from critical illness or steroid use, the following is appropriate:

Amount of dextrose in TPN is restricted to 100–150 g on the first day

Add half of the home daily insulin requirement to the TPN admixture for patients on insulin at home or two thirds of the insulin required in the past 24 hours for patients with abnormal glucose tolerance from critical illness or steroid use receiving insulin in the hospital

Monitor blood glucose level every 6 hours

Sliding-scale insulin

200–250 mg/dL	2–3 U
251–300 mg/dL	4–6 U
301–350 mg/dL	6–8 U
>350 mg/dL	8–12 U

Add two thirds of the sliding-scale insulin to the next TPN admixture

When blood glucose level is consistently <200 mg/dL, the amount of dextrose should be advanced by 50–100 g/d, with the insulin dose increased in proportion of the amount of dextrose increased

Increase calories provided by fat when blood glucose level is consistently high

FIGURE 14-23. A practical technique to provide total parenteral nutrition (TPN) to patients with diabetes mellitus [40–43].

Enteral Nutrition

INDICATIONS FOR ENTERAL FEEDING

In the following clinical settings, enteral nutrition should be a part of routine care:

  Protein–calorie malnutrition (>10% loss of usual weight or serum albumin levels <3.5 g/dL) with inadequate intake of nutrients for the previous 5 days

  Normal nutritional status with less than 50% of required nutrient intake orally for the previous 7–10 d

  Severe dysphagia

  Major full-thickness burns

  Small bowel resection in combination with administration of total parenteral nutrition

In the following clinical settings, enteral nutrition would usually be helpful:

  Major trauma (enteral nutrition would be contraindicated if paralytic ileus ensues)

  Radiation therapy

  Mild chemotherapy

  Liver failure and severe renal dysfunction

In the following clinical settings, enteral nutrition is of limited or undetermined value:

  Intensive chemotherapy (parenteral nutrition may be indicated for individuals with severe symptoms)

  Immediate postoperative period if patient is expected to resume oral intake within 5–7 d

  Acute enteritis

  <10% of the small intestine remaining

Enteral nutrition should not be used in the following clinical settings:

  Complete mechanical intestinal obstruction

  Ileus or intestinal hypomotility

  Severe diarrhea (resistance to pharmacologic therapy)

  High-output external fistula (>500 mL/d)

  Severe acute pancreatitis

  Patients with hypovolemic or septic shock

  Not desired by patients or legal guardian

  Prognosis does not warrant aggressive nutritional support

FIGURE 14-24. Indications for enteral feeding [18]. (*Adapted from* the American Society for Parenteral and Enteral Nutrition Board of Directors [18].)

TYPES OF AND USES FOR ENTERAL FEEDING TUBES

Type of Tube	Clinical Uses	Disadvantages
Nasoenteric	For short-term use (<30 d)	
Nasogastric	Large caliber can be used to decompress stomach, monitor gastric pH, provide medication or feeding; small caliber is used for feeding only	Aspiration, nasal and esophageal irritation, sinusitis
Nasojejunal	Patients at risk for aspiration, gastroparesis	Clogging, diarrhea more common
Enterostomy	For long-term use (>30 d)	
Gastrostomy	Swallowing disorders	Aspiration
Jejunostomy	Patients with tracheal aspiration, reflux esophagitis, gastroparesis, insufficient stomach from previous resection	Clogging, tube placement, diarrhea
Gastrojejunostomy	Patients with gastroparesis, pancreatitis, or proximal leak	Clogging

FIGURE 14-25. Types of and uses for enteral feeding tubes [6].

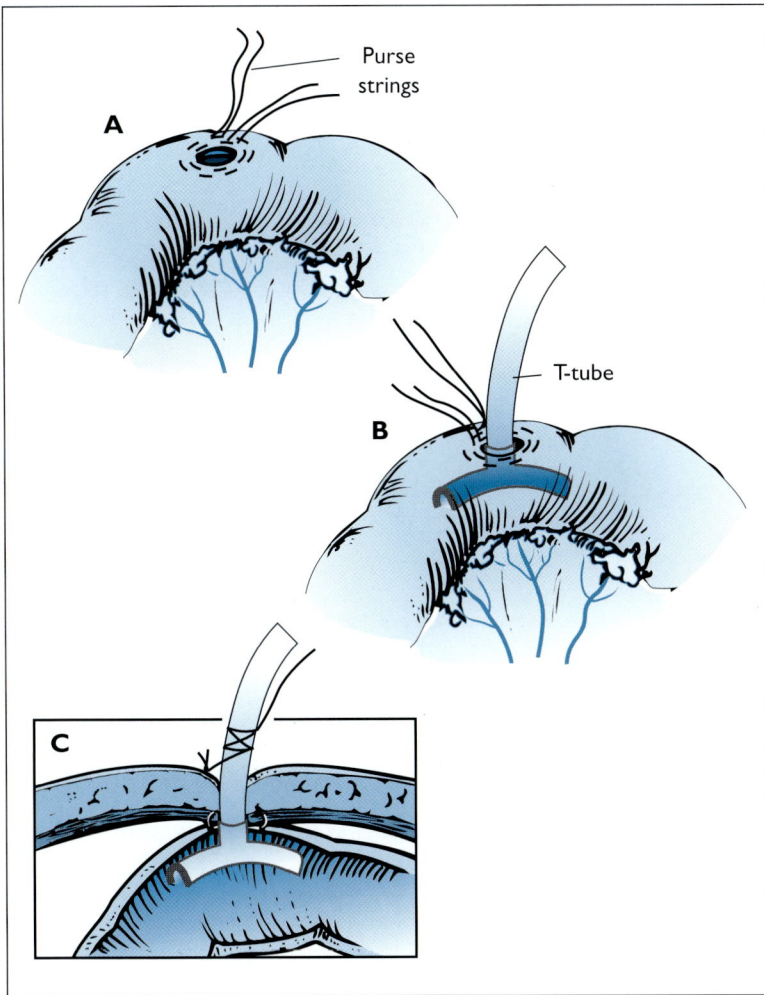

FIGURE 14-26. Jejunostomy tube insertion (A–C) [44]. An enterostomy tube can be placed endoscopically, radiologically, or surgically. Each technique has its own risks, benefits and complications. (Adapted from Bradley et al. [44].)

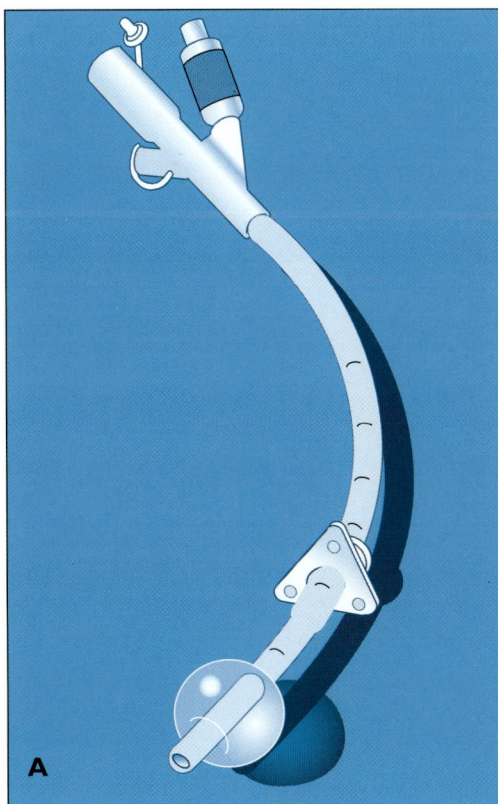

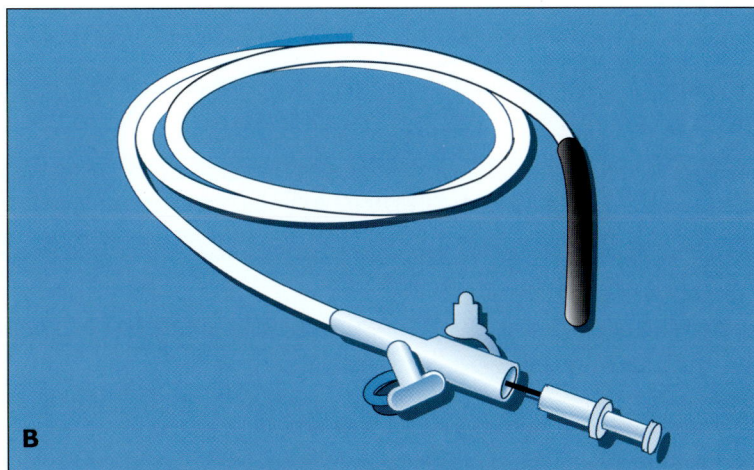

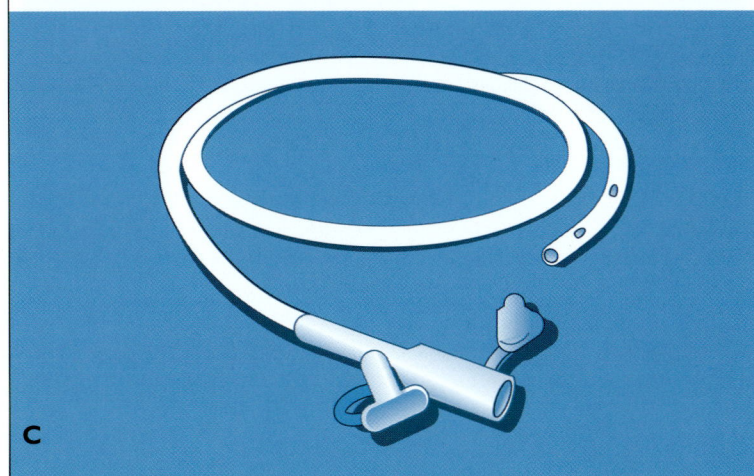

FIGURE 14-27. Enterostomy tubes. Enterostomy tubes are used for long-term enteral feeding (>1 month). A, Gastrostomy tube. B, Jejunostomy tubes.

ENTERAL FORMULAS

	Nutritionally Complete Formula	Elemental Formula
Description	Polymeric	Monomeric
General characteristics	Complete meal replacements	Protein as amino acid or peptides low in fat
Protein	15%–25% of claories from casein, soy, beef	8%–18% of calories from hydrolysed casein, whey, meat
Carbohydrate	50%–58% of calories from cornstarch, sucrose, corn syrup	70%–90% of calories from glucose, oligosaccharides, sucrose
Fat	21%–36% of calories from corn oil, soy oil, MCT oil	1%–2% of calories from sunflower oil, MCT oil
Osmolality range, *mOsm/kg water*	290–625	460–810
Caloric density, *kcal/mL*	1, 1.5, or 2	1
Na/K, *mmol/L*	15–40/26–25	15–30/30–35
Patient characteristics suitable for the formula	Anorexia, cancerous cachexia postoperative phase, burns	Enterocutaneous fistula, short-bowel syndrome, pancreatic insufficiency, inflammatory bowel disease

Special Enteral Formula

Hepatic encephalogpathy	Renal failure	State of severe metabolic stress
High in branched-chain amino acids and low in aromatic amino acids	Contains all essential amino acids	High in branched-chain amino acids but not low in aromatic amino acids
15%–25% of calories from free amino acids	8%–12% of calories from free amino acids	20%–25% of calories from free amino acids
50%–58% of calories from glucose, sucrose, oligosaccharides	60%–70%of calories from sucrose, oligosaccharides	6%–8% of calories from glucose, sucrose, oligosaccharides
20%–25% of calories from MCT oil, sunflower oil	10%–15% of calories from MCT oil, sunflower oil	6%–8% of calories from MCT oil, sunflower oil
500–600	590–1000	600–700
1–1.5	1.5	1
Generally electrolyte-free	10–15/<5	25/30
Patients with acute or chronic hepatic encephalopathy	Patients with acute renal failure	Multiple trauma, severe burns, severe sepsis

FIGURE 14-28. Enteral formulas [46]. MCT—medium-chain triglyceride. (*Adapted from* Shanbhogue *et al.* [46].)

ENTERAL FEEDING ADMINISTRATION GUIDELINES

Begin at low rate of full-strength formula (10–20 mL/hr).

Increase rate gradually (ie, 10 mL/hr every 24 h in the most critically ill and every 8–12 h for less severely ill patients)

Monitor for tolerance (eg, diarrhea, refeeding syndrome)

Aspirate stomach contents to check residual volume every 4–6 hr (for intragastric tube feeding only), hold or reduce the rate of the formula in half if residual >150 mL. Do not check for residual in postpyloric fed patients.

Elevate the top of the patient's bed to at least 30° to reduce the risk of aspiration.

FIGURE 14-29. Enteral feeding administration guidelines [45,46].

MONITORING DURING ENTERAL NUTRITION SUPPORT

Baseline	Serum albumin
	Weight
	Electrolytes, BUN, creatinine
	Ca^{++}, Mg^{++}, PO_4
	Blood glucose
	Liver function test
Daily	Fluid status (intake/output)
	Weight
	Blood glucose (as needed)
	Site of feeding tube
Weekly	Electrolytes, BUN, creatinine (more frequent if indicated)
	Ca^{++}, Mg^{++}, PO_4
	24-h urine urea nitrogen/creatinine
Every 3 wk	Serum albumin

FIGURE 14-30. Monitoring during enteral nutrition support [47]. BUN—blood urea nitrogen.

COMPLICATIONS OF ENTERAL NUTRITION

Complication	Prevention/Treatment
Aspiration	Use constant infusion instead of intermittent bolus; elevate head of the bed while feeding; monitor for and avoid gastric distention; feed postpylorically
Diarrhea	Reduce rate and/or concentration of tube feeding; review and avoid all medications that might cause diarrhea; treat antibiotic-associated diarrhea; add bulking agents (eg, phyllium or antispasmodic agent)
High gastric residuals	Identify patients at risk for delayed gastric emptying (eg, sepsis, hyperglycemia, diabetic gastroparesis, trauma, myocardial infarction); add prokinetic agents (eg, metoclopramide, cisapride, erythromycin); feed postpylorically
Dehydration	Monitor fluid balance and daily weight; provide adequate free water, particularly for patients on high-density tube feeding and patients with uncontrolled fluid loss
Refeeding syndrome	Identify patients at risk (marasmic patients); monitor fluid balance, daily weight, electrolytes, Ca^{++}, Mg^{++}, PO_4, and blood sugar

FIGURE 14-31. Complications of enteral nutrition [47-49].

ETHICAL ISSUES OF NUTRITION SUPPORT

Guidelines in this section are not coded; clinical studies do not form the basis of these recommendations.

Patients or their legally authorized surrogates have the right to accept or refuse nutrition support.

Patients should be encouraged to make known (preferably in writing) their desires regarding the use of life-sustaining treatment, including nutrition support, before a crisis occurs and while they still have decision-making capabilities.

Nutrition support should be given when the patient or surrogate desires it and scientific evidence and prevailing standards of practice indicate that the patient will probably benefit.

If, from the patient's or surrogate's perspective, the burdens of nutrition support outweigh the benefits, it is ethical to withhold or withdraw treatment. The oral or written refusal of a competent patient should be honored in any event, as should the refusal of a legally authorized surrogate.

When the benefits and burdens of nutrition support are unclear, time-limited trials are highly recommended.

Providers who are unwilling or unable to honor a valid request to forgo nutrition support (because of personal beliefs or institutional policy) should make reasonable efforts to arrange for prompt transfer of the patient's care to a practitioner or facility willing to implement the instructions.

Because of the difficult and often controversial nature of decisions to withhold or withdraw nutrition support and because of the perceived potential for abuse, health care institutions should develop written policies governing such decisions. Once adopted, these policies must be made known to patients at the time of admission, as required by the Patient Self-Determination Act. The policies should be subject to periodic review. In addition, institutions should monitor and periodically review surrogate decisions to withhold or withdraw nutrition support from incapacitated patients.

Health care providers should not make unilateral decisions to provide, withhold, or withdraw nutrition support on the basis of limiting costs or rationing scarce resources for the benefit of society, unless required by law. No such laws exist at this time.

A bioethics committee should be available to help surrogates make decisions on behalf of incapacitated patients. The patient's privacy should be protected throughout the decision-making process.

FIGURE 14-32. Ethical issues of nutrition support [18]. (*Adapted from* the American Society for Parenteral and Enteral Nutrition Board of Directors [18].)

References

1. Elmer R, Weiner DO: Intravenous alimentation with special reference to protein (amino acid) metabolism. *JAMA* 1939, 122:796.

2. Aubaniac R: L'injection intraveineuse sous claviculaire: avantage et technique. *Presse Med* 1952, 60:1456.

3. Dudrick SJ: The genesis of intravenous hyperalimentation. *JPEN* 1977, 1:23.

4. Dudrick SJ, Wilmore DW, Vars HM, Rhoads JR: Long term total parenteral nutrition with growth, development and positive nitrogen balance. *Surgery* 1968, 64:134–142.

5. Wilmore DW, Dudrick SJ: Growth and development of an infant receiving all nutrients exclusively by vein. *JAMA* 1968, 203:S60.

6. Shike M. Enteral nutrition. In *Modern Nutrition in Health and Disease*. Edited by Shils M, Olson J, Shike M, Ross AC. Baltimore: Williams & Wilkins; 1999:1643–1656.

7. Ham RJ: The signs and symptoms of poor nutritional status. *Prim Care* 1994, 21:33–54.

8. Blackburn GL, Bistrian BR, Baltej SM, et al.: Nutritional and metabolic assessment of the hospitalized patient. *JPEN J Parenter Enteral Nutr* 1977, 1:11–22.

9. Bistrian BR: Nutritional assessment of the hospitalized patient: a practical approach. In *Nutritional Assessment*. Edited by Wright RA, Heymsfield S, McManus III CB. Boston: Blackwell; 1984:183–205.

10. Stack JA, Babineau TJ, Bistrian BR: Assessment of nutritional status in clinical practice. *Gastroenterologist* 1996, 4(suppl 1):S8–S15.

11. Smith LC, Mullen JL: Nutritional assessment and indications for nutritional support. *Surg Clin North Am* 1991, 71:449–457.

12. McMahon MM, Farnell MB, Murray MJ: Nutritional support of critically ill patients. *Mayo Clin Proc* 1993, 68:911–920.

13. Van Way III CW: Nutritional support in injured patients. *Surg Clin North Am* 1991, 71:537–548.

14. Reinhardt GF, Myskofsky JW, Wilkens DB, et al.: Incidence and mortality of hypoalbuminemic patients in hospitalized veterans. *JPEN* 1980, 4:357–359.

15. Bray GA: Obesity: Definition, diagnoses and disadvantages. *Med J Aust* 1985, (suppl 142):S2–S8.

16. Hardy JD: Nutrition and cancer. In *American College of Surgeons, Committee on Pre and Postoperative Care Manual of Surgical Nutrition*. Edited by Balinger WF, et al. Philadelphia: WB Saunders Co; 1975:369–385.

17. Babineau TJ, Borlase BC, Blackburn GL: Applied total parenteral nutrition in the critically ill. In *Intensive Care Medicine*. Edited by Rippe JM, Irwin RS, Alpert JS, Fink MP. Boston: Little Brown; 1991:1675–1691.

18. American Society for Parenteral and Enteral Nutrition Board of Directors: Guidelines for the use of parenteral and enteral nutrition in adult and pediatric patients. *JPEN* 1993, 17(suppl):1SA–52SA.

19. Kenler AS, Blackburn GL, Babineau TJ: Total parenteral nutrition: priorities and practice. In *Textbook of Critical Care*. Edited by Ayres SM, Grenvik A, Holbrook PR, Shoemaker WC. Philadelphia: WB Saunders Co; 1995:1116–1126.

20. Cerra FB, Benitez MR, Blackburn GL, et al.: A consensus statement of the American College of Chest Physicians. *Chest* 1997, 111:769–778.

21. Driscoll DF, Blackburn GL: Total parenteral nutrition 1990: a review of its current status in hospitalized patients, and the need for patient-specific feeding. *Drugs* 1990, 40:346–363.

22. American Medical Association Department of Foods and Nutrition: Multivitamin preparations for parenteral use: a statement by the Advisory Group. *JPEN J Parenter Enteral Nutr* 1979, 3:258–262.

23. Howard L: Enteral and parenteral nutrition therapy. In *Harrison's Principles of Internal Medicine*. Edited by Fauci AS, Braunwald E, Isselbacher KJ, et al. New York: McGraw-Hill; 1998:472–480.

24. Latifi R, Dudrick SJ: Nutrition in surgical patients. In *Practical Handbook of Nutrition in Clinical Practice*. Edited by Kirby DF, Dudrick SJ. Boca Raton, FL: CRC Press; 1994:151–152.

25. Bistrian BR: Total parenteral nutrition solution requirements. In *APEX: The Perceptorship for Excellence in Parenteral Nutrition Support*. Edited by Bistrian BR. Norwalk, CT: Health Management Solutions; 1996: 5.1–5.20.

26. Hickey MS: Parenteral nutrition therapy guidelines. In *Handbook of Enteral, Parenteral, and ARC/AIDS Nutrition Therapy*. Edited by Hickey MS. St. Louis: Mosby–Year Book; 1992: 110–173.

27. Van Way III CW, Allen JA: Intravenous nutrition. In *Handbook of Surgical Nutrition*. Edited by Van Way III CW. Philadelphia: JB Lippincott; 1992:73–92.

28. Band JD: Central venous catheter-related infection: Types of devices and definition. *UpToDate* 1998, CD ROM ed, 6–3.

29. Flower JF, Ryan JA, Gough JA: Catheter-related complications of total parenteral nutrition. In *Total Parenteral Nutrition*. Edited by Fischer JE. Boston: Little, Brown; 1991:25–46.

30. Bistrian BR: Interaction of metabolic and infectious complications in total parenteral nutrition. ASPEN 20th Clinical Congress Proceedings 1996, Washington, DC, 1996:58–62.

31. Manfield PF, Hohn DC, Fornage BD, et al.: Complications and failures of subclavian vein catheterization. *N Engl J Med* 1994, 331:1735–1738.

32. Lowell JA, Bothe A: Central venous catheter related thrombosis. *Surg Oncol Clin N Am* 1995, 4:479–492.

33. Harre WD: Catheter induced upper extremity venous thrombosis. *UpToDate* 1998, CD ROM ed, 6–3.

34. Imperial J, Bistrian BR, Both AJ, et al.: Limitation of central vein thrombosis in total parenteral nutrition by continuous infusion of low dose heparin. *J Am Coll Nutr* 1983, 2:63–73.

35. Lowel JA, Bothe AJ: Venous access: preoperative, operative, and post-operative dilemmas. *Surg Clin North Am* 1991, 71:1231–1246.

36. Maki DG: Infections due to infusion therapy. In *Hospital Infections*, edn 2. Edited by Bennett JV, Brachman PS. Boston: Little, Brown; 1992:849.

37. Adal KA, Farr BM: Central venous catheter-related infections: a review. *Nutrition* 1996, 12:208–213.

38. Apovian CM, McMahon MM, Bistrian BR: Guidelines for refeeding the marasmic patient. *Crit Care Med* 1990, 18:1030–1033.

39. Solomon SM, Kirby DF: The refeeding syndrome: a review. *JPEN J Parenter Enteral Nutr* 1990, 14:90–97 .

40. Ahmad A, Bistrian BR: Providing nutritional support for critically ill diabetic patients. *J Crit Illness* 1995, 616–625.

41. McMahon MM, Rizza RA: Nutrition support in hospitalized patients with diabetes mellitus. *Mayo Clin Proc* 1996, 71:587–594.

42. Hongsermeier T, Bistrian BR: Evaluation of a practical technique for determining insulin requirement in diabetic patients receiving total parenteral nutrition. *JPEN J Parenter Enteral Nutr* 1993, 17:16–19.

43. Pomposelli J, Bistrian BR: Is TPN immunosuppressive? *New Horiz* 1994, 2:224–229.

44. Bradley C, Borlase, BC, Forse RA: Feeding tube placement. In *Enteral Nutrition*. Edited by Borlase BC, Bell SJ, Blackburn GL, Forse RA. New York: Chapman & Hall; 1994:193–198.

45. American Gastroenterological Association Medical Position Statement: guideline for the use of enteral nutrition. *Gastroenterology* 1995, 108:1280–1281.

46. Shanbhogue LKR, Bistrian BR, Blackburn GL: Trends in enteral nutrition in surgical patients. *J R Coll Surg Edinb* 1986, 31:267–273.

47. Rombeau JL, Caldwell MD, eds: *Clinical Nutrition: Enteral and Tube Feeding*. Philadelphia: WB Saunders Co; 1990.

48. Benya R, Mobarhan S: Enteral alimentation: administration and complications. *J Am Coll Nutr* 1991, 10:209–219.

49. Heimburger DC, Weinsier RL, eds: *Handbook of Clinical Nutrition*. St. Louis: Mosby–Year Book; 1997.

Index

mortality risk with, 72-73
office visit components in treating, 98
with overgrowth, 21
pharmacologic treatments for, 103-105
phenotypic expression of in adult men, 126
physician as agent of change for, 97
recommended diet for hypercholesterolemia
in, 131
reproductive function and, 133
sarcopenic, 99
surgical treatment for, 105-106
systolic and diastolic blood pressures with, 78
vertically integrated management of, 97-106
visceral, 69
Obesity gene, 134
Ob/ob mouse, 71
Oils, 2
plant sterols in, 129
Oligopeptides, 156
Oligovulation, 143
Omega 3 fatty acids
in cytokine production, 61
structure of, 128
Omega 6 fatty acids, 128
Omega-3-rich oils, 1
Omeprazole, 161
Oncogenes
activation of, 173
in cancer cell growth, 167
Onion, organosulfides in, 175
Optico-septal dysplasia, 142
Organosulfides, 175
Orlistat
long-term effects of, 104
pharmacologic actions of, 103
weight loss with, 104, 105
Orthopedic problems, 26
Osteoarthritis
with obesity, 69
obesity and, 77
Osteoporosis, 34
with calcium deficiency, 34
with restrained eating in adolescents, 17
Overnutrition, 1
lack of adaptation to, 69, 81
metabolism with, 4
overgrowth and, 21
Overweight
age-adjusted prevalence of, 98
lean vs. fat, 97
Oxalic acid, 10
Oxidant stress processes, 1
Oxidation stress, 8-9
Oxindole alkaloids, 85
Oxygen
function and amount of in body, 10
saturation of in obesity, 79
Oxygen radicals, scavengers of, 8
Oxygenated ligands, 13

P

Panax ginseng, 88
Pancreas, exocrine and endocrine secretion of, 153
Pancreatic enzymes, 149
regulation of after meal, 153
therapeutic, 161
Pancreatic insufficiency, 161

Pancreatic lipase, 154
Pancreatic proteases, 156
Pancreatitis, 161
Pantothenic acid
in energy metabolism, 32
neurologic and behavioral effects of, 46
recommended levels for, 187
Paranoia, 46
Parasitism, 163
Parathyroid hormone, 44
Parenteral nutrition, 199
catheter positioning for, 206
chest radiography of catheter in, 206
considerations with, 207
guidelines for, 204
indications for, 204
infectious complications of, 208
mechanical complications of, 207-208
metabolic complications of, 209
micronutrient administration guidelines in, 205
practical technique with diabetes mellitus, 209
routes of, 203
starting, 205
venous access for, 206
Parenting, in childhood obesity, 17
Parthenolide, 87
Patient Self-Determination Act, 213
Peal flour, 5
Peanut meal, 5
Peas, fiber in, 127
Pellagra, 33
with vitamin deficiency, 46
Pepsins, 156
Peptidase, 156
Peptide neurotransmitters, 151
Peptide YY, 151
Peripheral axonopathy, 46
Peripheral neuropathy, 46
Peripheral parenteral nutrition, 203
Pesticides, carcinogenic, 14
Phenolic acids, 175
Phenolphthalein, 45
Phentermine, 103
Phenylalanine, 5
Phenytoin, 45
Phospholipids, 5
Phosphorus
in bone remodelling, 44
function and amount of in body, 10
RDA requirements for, 34
recommended dietary intake of, 33
recommended levels for, 187
Photomedicines, prescriptions of in Germany, 83
Photooxidative vision damage, 47
Phthalides, 175
Phytates, 175
Phytic acid, 10
Phytochemicals, 1, 13
antioxidant, 8
in carcinogen activation, 172
in diet, 2
in fruits and vegetables, 9
Phytoestrogens, 177
Phytosterols, 124
characteristics of, 129
in cholesterol reduction, 119, 130
in common foods, 129
Pima Indians

gene-environment interaction in, 15
obesity in, 74
Pinto beans, protein value of, 5
Plants. *See also* Botanical supplements
anticancer agents in, 175
in diet, 1
hormone-like substances in, 13
natural antioxidants in, 1
phytochemicals of, 1
stanols of, 130
sterols of, 129
Plasma membrane, lipid peroxidation of, 125
Plasminogen activator inhibitor I, 131
Polyacetylenes, 175
in echinacea, 86
Polycyclic aromatic hydrocarbons, 14
Polycystic ovary syndrome
androgen levels with, 144
body composition changes and hyperandrogenemia in, 143
with obesity, 73
obesity and, 133
with upper-body obesity, 69
Polypeptides, 156
Polyphenols, 9
in green tea, 89
protective action of, 14
Polysaccharides, 6
in astragalus, 84
Polyunsaturated fats
in cholesterol oxidation, 125
in cholesterol reduction, 125
impaired immune function and, 53
Polyunsaturated fatty acids, 34
Postmenopausal obesity, breast cancer and, 75
Potassium
deficiency of, 34
function and amount of in body, 10
in hypertension, 41
PPAR-gamma receptor, 174
PPN. *See* Peripheral parenteral nutrition
Prader-Willi syndrome, 142
Prepubertal nutrition, 168
Primrose oil, 87
Proanthocyanidins
in grape seed, 89
in St. John's wort, 91
Procyanidin oligomers, 89
Product labeling, herbal, 83, 92-93
Proline, 5
Prostate cancer
arachidonic acid metabolites in, 174
diet and, 167
incidence of in men, 170
obesity and, 169
sex hormone interconversions in, 171
Protein, 2
in American diet, 150
amino acids of, 5
brush-border digestion and transport of, 156
calories stored as, 3
depletion of with starvation or semi-
starvation, 100
in dietary recommendations, 1
dietary recommendations of, 16
digestion of, 8
metabolism of, 4
quality of, 1, 5

Temperature stability, 18
Terpenoids, 9
    protective action of, 14
Testosterone
    interconversions of in cancer, 171
    levels of
        in acute illness, 146
        in polycystic ovary syndrome, 144
        sex hormone-binding globulin and, 143
    obesity and, 141-142
Tetany, 34
Texture, food, 6
T-helper cells, 59
    diet and, 61
Thermogenesis
    hypothalamus in, 70
    impaired, 28
Thiamin, 9
    deficiency of, neurologic and behavioral effects
        of, 46
    recommended levels for, 187
Thiamin pyrophosphate, 32
Threonine, 5
Thrifty gene hypothesis, 15
Thrombosis, catheter-related, 208
Thymic involution, 58
Thymus
    in malnourished children, 62
    size of with age, 58
    T cells in, 59
Thyroid hormone, neonatal, 25
Thyroxine, 55
Tin, 10
Tobacco smoke, carcinogenic, 14
Tolerable upper intake level, 188
Total parenteral nutrition, 203
    catheter positioning for, 206
    considerations with, 207
    indications for, 204
    infectious complications of, 208
    macronutrient guidelines in, 204
    mechanical complications of, 207-208
    metabolic complications of, 209
    micronutrient guidelines for, 205
    practical technique with diabetes mellitus, 209
    starting, 205
    venous access for, 206
TPN. See Total parenteral nutrition
Transcobalamin, 157
Transferrin receptor, 159
    production of, 12
Triceps skinfold test, 179, 180
Triceps skinfold thickness, 181
    genetics in, 26
Trigger foods, 101
Triglycerides
    breakdown of, 123
    in diabetes type 2, 110
    diet and plasma concentrations of, 112, 115, 126
    dietary fats and sugars and, 126
    dietary fiber and, 115
    digestion and absorption of, 154
    endogenous, 123
    functions of, 5
    long-chain and medium-chain, 154
    metabolism of, 122
    plasma clearance of, 113
    storage of, 8
    structure of, 128
Triiodothyronine, 55

Triterpenes, 175
    in valerian, 92
Tropical sprue, 163
Trypsin, 156
Tryptamine, 15
Tryptophan, 5
Tube feeding, routes of, 203. See also Enteral
        nutrition; Parenteral nutrition
Tumor suppressor genes, 167
Tumors
    host metabolism and, 177
    phytochemicals inhibiting, 13
    in rats, 177
Tyrosine, 5
Tyrosine kinase inhibitors, 13

U

UI. See Tolerable upper intake level
Undernutrition
    chronic, in reproductive dysfunction, 136-139
    maternal, 138
    sexual maturation and, 133
Uniparental disomy, 142
Upper-body fat measurement, 73
Urinary tract infections
    cranberry for, 86
    uva-ursi for, 91
Uva-ursi, 91

V

Vaccinium myrtillus, 84
Vagal nerves, 152
Vagus nerve, 150
Valerian, 92
    sales of, 83
Valine, 5
Vanadium
    in diabetes, 49
    function and amount of in body, 10
Vascular disease, 37
Vasoactive intestinal peptide, 151
Vegetable oils, 125
Vegetables
    anticancer agents in, 175
    cruciferous, 167
    dietary recommendations of, 1, 16
    fiber in, 7
    plant sterols in, 129
    soluble and insoluble fiber in, 127
    vitamins and phytochemicals in, 9
Vegetarian Food Guide Pyramid, 195
Venous thrombosis, 208
Vertical banded gastroplasty
    for obesity, 105
    results of, 106
Very-low-density lipoproteins
    in diabetes type 2, 110
    particles of, 122
    particles of in hypercholesterolemia, 122
    plasma levels of, 112, 120
Vision, 47-48
Vitamin A, 9
    absorption and metabolism of, 160
    beta-carotene conversion to, 176
    deficiency of, 64
    in immune function, 50

lung cancer and, 42
    RDA requirements for, 34
Vitamin B, 9
    in energy metabolism, 32
    heart disease and, 37-40
Vitamin B6
    function and deficiency of, 33
    homocysteine and, 38, 39-40
    in immune function, 50
    neurologic and behavioral effects of, 46
    RDA requirements for, 34
    recommended levels for, 187
Vitamin B12
    absorption of, 11, 149, 157
    deficiency of, 33, 156
    homocysteine and, 38, 39-40
    in immune function, 50
    metabolic interaction with folate, 158
    neurologic and behavioral effects of, 46
    recommended levels for, 187
    structure of, 156
    uptake and transfer of, 157
Vitamin C, 9
    antioxidant properties of, 9
    in bone remodelling, 44
    in cancer prevention, 41
    cataracts and, 48
    in cranberry, 86
    deficiency of, 33
        immune function with, 65
    in diabetes, 49
    dietary sources of, 1
    in energy metabolism, 32
    in immune function, 50
    in nutrient metabolism, 1
Vitamin D, 9
    absorption of, 160
    in bone mineral density, 44
    in bone remodelling, 44
    deficiency of, 33
    in diabetes, 49
    in fracture incidence, 45-46
    recommended levels for, 187
    synthesis and activation of, 11
Vitamin D-binding protein, 160
Vitamin D-stimulated pump, 159
Vitamin E
    antioxidant properties of, 9, 33
    in cancer prevention, 41
    cataracts and, 48
    coronary heart disease and, 37
    deficiency of, 33, 34
        immune function with, 64
    in diabetes, 48, 49
    glucose tolerance and, 49
    in hepatitis B in elderly, 65
    in immune function, 50, 51
    neurologic and behavioral effects of, 46
    RDA requirements for, 34
    removal of in food processing, 125
Vitamin K, 9
    in energy metabolism, 32
Vitamins, 2
    absorption of, 149
    in bone health, 44-46
    deficiencies of, 33
        in celiac disease, 163
        in immune function, 50
        impaired immune function and, 53

Color Plates

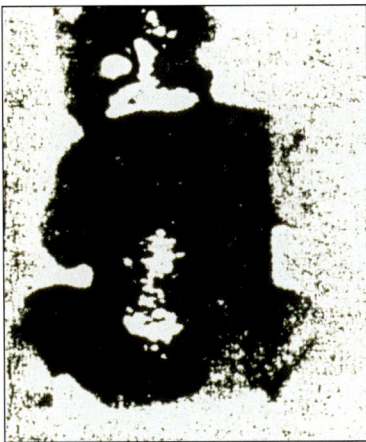

FIGURE 2-3A. Page 18

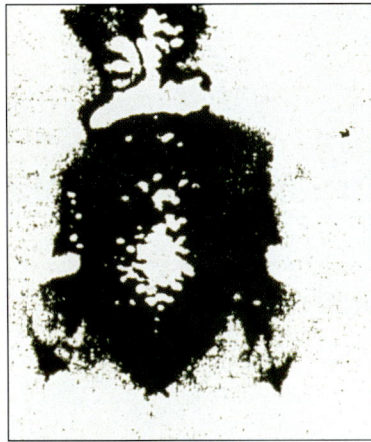

FIGURE 2-3B. Page 18

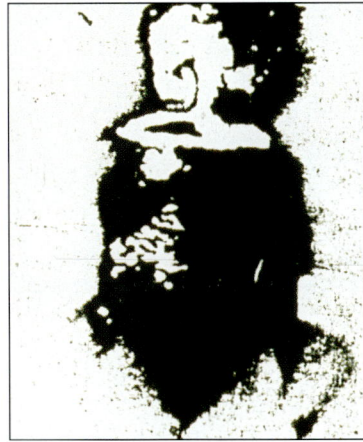

FIGURE 2-3C. Page 18

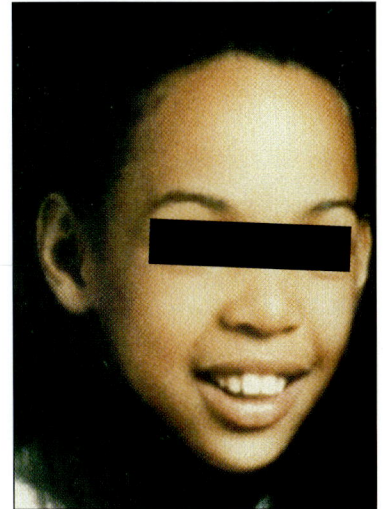

FIGURE 2-19A. Page 26

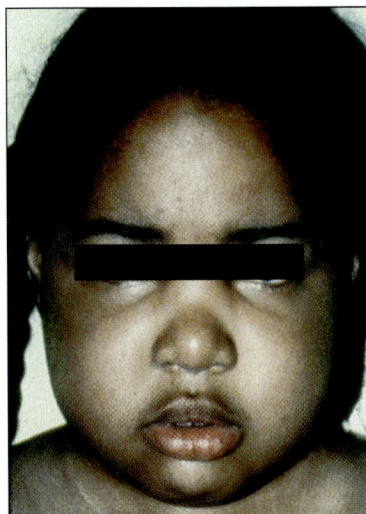

FIGURE 2-19B. Page 26

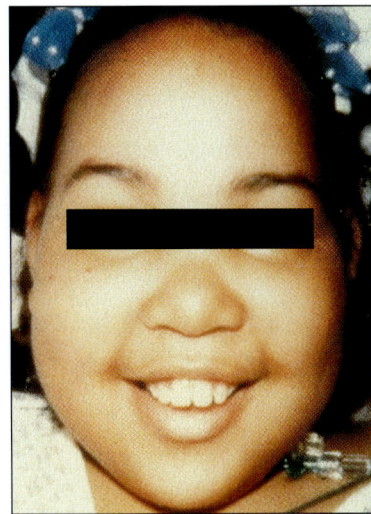

FIGURE 2-19C. Page 26

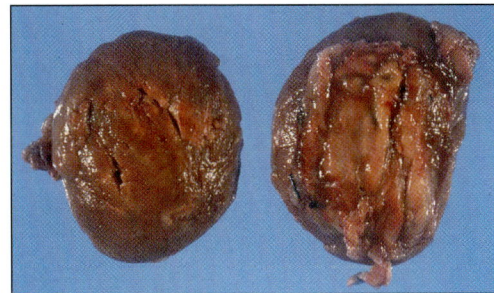

FIGURE 2-19D. Page 26

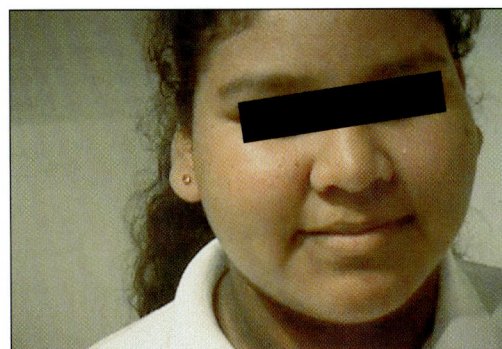

FIGURE 2-25. Page 28

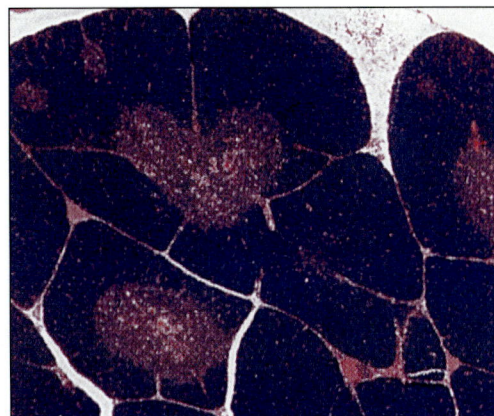

FIGURE 4-12A. Page 58

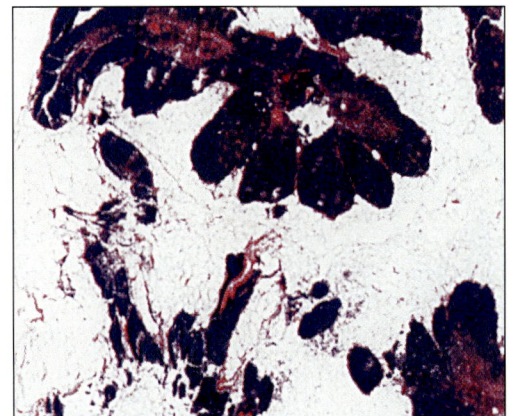

FIGURE 4-12B. Page 58

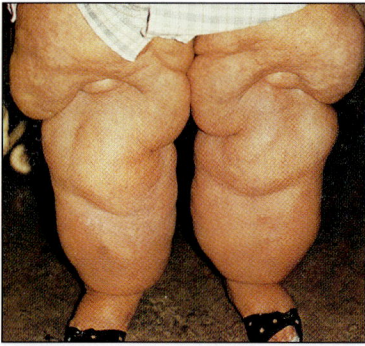

FIGURE 7-30. Page 106

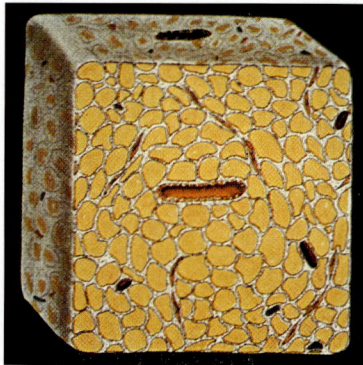

FIGURE 12-21. Page 175

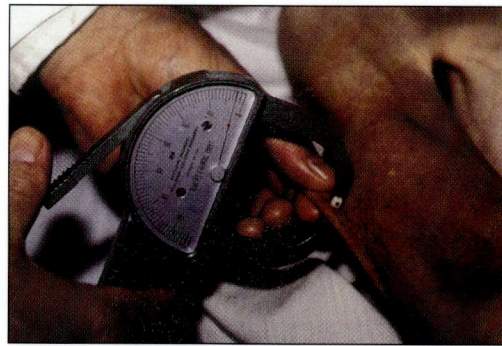

FIGURE 13-3. Page 180

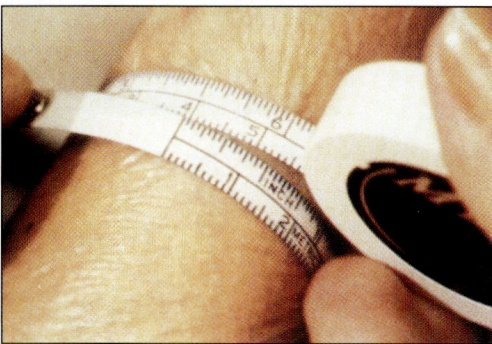

FIGURE 13-5. Page 181